Experimental Neuroanatomy

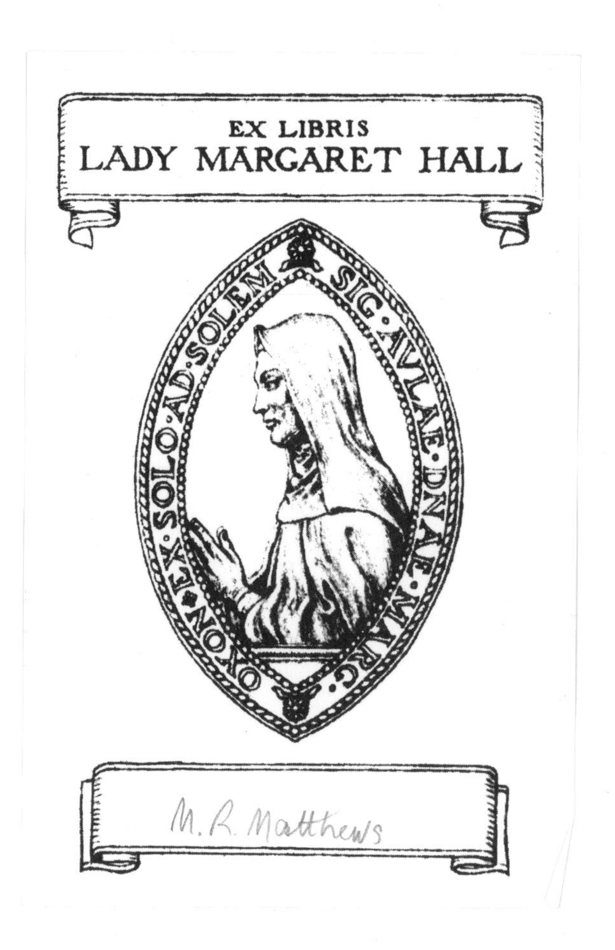

The Practical Approach Series

Affinity Chromatography
Anaerobic Microbiology
Animal Cell Culture (2nd Edition)
Animal Virus Pathogenesis
Antibodies I and II
Biochemical Toxicology
Biological Data Analysis
Biological Membranes
Biomechanics—Materials
Biomechanics—Structures and Systems
Biosensors
Carbohydrate Analysis
Cell-Cell Interactions
Cell Growth and Division
Cellular Calcium
Cellular Neurobiology
Centrifugation (2nd Edition)
Clinical Immunology
Computers in Microbiology
Crystallization of Nucleic Acids and Proteins
Cytokines
The Cytoskeleton
Diagnostic Molecular Pathology I and II
Directed Mutagenesis
DNA Cloning I, II, and III
Drosophila
Electron Microscopy in Biology
Electron Microscopy in Molecular Biology
Electrophysiology
Enzyme Assays
Essential Molecular Biology I and II
Eukaryotic Gene Transcription
Experimental Neuroanatomy
Fermentation
Flow Cytometry
Gel Electrophoresis of Nucleic Acids (2nd Edition)
Gel Electrophoresis of Proteins (2nd Edition)
Genome Analysis
Growth Factors
Haemopoiesis
Histocompatibility Testing
HPLC of Macromolecules
HPLC of Small Molecules
Human Cytogenetics I and II (2nd Edition)
Human Genetic Diseases
Immobilised Cells and Enzymes

Immunocytochemistry
In Situ Hybridization
Iodinated Density Gradient Media
Light Microscopy in Biology
Lipid Analysis
Lipid Modification of Proteins
Lipoprotein Analysis
Liposomes
Lymphocytes
Mammalian Cell Biotechnology
Mammalian Development
Medical Bacteriology
Medical Mycology
Microcomputers in Biochemistry
Microcomputers in Biology
Microcomputers in Physiology
Mitochondria
Molecular Genetic Analysis of Populations
Molecular Neurobiology
Molecular Plant Pathology I and II
Monitoring Neuronal Activity
Mutagenicity Testing
Neural Transplantation
Neurochemistry
Neuronal Cell Lines
Nucleic Acid and Protein Sequence Analysis
Nucleic Acid Hybridisation
Nucleic Acids Sequencing
Oligonucleotides and Analogues
Oligonucleotide Synthesis
PCR
Peptide Hormone Action
Peptide Hormone Secretion
Photosynthesis: Energy Transduction
Plant Cell Culture
Plant Molecular Biology
Plasmids
Pollination Ecology
Postimplantation Mammalian Embryos
Preparative Centrifugation
Prostaglandins and Related Substances
Protein Architecture
Protein Engineering
Protein Function
Protein Phosphorylation
Protein Purification Applications
Protein Purification Methods
Protein Sequencing
Protein Structure
Protein Targeting
Proteolytic Enzymes
Radioisotopes in Biology
Receptor Biochemistry
Receptor–Effector Coupling
Receptor–Ligand Interactions
Ribosomes and Protein Synthesis
RNA Processing
Signal Transduction
Solid Phase Peptide Synthesis
Spectrophotometry and Spectrofluorimetry
Steroid Hormones
Teratocarcinomas and Embryonic Stem Cells
Transcription Factors
Transcription and Translation
Tumour Immunobiology
Virology
Yeast

Experimental Neuroanatomy

A Practical Approach

Edited by

J. P. BOLAM

MRC Anatomical Neuropharmacology Unit
Mansfield Road
Oxford

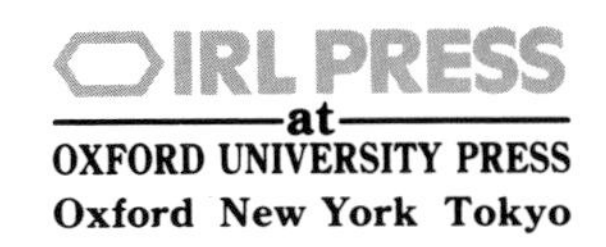

Oxford New York Tokyo

Oxford University Press, Walton Street, Oxford OX2 6DP
Oxford New York Toronto
Delhi Bombay Calcutta Madras Karachi
Kuala Lumpur Singapore Hong Kong Tokyo
Nairobi Dar es Salaam Cape Town
Melbourne Auckland Madrid
and associated companies in
Berlin Ibadan

Published in the United States
by Oxford University Press Inc., New York

A catalogue record for this book is available from the British Library

Library of Congress Cataloging in Publication Data
Experimental neuroanatomy : a practical approach / edited by J. P. Bolam.—1st ed.
(The Practical approach series)
includes bibliographical references and index.
1. Neuroanatomy—Laboratory manuals. I. Bolam, J. P. II. Series.
[DNLM: 1. Neuroanatomy—methods—laboratory manuals. WL 25 E96]
QM451.E96 1992 611.8'078—dc20 92–49818
ISBN 0–19–963326–6 (hbk.)
ISBN 0–19–963325–8 (pbk.)

Typeset by Footnote Graphics, Warminster, Wilts
Printed in Great Britain by Information Press Ltd, Eynsham, Oxon

Preface

The past 10–15 years has seen an explosion in the number of techniques available to the experimental neuroanatomist to enable the study of both connections and chemical characteristics of neurones and their processes. There is an ever-increasing trend to apply techniques at the electron microscopic level so that synaptic connections of neuronal structures of known connectivity and/or chemistry can be established. These procedures can be combined in a bewildering number of ways to elucidate complex neuronal interactions and their application, either alone or in combination, leading to major advances in our knowledge and understanding of the nervous system. This book is designed to be a basic laboratory manual for experimental neuroscientists and contains detailed protocols of the major experimental neuroanatomical techniques that are available today. It covers the very first steps in experimental neuroanatomy, i.e. preparation of the animals, perfusion-fixation, sectioning, and preparation of the sections for light and electron microscopy, through many of the 'modern' neuroanatomical techniques including the most up-to-date procedures for tract-tracing and chemical characterization of neurones, to combinations of these techniques. There is an emphasis on ultrastructural analysis so that synaptic connections between different neuronal structures can be identified. Chapter 1 deals with the basic procedures that are used throughout the book for the preparation of neural tissue for light and electron microscopy. Chapters 2–5 describe methods for tracing neuronal connections and Chapters 6–8 cover methods for the chemical characterization of neurones. Chapters 9 and 10 deal with more specialized techniques for the morphological characterization of neurones involving the intracellular injection of dyes. The final chapter (11) describes the ways in which many of the techniques can be used in combination with each other. This book is aimed at experienced neuroanatomists, and postgraduates and neuroscientists in other fields who wish to make use of experimental neuroanatomical techniques. As stated above, this book is a laboratory manual that will enable those with only a minimum of experience to carry out techniques and generate experimental data. It should be remembered, however, that to interpret correctly or accurately experimental data is not a skill that can be included in a laboratory manual or written in a protocol, but comes with experience and a wide knowledge of the system within which one is working.

Oxford J.P.B.
March 1992

Contents

Contributors

J. P. BOLAM
MRC Anatomical Neuropharmacology Unit, Mansfield Road, Oxford, OX1 3TH, UK.

EBERHARD H. BUHL
MRC Anatomical Neuropharmacology Unit, Mansfield Road, Oxford, OX1 3TH, UK.

J. PATRICK CARD
Viral Diseases Research, DuPont Merk Pharmaceutical Co., Wilmington, Delaware 19880, USA.

PIERS EMSON
MRC Neuroendocrinology Unit, Institute of Animal Physiology, Babraham, Cambridge, UK.

CHARLES R. GERFEN
Laboratory of Cell Biology, National Institute of Mental Health, Bethesda, MD 20892, USA.

C. A. INGHAM
Department of Preclinical Veterinary Sciences, Royal (Dick) School Veterinary Studies, Edinburgh University, Summerhall, Edinburgh, EH9 1QH, UK.

IDA J. LLEWELLYN-SMITH
Department of Medicine and Centre for Neuroscience, Flinders University, Bedford Park, South Australia 5042, Australia.

D. J. MAXWELL
Department of Preclinical Veterinary Sciences, Royal (Dick) School Veterinary Studies, Edinburgh University, Summerhall, Edinburgh, EH9 1QH, UK.

JANE B. MINSON
Department of Medicine and Centre for Neuroscience, Flinders University, Bedford Park, South Australia 5042, Australia.

PAUL PILOWSKY
Department of Medicine and Centre for Neuroscience, Flinders University, Bedford Park, South Australia 5042, Australia.

YOLAND SMITH
Centre de Recherche en Neurobiologie, Hôpital de l'Enfant-Jesus, 1401, 18ième Rue, Quebec, G1J 1Z4, Canada.

PETER L. STRICK
Departments of Neurosurgery and Physiology, SUNY Health Science Center, VA Medical Center, Syracuse, NY 13210, USA.

S. TOTTERDELL
Department of Pharmacology, Mansfield Road, Oxford, OX1 3QT, UK.

STEVEN R. VINCENT
Division of Neurological Sciences, Department of Psychiatry, University of British Columbia, 2255 Westbrook Mall, Vancouver, BC, Canada.

W. SCOTT YOUNG III
Laboratory of Cell Biology, National Institute of Mental Health, Bethesda, MD 20892, USA.

Abbreviations

ABC	avidin–biotin–peroxidase complex
AC	alternating current
AOAA	amino-oxyacetic acid
BCIP	5-bromo-4-chloro-3-indoyl phosphate toluidinium salt
BDHC	benzidine dihydrochloride
β-NADPH	nicotinamide adenine dinucleotide phosphate, reduced form
BSA	bovine serum albumin
BSL II	biosafety level II
CNS	central nervous system
c.p.m.	counts per minute
CT	cholera toxin
cTT	fragments of tetanus toxin
CTB	cholera toxin subunit B
CTB-HRP	cholera toxin subunit B conjugated to horseradish peroxidase
CTB-gold	cholera toxin subunit B conjugated to colloidal gold
DAB	3,3′-diaminobenzidine tetrahydrochloride
DAB-Co	3,3′-diaminobenzidine tetrahydrochloride intensified with cobalt
DAPI	4,6-diamidino-2-phenylindole
DC	direct current
DDSA	dodecenyl succinic anhydride
DFP	diisopropylphosphofluoridate
DiI	1,1′-dioctadecyl-3,3,3′,3′-tetra-methylindo-carbocyanine perchlorate
DiO	3,3′-dioctadecyloxa-carbocyanine perchlorate
DMP	dimethyl phthalate
DMSO	dimethyl sulphoxide
DMX	dorsal motor nucleus of the vagus
DTT	dithiothreitol
EA	epon/araldite
EDTA	ethylenediaminetetra-acetic acid
EM	electron microscopy
FB	fast blue

FITC	fluorescein isothiocyanate
FRAP	fluoride-resistant acid phosphatase
GABA	gamma aminobutyric acid
GABA-T	gamma aminobutyric acid transaminase
HRP	horseradish peroxidase
HSV	*herpes simplex* virus
ISHH	*in situ* hybridization histochemistry
iso-OMPA	*N*,*N′*-bis-(1-methylethyl)-pyrophosphorodiamidic anhydride
LM	light microscopy
LY	Lucifer Yellow
MAO	monoamine oxidase
MPTP	1-methyl-4-phenyl-1,2,3,6-tetrahydropyridine
NAD	nicotinamide adenine dinucleotide
NAD(H)	nicotinamide adenine dinucleotide, reduced form
NBT	nitroblue tetrazolium
NGS	normal goat serum
NHS	normal horse serum
NS	normal serum
NTS	nucleus tractus solitarius
PAP	peroxidase anti-peroxidase complex
PB	phosphate buffer
PBGT	phosphate buffer, 1% goat serum, 0.3% Triton
PBHT	phosphate buffer, 1% horse serum, 0.3% Triton
PBS	phosphate-buffered saline
PEG	polyethylene glycol
PEG/TB	polyethylene glycol in Tris-buffer
p.f.u.	plaque-forming units
PHA	phytohaemagglutinin
PHA-L	*Phaseolus vulgaris*–leucoagglutinin
PMS	phenazine methosulphate
PMSH	phenazine methosulphate, reduced form
PRV	pseudorabies virus
SCG	superior cervical ganglion
SDS	sodium dodecyl sulphate
SNr	substantia nigra pars reticulata
SSC	sodium chloride sodium citrate buffer
TB	Tris-buffer
TBS	Tris-buffered saline
TBS-TX	Tris-buffered saline containing Triton X-100
TdT	terminal deoxitidyl transferase
TE	Tris-EDTA buffer
TEM	transmission electron microscopy
TF	transitional fluid

Tris	Tris(hydroxymethyl)methylamine
TRITC	tetramethylrhodamine isothiocyanate
TPBS	Tris and phosphate-buffered saline
TMB	tetramethylbenzidine
TMB-N	tetramethylbenzidine stabilized with sodium nitroprusside
TMB-T	tetramethylbenzidine stabilized with tungstate
WGA-apo-HRP-gold	wheatgerm agglutinin conjugated to enzymatically inactive horseradish peroxidase and colloidal gold
WGA	wheatgerm agglutinin
WGA-gold	wheatgerm agglutinin conjugated to colloidal gold
WGA-HRP	wheatgerm agglutinin conjugated to horseradish peroxidase
WGA-HRP-gold	wheatgerm agglutinin conjugated to horseradish peroxidase and colloidal gold

1

Preparation of central nervous system tissue for light and electron microscopy

J. P. BOLAM

1. Introduction

Techniques of experimental neuroanatomy are those that enable one to characterize the position of neurones in the microcircuits of the nervous system on the basis of their morphology, chemistry, and connections. The essence of the techniques are that the morphology, chemistry, and output region of neurones are identified first at the light microscopic level and then the chemistry, origin, and pattern of afferent synaptic input are identified at the electron microscopic level. Information of this nature is a pre-requisite to the characterization of the microcircuitry or neuronal networks of a region and provides a framework within which functional data can be interpreted. For the analysis of individual neuronal elements or populations of neurones in the microcircuitry of an area it is necessary to examine the tissue at the light microscopic level. For the analysis of *synaptic* interactions of individual neurones or populations of neurones, it is necessary to examine the tissue at the ultrastructural level with an electron microscope. The object of this chapter is to introduce to the reader the basic techniques used in the preparation of tissue from neuroanatomical experiments for light and electron microscopy. Since a high proportion of modern experimental neuroanatomical procedures can be applied to ultrastructural analysis and it is by electron microscopy alone that synaptic connections between neurones can be identified, the main emphasis of this chapter will be on the preparation of the material for *electron microscopy*. However, in the use of modern experimental neuroanatomical techniques, material is generally prepared for light microscopy first, and then the same material is examined at the electron microscopic level. The techniques for the preparation of material for light and electron microscopy will not be dealt with in an exhaustive manner but will be confined to those that have proved successful in the hands of the author and his close colleagues for the analysis of many areas of the central nervous system.

1.1 Sequence of procedures in experimental neuroanatomy

The sequence of events or procedures for the preparation of material for light and/or electron microscopy in neuroanatomical experiments are virtually the same no matter what the system or experimental manipulation that has been performed.

(a) Carry out experimental manipulation on animal, for example injection of retrograde tracers (Chapter 2) or injection of anterograde tracers (Chapter 3).

(b) After the appropriate survival time fix the CNS, preferably by perfusion (*Protocol 3*).

(c) Remove the fixed brain from the animal, dissect out areas of interest, and cut sections preferably on a vibrating microtome (*Protocol 4*).

(d) Carry out histochemical or immunohistochemical procedure to reveal injected or endogenous substances (see individual chapters).

(e) Mount the sections prepared for light microscopy on coated slides, dehydrate, clear, and apply coverslips (*Protocols 5* and *6*).

(f) Post-fix the sections prepared for electron microscopy in osmium tetroxide (*Protocol 7*).

(g) Carry out single section Golgi-impregnation if required (*Protocol 12*).

(h) Dehydrate sections and flat-embed in an electron microscopic resin on microscope slides (*Protocol 8*).

(i) Examine the sections in the light microscope, select, record, and re-embed neurones and regions of interest in blocks of resin suitable for ultrathin sectioning (*Protocol 9*).

(j) Cut ultrathin sections at 60–90 nm on an ultramicrotome and collect on coated single-slot grids (*Protocol 10*).

(k) Carry out post-embedding immunocytochemistry (Chapter 6).

(l) Stain the ultrathin sections (*Protocol 11*) and examine in the electron microscope.

2. Fixation

The first step in the preparation of tissue from neuroanatomical experiments for light and electron microscopy is fixation. The process of fixation is in effect the preservation of tissue so that it will survive in its natural state or near-natural state during subsequent processing, during storage, and during examination in the light and/or electron microscopes. The functions of fixation are thus to stabilize the cellular organization such that:

- the tissue will no longer undergo degradation in response to endogenously released enzymes or as a response to the action of micro-organisms
- subsequent processing steps do not extract tissue components
- the tissue is hardened or strengthened to aid sectioning

Furthermore, an ideal fixative is one that penetrates into the tissue rapidly, acts rapidly, and is essentially irreversible.

Although many different substances may be used for fixation of biological tissue for light and electron microscopic analyses (1, 2) the most commonly used system in electron microscopic experimental neuroanatomy is a double fixation, initially with a buffered aldehyde (specifically paraformaldehyde and glutaraldehyde) solution followed by post-fixation in osmium tetroxide (3). For light microscopy only the primary fixation in aldehydes is necessary. The aldehydes react primarily with proteins, stabilizing the tissue by cross-linkage whereas the osmium tetroxide, exposed to the tissue at a later time, reacts with various tissue components but especially unsaturated lipids. The osmium tetroxide has the added advantage that it also stains the tissue providing extra contrast at the electron microscopic level. Aldehyde fixatives are generally prepared and used in a buffered solution at physiological or slightly higher pH. The most commonly used buffers for the preparation of aldehyde fixatives and the most commonly used in histochemical or immunohistochemical techniques are phosphate buffers, the preparation of which is described in *Protocol 1*.

Protocol 1. Preparation of phosphate buffer (PB) and phosphate-buffered saline (PBS)

1. Prepare stock solution of 0.2 M $Na_2HPO_4{\cdot}2H_2O$, (35.6 g/litre): solution A.[a]
2. Prepare stock solution of 0.2 M $NaH_2PO_4{\cdot}2H_2O$, (31.2 g/litre): solution B.[a]
3. For a stock solution of 0.2 M phosphate buffer at pH 7.4 mix solutions A and B in a ratio of 4:1. Check pH, adjust with solutions A or B as necessary. Stock may be kept up to one week at 4°C. Different pH values are prepared by mixing solutions in different ratios.
4. For a working solution of 0.1 M dilute stock one in two with distilled water. For 0.05 M dilute the stock 1 in 24 in distilled water.
5. Phosphate-buffered saline is prepared by mixing:
   - 0.2 M PB 50 ml
   - NaCl 8.76 g
   - KCl 0.2 g
   - distilled water up to 1 litre

[a] The stock solutions may be stored for long periods at 4°C, but should be warmed to ensure that all crystals are dissolved before use.

The preparation of buffered paraformaldehyde/glutaraldehyde fixatives are described in *Protocol 2*. The concentration of aldehydes in the fixative depends upon the procedures that are to be applied to the tissue and the reader is referred to individual chapters. In general terms the higher the concentrations of aldehydes, the better preserved is the tissue and in particular the higher the concentration of glutaraldehyde the better the ultrastructural preservation. For light microscopy it is often only necessary to use paraformaldehyde (~ 4%) alone. It should be remembered however, that the process of fixation may also reduce the activity of endogenous or exogenous enzymes that are subjects of histochemical reactions and may obscure or denature antigenic sites. Strong fixation with high concentrations of glutaraldehyde may also hinder penetration of reagents into the tissue. It is therefore necessary to attain a balance between the degree of preservation of the tissue and the maintenance of antigenic sites or of an enzyme activity. Thus in immunocytochemistry it is generally necessary to use only low concentrations of glutaraldehyde (although there are notable exceptions see Chapters 5 and 6). Some enzymes, both exogenous and endogenous tolerate high concentrations of glutaraldehyde and their histochemical detection can be carried out in well fixed tissue. For the specific requirements of fixation for different histochemical procedures see individual chapters.

Protocol 2. Preparation of paraformaldehyde–glutaraldehyde fixative in phosphate buffer[a]

Materials

- paraformaldehyde (Aldrich or TAAB)
- glutaraldehyde (supplied as a 25% aqueous solution from all EM suppliers, stored at 4°C)
- 0.5 M NaOH
- 0.2 M phosphate buffer (*Protocol 1*)

Method

All steps should be carried out in a fume hood.

1. Heat distilled water (just under half of the final volume of fixative required) to 65–70°C.
2. Weigh out the paraformaldehyde powder and add to the water in a fume hood. Stir continuously with a magnetic stirrer.
3. Add 0.5 M NaOH dropwise, until the solution clears. There is a slight delay in this so do not add too much sodium hydroxide.
4. Filter the paraformaldehyde solution.

5. Add 0.2 M phosphate buffer (half final volume). The fixative can be prepared to this step the evening before fixation (stored at 4°C) if being used immediately, cool to appropriate temperature.
6. Add appropriate volume of the 25% glutaraldehyde to give the desired final concentration (see *Table 1*).
7. Make up to final volume with distilled water.

Examples

For 500 ml of 4% paraformaldehyde/0.5% glutaraldehyde: dissolve 20 g paraformaldehyde in 200 ml of water, add 250 ml 0.2 M phosphate buffer, add 10 ml of 25% glutaraldehyde solution, and make up to 500 ml with distilled water.

For 250 ml of 3% paraformaldehyde/0.1% glutaraldehyde: dissolve 7.5 g paraformaldehyde in 100 ml of water, add 125 ml 0.2 M phosphate buffer, add 1.0 ml of 25% glutaraldehyde solution, and make up to 250 ml with distilled water.

See *Table 1* for volumes of 25% glutaraldehyde solution to give selected final concentration.

[a] **Safety note 1**. Paraformaldehyde and glutaraldehyde are both extremely toxic by ingestion, inhalation, and contact with the skin. Wear appropriate protective clothing and avoid contact with the skin. *All* manipulations with the aldehydes, including perfuse–fixation, should be carried out in a fume cupboard. Waste should be washed away with large volumes of water. Aldehydes should be stored away from 'fixable' reagents, e.g. antisera.

Table 1. Volume of 25% glutaraldehyde solution required to prepare fixatives

	Volume of fixative (ml) required						
Conc. of glutaraldehyde required	**100**	**200**	**300**	**400**	**500**	**750**	**1000**
0.01%	0.04	0.08	0.12	0.16	0.2	0.3	0.4
0.05%	0.2	0.4	0.6	0.8	1.0	1.5	2.0
0.1%	0.4	0.8	1.2	1.6	2.0	3.0	4.0
0.2%	0.8	1.6	2.4	3.2	4.0	6.0	8.0
0.5%	2.0	4.0	6.0	8.0	10.0	15.0	20.0
1.0%	4.0	8.0	12.0	16.0	20.0	30.0	40.0
2.0%	8.0	16.0	24.0	32.0	40.0	60.0	80.0
2.5%	10.0	20.0	30.0	40.0	50.0	75.0	100.0
5.0%	20.0	40.0	60.0	80.0	100.0	150.0	200.0

2.1 Perfusion–fixation

Fixatives are exposed to the tissue by either vascular perfusion (*Protocol 3*) or by immersion. The former, perfusion–fixation, is by far the superior since it is possible to remove blood from the vasculature, fixation is more rapid and is more even, and excess fixative can be removed by perfusion with buffer. If it is necessary to perform immersion fixation, say for human post-mortem or biopsy tissue, then the tissue should be cut as thinly as possible to aid penetration of the fixative, and at least the initial fixative solution should be cold to slow down any degradation of the tissue. For most purposes, especially when experimental manipulations have been performed on the animal, perfusion–fixation will be the method of choice. The technique of perfusion–fixation is essentially the same for different experimental procedures and species, the exact details for the individual procedures are given in the appropriate chapters. The essence of perfusion–fixation is that the fixative is administered to a deeply anaesthetized animal directly into the vasculature by means of a cannula inserted through the heart into the aorta. The fixative is pumped around the circulation by means of a peristaltic pump or a gravity feed mechanism, and a mixing chamber is included to give a gradual change from the vascular rinse to the fixative.

Protocol 3. Perfusion–fixation (see also Chapter 10, *Protocol 2*)

The following are required:

- anaesthetic
- peristaltic pump or gravity feed system
- mixing chamber
- dissection instruments (large and small scissors, clamps, arterial clip)
- wide bore (approximately 2 mm internal diameter) blunt-ended needle
- vascular rinse solution, (e.g. Tyrode's solution (see Appendix, this chapter) or 0.9% NaCl solution)
- fixative
- dissection board

Method

See *Safety note 1* in *Protocol 1*.
The following method is for a 200–300 g rat.

1. Deeply anaesthetize the animal. We use 350 mg/kg chloral hydrate (intraperitoneally) as a 3.5% solution in 0.9% NaCl solution, but any suitable anaesthetic will be adequate.
2. Pin out the deeply anaesthetized rat on a dissection board either in a large

tray in a fume cupboard or over a ventilated down-draught sink. Set perfusion apparatus flowing with vascular rinse at a rate of approximately 20 ml/min.

3. Open abdominal cavity, take hold of xyphoid cartilage with clamp, and lift to expose the diaphragm. Cut away connections between the liver and the diaphragm.
4. With blunt-ended scissors cut the diaphragm away from the rib cage and cut along sides of the rib cage, lift the cut rib cage to expose the heart, and cut away the pericardium if necessary. Once the thoracic cavity is opened then speed is of the utmost importance as the brain is no longer oxygenated.
5. Grasp the heart between thumb and forefinger and insert the cannula into the base of the left ventricle, push gently into the aorta, and clamp (with arterial clip) in position above the heart.
6. Immediately cut the right atrium with scissors. Blood should flow freely. After 60–90 sec change to the fixative.[a] Move lungs to one side and clamp the descending aorta.[b]
7. Continue the perfusion at the rate and for the time recommended in individual procedures. An average rate and time for a rat is 10 ml/min over a period of 20–30 min.[c]
8. Post-perfuse with buffer if indicated in the individual procedures.

[a] If the lungs turn white and become bloated, then the cannula is in the wrong position, i.e. it has been pushed into the left atrium and not the aorta.
[b] Should the hind legs stiffen it implies that the clamping of the descending aorta is ineffective.
[c] A good perfusion is characterized by fasciculations of muscles when first exposed to the fixative, followed by a rapid hardening.

On completion of the perfusion the head of the animal is removed, the skin and muscle are cut away from the top of the skull, and with the aid of bone snippers, the brain is carefully removed. The brain should be firm to the touch and creamy-white in colour when a low concentration of glutaraldehyde is used, and yellow when a high concentration is used. Any pink coloration indicates the presence of blood and a poor perfusion and hence poorly fixed tissue. Slightly soft brains can be hardened by post-fixation in paraformaldehyde solutions at 4°C and indeed it is recommended in some histochemical procedures to do so. Once the brain is removed, the areas of interest are cut into blocks or slices of about 5 mm thickness. This can be carried out freehand with a single or double-edged razor blade, or using a perspex guide into which the brain is placed and cut along guide lines. Alternatively, when a specific plane of section is required, for instance in relation to an atlas, a stereotaxic frame can be used to make guide cuts. To do this the top of the brain is exposed and the head is placed in a stereotaxic frame, a razor blade held in a micromanipulator is then used to produce guide cuts in the required plane and thickness.

3. Sectioning of the brain

Sections suitable for histochemical reactions and histological analysis by light microscopy can be prepared using frozen tissue cut on a cryostat or freezing microtome or alternatively, non-frozen tissue cut on a vibrating microtome (*Protocol 4*). In the electron microscope, however, frozen sections have very poor ultrastructure and they are generally not used for preparation of sections for electron microscopy. The most commonly used system to prepare sections for electron microscopy is the vibrating microtome (*Protocol 4*). Several models of vibrating microtomes are available on the market (Vibratome; Vibroslice). The essential features are that the tissue (which can be of almost any hardness from fresh to well-fixed), is glued to the stage, a razor blade then advances over the tissue whilst vibrating in the plane of section but at 90° to the direction of advance (i.e. a sawing motion), and the thickness of the sections adjusted by raising the stage. The vibration of the blade enables it to cut through even quite soft tissue. In general terms the higher the frequency or amplitude of vibration and the slower the speed of advance, the better the sections are.

For light microscopy, whole brain sections or hemisections are cut. The same may also be applied to electron microscopic sections, however it may be necessary to trim the blocks down to include only the area of interest, as large sections often become damaged during subsequent processing and it is often difficult to keep them flat.

Protocol 4. Vibrating microtome sections

Materials

- vibrating microtome
- cyanoacrylate adhesive
- phosphate buffer or phosphate-buffered saline (see *Protocol 1*)
- labelled glass vials (or some other receptacle for collecting the sections)
- artist's paint brush
- agar (5% in distilled water)

Method

1. Gently dry the block or slice of fixed brain by dabbing on absorbent paper and glue to the stage of the microtome with cyanoacrylate glue.
2. If tissue requires support, surround it with agar that has been melted in a water bath and allow it to set.

3. Mount the stage in the microtome and fill the bath with cold PBS or PB.
4. Cut sections at 20–100 μm (usually 50–70 μm) using maximum amplitude of vibration and slow speed of advance.
5. Pick up sections with a paint brush and place in a vial containing PB or PBS.
6. Wash sections several times in PB or PBS by pipetting the solutions from the vials with a disposable Pasteur pipette.
7. Carry out the histochemical procedure or store at −23°C after equilibration in a cryoprotectant solution consisting of: 160 ml 0.05 M phosphate buffer (pH 7.4), 120 ml ethylene glycol, and 120 ml glycerol.

Failure to cut sections or the cutting of irregular sections can be due to several reasons:

- blunt or damaged blade
- tissue not adequately stuck to the microtome stage
- tissue block is too high which results in its movement before the advancing blade
- insufficient support for tissue

4. Processing of sections

It is at this stage that histochemical or immunohistochemical procedures are carried out and the reader is referred to individual chapters. The reactions are generally carried out on free-floating sections in the scintillation vials (or similar) of about 15 ml capacity and subjected to constant, gentle, shaking although sections for light microscopy can be incubated by the various histochemical procedures after mounting on slides (see below). The most effective shakers are those that move in a rotary fashion, (e.g. IKA-Vibrax VKR). For individual shakers and vials, the optimum volume of solution should be determined that results in gentle 'wafting' of the sections when put on the shaker. For 15 ml glass vials and a IKA-Vibrax VKR shaker, the optimum volume is 1–3 ml. It is at this stage that the paths divide for sections prepared for light microscopy and those prepared for electron microscopy since the conditions of incubation are often different and the subsequent procedures are different.

5. Mounting of sections for light microscopic analysis

Those sections that are prepared from tissue that is to be used for light microscopy alone, and those sections in electron microscopic studies that will only be used for light microscopic analysis, i.e. injection sites, are then mounted on to microscope slides. The sections can of course be mounted on to slides first and then reacted on the slides, however it is generally more economical in reagents and convenient to carry out the reactions on free-floating sections, and in general, the quality of staining is better. The microscope slides are coated or subbed with a substance, (e.g. gelatin, egg albumin) that aids the adherence of the sections to the glass (*Protocol 5*, see also Chapter 8, *Protocol 1* and Chapter 6, *Protocol 1*). The sections are mounted by gently rolling them around a soft artist's paint brush and then 'unrolling' them on to the slide. Alternatively, the sections can be placed in a trough of buffer, the microscope slide dipped into the trough at an angle of 20–45°, the sections gently moved into position above the slide with an artist's paint brush, and the slide gently lifted out while keeping the section relatively still. The section can be moved around and correctly positioned with the paint brush whilst they are still wet. Several sections are generally placed on each slide and they are then left to air-dry at room temperature for about 12–18 h. This time may be reduced by the use of a cold air blower.

Protocol 5. Coating glass microscope slides

Materials

- acid alcohol (a few drops of glacial acetic acid added to absolute ethanol)
- microscope slides
- chrome alum (chromic potassium sulphate)
- gelatin

Method

1. Soak slides in acid alcohol for several hours.
2. Remove slides from acid alcohol using forceps and place in slide carriers.
3. Wash under running water (preferably hot) for several minutes and then wash in several changes of distilled water.
4. Dry in an oven away from dust.
5. Prepare slide coating medium by mixing:
   - chrome alum 0.1 g
   - gelatin 1.0 g
   - distilled water 200 ml

   Heat gently to dissolve. Cool before use. This solution may be stored up to several weeks at 4°C.
6. *Either*: take slides one at a time, hold by edges in thumb and forefinger,

and dip into the cold coating solution. Allow to dry in the upright position in a dust-free environment.
Or: immerse slide carrier containing slides in staining dish containing the gelatin solution. Drain on absorbent paper and dry in a dust-free environment.

7. Store coated slides in a closed container to avoid contamination with dust.

In order to examine sections in the light microscope it is necessary to infiltrate them with a medium that 'fills' all spaces in the tissue, in effect, it evens out the changes in refractive index of the tissue (clearing). Most mounting media are not miscible with water, so in order to completely infiltrate the tissue it is necessary to remove water or dehydrate the tissue prior to exposure to the medium. The tissue is dehydrated in graded dilutions of ethanol before soaking in a link reagent (a substance in which both the alcohol and mounting medium dissolve), e.g. xylene, and infiltrating with the mounting medium. Coverslips are then applied to the section, the remaining link reagent and the solvent of the mounting medium evaporate, and the medium sets hard (*Protocol 6*). In this form the sections can be stored indefinitely and can be examined in the light microscope.

Protocol 6. Dehydration, clearing, and mounting light microscopic sections

Materials

- graded series of volume for volume dilutions of ethanol in water (50%, 70%, 90%, 100%)
- dry absolute ethanol (ethanol stored over anhydrous cupric sulphate)
- xylene
- mounting medium such as XAM or DPX (BDH)
- coverslips
- staining dishes and slide carriers (alternatively Coplin jars may be used)

Method

1. Place the slides with dried-on sections in the slide carrier. Place the slide carrier in the dishes containing the increasing concentrations of ethanol, removing excess ethanol solutions from the slide carrier between each dilution by dabbing on absorbent paper.

2. 50% ethanol for 10–15 min.

3. 70% ethanol for 10–15 min.

4. 90% ethanol for 10–15 min.

Protocol 6. *Continued*

5. 100% ethanol for 10–15 min.
6. Dry absolute ethanol for 10–15 min.
7. Two changes of xylene for 10–15 min each.[a,b]
8. Apply a 'line' or 'blob' of mounting medium, (e.g. XAM or DPX) on a coverslip using a glass rod.
9. Remove one slide from the xylene and place it, sections down, on the coverslip. Turn the slide with adhering coverslip over and apply gentle pressure to the coverslip to spread mounting medium completely over the sections. Do not allow the sections to dry out before they are exposed to the mounting medium.
10. Leave the slides to set dry.[c]

[a] **Safety note 2.** Xylene and xylene-based mounting media are toxic and inflammable, all manipulations should therefore be carried out in a fume cupboard.
[b] Do not use solvent-based markers to label slides as these wash off in the xylene. Use a diamond marker or pencil if slides have frosted ends.
[c] Coverslips can be removed, even after the mounting medium is set, by soaking for several hours (up to days) in xylene. This may be necessary if the sections partially dry out during mounting or insufficient medium was put on the coverslip.

5.1 Counterstaining of light microscopic sections

It is sometimes desirable to counterstain sections that are prepared for light microscopy to enable injection sites, sites of transport of axonal tracers, and immunocytochemically stained structures to be correctly identified.

5.1.1 Nissl staining

A most effective and reliable stain for light microscopic sections is the Nissl stain using cresyl violet. The sections are mounted on to coated slides and allowed to dry, as described above. Prior to staining they are 'defatted' by passing through graded dilutions of ethanol for about three minutes each in a manner similar to that described in *Protocol 6*, after which they are rehydrated by passing back through decreasing concentrations of ethanol, and finally back into water. Place the sections in cresyl violet solution for 10 to 30 minutes consisting of:

- 1 M sodium acetate 15 ml
- 0.2 M formic acid 75 ml
- 0.5% aqueous cresyl violet 150 ml

When the sections have an overall, even blue appearance dehydrate, infiltrate with a mounting medium and apply a coverslip as described in *Protocol 6*. The ethanol solutions act to differentiate the stain, causing myelin and other components to lose colour whereas perikarya retain the colour. Differentiation can be accelerated by slightly acidifying the 70% and 90% ethanol with acetic acid.

6. Preparation of sections for electron microscopic analysis

6.1 Post-fixation in osmium tetroxide

After processing for the histochemical and immunohistochemical procedures described in the individual chapters, sections that have been selected for electron microscopy are post-fixed in a buffered osmium tetroxide solution (*Protocol 7*). During treatment with osmium the sections will turn black, will harden considerably, and will become brittle. Any unevenness or folds in the sections will be difficult to remove after osmium treatment and even more so after subsequent treatments, it is therefore important to ensure that the sections are completely flat before treatment.

Safety note 3. Osmium tetroxide is a powerful oxidizing agent, it is extremely toxic, and is volatile. *All* manipulations should be carried out in a fume hood and wearing protective gloves and clothing. Stock osmium solutions should be stored in ground glass-stoppered bottles, preferably *double* ground glass-stoppered, at 4°C in a fridge dedicated to toxic substances. Waste osmium solutions can be rendered less hazardous by placing in a strongly alkaline solution. All waste and washings are therefore placed in a bottle containing sodium hydroxide pellets from which the metal can be reclaimed.

Protocol 7. Post-fixation with osmium tetroxide

A. *Preparation of stock and working solutions of osmium tetroxide*

Materials

- osmium tetroxide (usually supplied as 1 g solid in sealed ampoules; OXKEM Ltd. or Electron Microscope Suppliers)
- 0.2 M phosphate buffer (*Protocol 1*)
- ground glass-stoppered bottles (preferably double stoppered)
- laboratory film, e.g. Parafilm (made by American Can Company)

Method

1. To prepare a 4% stock solution, open 1 g ampoule of osmium tetroxide and dissolve in 25 ml of distilled water in ground glass-stoppered bottle. This may take up to 24 h without stirring but the time is considerably shortened with stirring. The stock solution is stored at 4°C for several months, but should be in a fridge dedicated to toxic substances since even with ground glass stoppers and several layers of Parafilm, the osmium escapes.

Protocol 7. *Continued*

2. To prepare a working solution of 1% in 0.1 M phosphate buffer (pH 7.4) mix 4% stock solution, 0.2 M phosphate buffer, and distilled water in the ratios 1:2:1. Thus for 20 ml mix the following:
   - stock 4% osmium tetroxide 5 ml
   - 0.2 M phosphate buffer (pH 7.4) 10 ml
   - distilled water 5 ml

B. *Post-fixation with osmium tetroxide*

Materials

- 1% osmium tetroxide in 0.1 M phosphate buffer, pH 7.4
- 0.1 M phosphate buffer, pH 7.4 (*Protocol 1*)
- Petri dishes (if the number of sections is large)
- artist's paint brush

Method

1. Equilibrate sections with 0.1 M phosphate buffer (pH 7.4).
2. Pipette off the phosphate buffer and ensure that the sections are flat using a paint brush. If there are many sections, transfer to a Petri dish.
3. Carefully pipette 1–2 ml of the 1% osmium tetroxide solution using a glass Pasteur pipette and cover. (Sections in Petri dishes will require a greater volume.) Ensure that the sections do not float on the solution. The sections will rapidly turn black and become very brittle, any sections that are folded will remain so. Caps of the vials will also become black and should therefore be saved only for osmium treatment or discarded after use.
4. The incubation time depends on the thickness of the sections:[a]
   - for sections of 50 μm incubate for approximately 20–25 min
   - for sections of 70 μm sections incubate for 30 min
   - for sections of 100 μm incubate for 40 min
   - for 1 mm cubes of tissue incubate for 1 h
   - for slabs of tissue (approximately 5 × 5 × 1 mm) incubate for up to 4 h
5. Pipette off the osmium solution and place in waste osmium bottle.
6. Wash sections at least three times for 15 min each in phosphate buffer. If the sections are not to be subjected to further processing, e.g. Golgi-impregnation, it is preferable to dehydrate and embed in an electron microscopic resin immediately (*Protocol 8*).

[a] If the osmium solution changes from straw colour to a deep purple it should be replaced with fresh solution.

6.2 Dehydration and embedding in resin

Following post-fixation with osmium tetroxide the sections may be subjected to Golgi-impregnation (see *Protocol 12*), but if this is not required they should be embedded in an electron microscopic resin. The main reason for embedding tissue for electron microscopy in resin is to provide support during the preparation of ultrathin sections. However, one of the advantages is that the procedures, as with light microscopic preparations, clears the tissue and results in a preparation that is suitable for high resolution light microscopic analysis. Also, as is the case with light microscopic preparations, most resins are not miscible with water; in order to obtain complete infiltration of the tissue it is first necessary to dehydrate the tissue with ethanol to remove all water. Once all the water is removed and the tissue equilibrated in an appropriate link reagent, (i.e. a substance that is miscible with both ethanol and the resin) it is infiltrated with the resin in a liquid form, this is then allowed to polymerize. The ideal resin is one that is soluble in the dehydrating agent, does not change volume on polymerization and polymerizes evenly, is easy to cut with an ultramicrotome, has good optical qualities, and is stable in the electron beam of the electron microscope. The most commonly used resins in the preparation of neural tissue for electron microscopy are epoxy resins but several other types are available including those that are miscible with water prior to polymerization (1, 2).

Protocol 8. Dehydration and embedding in resin

Materials

- graded series of volume for volume dilutions of ethanol in water (50%, 70%, 90%, 100%)
- dry absolute ethanol (ethanol stored over anhydrous cupric sulphate)
- propylene oxide[a]
- electron microscopic resin (e.g. Durcupan ACM, Fluka)
- aluminium foil for making boats

Method

Osmium-treated and washed sections are treated sequentially in glass vials with the following.

1. 50% ethanol for 15 min. Use a large volume (~ 10 ml) to ensure that all the phosphate is removed since any remaining phosphate may react with the uranyl acetate in the following step to produce an electron dense precipitate in the tissue.

Protocol 8. *Continued*

2. 0.5–1.0% uranyl acetate[b] in 70% ethanol for 20–30 min. Prepare the uranyl acetate solution before it is required (~ 30 min) since it takes time to dissolve. Filter before use.
3. 95% ethanol for 15 min.
4. 100% ethanol for 10–15 min.
5. Dry absolute ethanol for 10–15 min.
6. Two changes of propylene oxide for 10–15 min each.[a]
7. During dehydration prepare aluminium boats using vials as a mould, attach these to an appropriate container (we use photographic paper boxes) with double sided adhesive tape.
8. Prepare resin[c] according to manufacturer's instructions. For Durcupan, mix the components A:B:C:D in the ratios 10:10:0.3:0.2 by weight, in a disposable plastic beaker. Mix thoroughly with a disposable glass pipette or wooden spatula and add 1–2 ml to each aluminium boat. The resin components should be weighed out in the fume hood.
9. Using a paint brush (dedicated) transfer the sections from the last propylene oxide to resin in the aluminium boats and leave overnight in the fume cupboard. Ensure that the sections do not dry out at this stage and that they are completely submerged in the resin. The label from the scintillation vial can be transferred to the aluminium boat, care should be taken to avoid the propylene oxide washing the writing off the labels.
10. Gently warm the boats containing the sections and the resin on a hot plate and transfer the sections, one at a time, with forceps to uncleaned microscope slides.[c] Allow them to settle for a few minutes.
11. Briefly examine the slides under a dissection stereo-microscope (protected from contamination with resin by covering in laboratory or kitchen film) to ensure that sections or fragments of sections are not overlying each other. The sections or fragments can be manoeuvred about the slide with cocktail sticks or a paint brush.
12. Place a coverslip on top of sections.[d] Allow to settle again and then press down gently to remove all air bubbles and any excess resin. The amount of resin should be sufficient to cover the sections and spread to the edge of the coverslip by capillary action but not to emerge from the sides when the coverslip is pressed. Excess resin can be removed by absorbing it on to filter paper and extra resin can be added by placing drops along the edge of the coverslip.
13. Place the slides in containers (photographic boxes lined with aluminium foil) and polymerize the resin by heating in oven at 60°C for 48 h. All materials contaminated with resin are heated under the same conditions

and then disposed of. The sections are now in a form suitable for light microscopic analysis prior to electron microscopy and can be stored indefinitely.

[a] **Safety note 4**. Propylene oxide is potentially extremely toxic by ingestion, inhalation or absorption through the skin, and is highly volatile and flammable, it should be handled *only* in a fume cupboard. Do not wear gloves as it will dissolve in them and concentrate next to the skin. Place waste propylene oxide in a 500 ml loosely stoppered bottle containing 200 ml ethanol and 200 ml of ammonia solution (35%). When full leave for approximately two days and then wash down the sink with large volumes of water. All materials contaminated with the propylene oxide should be left in the fume hood for at least one day to allow complete evaporation.

[b] **Safety note 5**. Uranyl acetate is toxic both because it is a heavy metal and is radioactive, protective clothing and gloves should be worn and it should only be handled in a fume hood.

[c] **Safety note 6**. Some components of epoxy resins are likely to be toxic. Wear protective clothing and gloves, only handle in a fume hood, and polymerize all contaminated materials.

[d] The slides and coverslips should not be cleaned and may in fact be passed gently through the fingers to coat them with grease or they may be silicon-coated. This aids the removal of the coverslip during the re-embedding of the sections at a later date (*Protocol 9*). Alternatively the sections may be embedded between acetate sheets (see Chapter 10) or plastic coverslips may be used.

6.3 Light microscopic analysis prior to electron microscopy

Once the resin has polymerized the sections are in a form in which they may be stored indefinitely. They are suitable for detailed light microscopic analysis and in fact the osmium treatment and embedding in an epoxy resin produces material of high quality and allows more detail to be resolved than material prepared for light microscopy alone. The main advantage however, of tissue flat-embedded on microscope slides is that the *same* sections that are examined in the light microscope are examined in the electron microscope, and indeed the *same neuronal structures* that are identified in the light microscope can be examined in the electron microscope (correlated light and electron microscopy). The sections are examined for structures that are stained by the histochemical or immunocytochemical protocols. Neurones, neuronal structures, or regions of interest are noted, sometimes drawn (with the aid of a drawing tube) and photographed. The region of interest, containing the neurones or neuronal structures that are to be examined in the electron microscope or that are to be subjected to post-embedding immunocytochemistry (Chapter 6), is then re-embedded in blank blocks of resin, or glued on to blank blocks of resin that are suitable for further sectioning for electron microscopy (*Protocol 9*).

Protocol 9. Re-embedding for electron microscopy

Materials

- dissection microscope
- single edged razor blades

Protocol 9. *Continued*

- scalpel with pointed blades
- blank tubes of resin or truncated electron microscopy embedding capsules
- cyanoacrylate glue or electron microscopy resin
- hot plate

Method

1. Ensure that all excess resin around the edge of the coverslip is removed.
2. Completely remove coverslip from the slide or remove just that part of the coverslip which overlies the neurones or regions of interest by gently inserting a razor blade between the coverslip and the resin and pushing until the coverslip is free. Once the coverslip is removed the slide can still be examined in the light microscope even using oil immersion lens, although care should be taken not to damage the tissue since it is no longer protected by the coverslip.[a]
3. Identify neurones or regions to be re-embedded in the light microscope and make guide cuts in the resin with a razor blade or pointed scalpel blade.
4. Warm slide gently on a hot plate to soften the resin,[b] cut around neurones or areas of interest with a scalpel blade under the dissecting microscope, and remove piece of tissue with forceps.
5. Flatten the small piece of resin-embedded tissue by placing it on a warm razor blade or slide and even sandwiching between two of them if necessary.
6. *Either*: glue to the end of a blank tube of resin[c] with cyanoacrylate glue (Superglue) or araldite.
   Or: place face down on a fresh microscope slide, place truncated embedding capsule over it, fill with resin, place label in, and seal with a coverslip. Polymerize the resin at 60°C for 48 h. Once polymerized, remove the coverslip and capsule with the aid of a razor blade. The block should come away from the slide easily.

[a] If a section is damaged after the coverslip has been removed it can be repaired by applying a small drop of resin and a new coverslip, and curing for 48 h at 60°C. Similarly, after cutting out the region of interest, the slide can be restored by the same method. Following removal of the coverslip, good optical qualities of the slide can be restored temporarily, by applying a drop of immersion oil and a new coverslip.

[b] The resin is brittle at room temperature: should it be cut without warming there is the possibility of splitting or cracking areas of interest. Furthermore once a piece of tissue is cut away from the slide it should only be further trimmed when warmed as trimmed pieces or, just as likely, the area of interest may 'flick' away.

[c] The blank tubes of resin are made either using a mould or by cutting off the pointed end of an embedding capsule, placing it on a slide, over-filling with resin, placing a coverslip over the end, and curing for 48 h at 60°C. The resultant blocks should have two optically good surfaces that allow the examination of the re-embedded tissue in the light microscope. The blank blocks measure 8 mm in diameter and about 10 mm in height.

6.4 Re-sectioning for electron microscopy

The sections prepared for examination in the light microscope prior to the electron microscope are in the region of 50–100 μm in thickness. For electron microscopy, however, it is necessary to have sections of a thickness in the region of 60–90 nm. In order to examine this material in the electron microscope or indeed material prepared for direct electron microscopic analysis, it is necessary to re-section at a thickness suitable for electron microscopy. Sectioning at this thickness can only be carried out on commercially available microtomes, referred to as ultramicrotomes (Leica). Tissue that has been re-embedded in blocks of resin in the manner described above are suitable for sectioning on an ultramicrotome. A precise description of sectioning on an ultamicrotome is beyond the scope of this volume, it is a difficult process that requires instruction in relation to a particular ultramicrotome. Only the basic principles will be briefly described here.

6.4.1 Principles of sectioning for electron microscopy

The essential features of all ultramicrotomes are:

- chuck to hold specimen
- knife holding block
- advance mechanism; either thermal feed or mechanical
- stereo-microscope
- system of illumination
- glass or diamond knife

A block with the re-embedded tissue is examined in the light microscope by placing on a glass microscope slide and treating as a normal light microscopic preparation; the neurones, neuronal structures, or regions of interest are located. The block is then placed in the ultramicrotome chuck which is put in a position for direct viewing of the block surface. The surplus resin and tissue are trimmed away with a razor blade under stereo-microscopic guidance. With frequent comparisons with the image seen in the light microscope, the block is trimmed to produce a face suitable for ultrathin sectioning (in the region of 1 mm^2 or less, and the top and bottom edges parallel). The chuck with trimmed block is placed in the cutting position. The chuck is adjusted to make the block surface parallel to the knife edge. The knife holding block, which is stationary during the operation of the microtome, is advanced to the block surface by a coarse and fine manual feed. Fine adjustments to make the block surface parallel to the knife edge are made; the chuck and the knife holder between them can be adjusted in all three planes. The close adjustment is aided by the special illumination system that gives a reflection of the knife edge on the block surface. Once 'lined-up' the boat, which is an integral part of a diamond knife but must be attached to a glass knife, is filled with water. The machine is turned on and the specimen passes the knife edge and is then advanced by either a mechanical or thermal feed. Sections float on the water; the thickness is monitored by their interference colours and adjusted accordingly. A well trimmed specimen with clean, parallel edges will result in a ribbon of sections of consistent thickness. Series of up to 100 sections are cut in a single session. If analysis of serial sections is to be carried out, which is usually the case in the analysis of synaptic connections, the sections are collected on single-slot coated grids (*Protocol 10*) rather than on mesh grids, as a significant area of the sections would be obscured by the bars of a mesh grid. The grids are dried and stored in a commercially available grid box (Agar Scientific Ltd. or Cambridge Instruments).

6.4.2 Some useful hints for ultrathin sectioning

(a) The smaller the block face the easier it is to cut long series of sections, and the easier it is to locate structures in correlated light and electron microscopic analyses.

(b) An asymmetric shape to the block surface makes orientation in the electron microscope easier.

(c) Dirt is easily picked up during sectioning so always clean forceps, syringe needles, eyelashes etc. with ethanol prior to any manipulation of sections or electron microscope grids.

(d) Always store sections in the grid boxes in the same way, i.e. sections either to the right or to the left.

6.4.3 Semi-thin sectioning on an ultramicrotome (see also Chapter 6, *Protocol 1*)

The ultramicrotome can be used to cut sections at 1–5 μm from resin embedded tissue (semi-thin sections). The same material that is prepared for electron microscopy can be cut, and indeed one of the main reasons for cutting semi-thin sections is that they aid in orientation of sections in the electron microscope and the localization of structures first identified in the light microscopic section. The sections are only cut with glass knives since sections of this thickness damage the cutting edge of a diamond knife. As with ultrathin sections the semi-thin sections are floated on water, picked up with a drop of water with the point of a hypodermic needle or a specially designed loop, and placed on a drop of water on coated microscope slides (*Protocol 5*). The sections are dried on to the slide with gentle heat on a hotplate. The sections can then immediately have a coverslip applied with a mounting medium (XAM or DPX) or they can be stained with a mixture consisting of:

- 50 ml 1% aqueous Azur II
- 50 ml 1% toluidine containing 0.5 g sodium tetraborate
- 6 g sucrose

Filter the stain before use, place a drop on the section, heat gently on a hotplate, and wash in running water. Alternatively, they can be subjected to post-embedding immunocytochemistry (see Chapter 6).

Protocol 10. Coating of single-slot electron microscope grids

Materials

- single-slot electron microscope grids (copper, nickel, or gold; from any EM supplier)
- chloroform
- grid-coating resin (Pioloform, Butvar or Formvar, Fisons Polaron)
- distilled water
- staining trough or dish
- grid-coating apparatus (from Agar Scientific Ltd.) or small vessel with tap at bottom
- laboratory film, e.g. Parafilm (made by American Can Company)
- Petri dishes

Method

1. Clean grids in chloroform, dry on filter paper, and store in Petri dish.
2. Prepare a 1% solution of grid-coating resin in chloroform, filter, and store at 4°C.
3. Fill coating apparatus with the resin solution. Put cleaned microscope slide in the solution in the upright position. The slide is then coated with the Pioloform by either opening the tap at the bottom of the vessel and allowing the solution to flow out, or by slowly lifting the slide vertically out of the vessel. The thickness of the film is dependent on the rate of removal of the slide from the solution or the rate of flowing out of the solution (the slower the rate the thinner the film).
4. Once all the chloroform has evaporated, remove the film from the slide by scoring the bottom edge of the slide with a razor blade and lowering it into the water at an angle of about 45°. The film should separate from the slide, and by continuing to lower the slide into the water, the film will float off completely. The.correct thickness of the film appears silver in colour when illuminated from a lamp above the surface of the water.[a]
5. Place grids on to the film, one at a time, with the matter side down. Cover the whole film with grids but take care that they do not overlap.
6. Remove the film with grids adhering from the water by placing a piece of laboratory film (Parafilm) on top of them and gently lifting. Place the Parafilm with coated grids in a clean Petri dish.

Protocol 10. *Continued*

7. Before using a batch of grids, examine a few from each film in the electron microscope to check for strength, evenness, and cleanliness.

[a] Cover water surface with foil when not in use to prevent dust falling on to it.

6.4.4 Manipulations of ultrathin sections

Ultrathin sections collected on coated *gold* or *nickel* grids are in a form that is suitable for immunocytochemistry by the immunogold method (post-embedding immunocytochemistry: see Chapter 7). For most applications *copper* grids are used. The sections can be immediately examined in the electron microscope but it is usually necessary to stain the sections with heavy metals to improve contrast. The two most commonly used stains are uranyl acetate and lead citrate (*Protocol 11*). It is usual to expose the tissue to uranyl acetate during the dehydration procedure (see *Protocol 8*), but this is not necessarily the case, and it can be performed on sections prior to the lead staining.

Protocol 11. Staining of ultrathin sections with Reynolds' lead citrate[a] (4)

Materials

- lead nitrate
- tri-sodium citrate
- 4 M sodium hydroxide
- sodium hydroxide pellets
- Petri dish
- laboratory film, (e.g. Parafilm)
- filter paper
- wash bottle containing distilled water
- hair dryer
- Pasteur pipettes

A. *Preparation of the lead citrate*

1. Weigh out 0.27 g of lead nitrate (we use glass vials).
2. Weigh out 0.35 g of tri-sodium citrate in a separate vial.
3. Add 9.6 ml of distilled water to the lead nitrate. Put cap on vial and shake to dissolve.

4. Add the tri-sodium citrate to the lead nitrate solution. Shake to dissolve. At this stage the solution is milky in appearance.
5. Add 0.4 ml of 4 M NaOH. Replace cap quickly[b] and shake.

B. *Staining of sections*[c]

1. Prepare a Petri dish containing a piece of laboratory film and sodium hydroxide pellets to absorb CO_2.
2. Take up some of the lead citrate solution in a Pasteur pipette, discard first drop, and place separate drops on to the Parafilm, only removing the cover of the Petri dish as far as is necessary.
3. Place grids, sections down on the drops of stain (one grid per drop) and leave for 1.5–5.0 min.
4. Pick grids up one at a time, wash in a stream of distilled water, dry excess water off with filter paper, particularly between the points of the forceps, and completely dry with warm air from a hair dryer.
5. Replace grid in grid box.

[a] **Safety note 7**. Lead and lead salts are toxic, appropriate precautions should be taken to prevent contact with the skin.

[b] This solution can be stored up to two weeks at 4°C. Prevent contact as far as possible between lead citrate and the air as atmospheric carbon dioxide reacts to form an insoluble, electron dense precipitate.

[c] The same method can be applied to staining of sections with uranyl acetate (1% aqueous solution that is filtered before use), except that the precautions to avoid contact with CO_2 are not necessary, and the staining time is 20–60 min (see *Safety note 4, Protocol 8*).

7. Examination of sections in the electron microscope

If the tissue has not been subjected to any histochemical or immunocytochemical staining procedure then the sections are examined in the electron microscope by standard procedures. Similarly, if the material contains a high density of labelled structures, for instance anterogradely labelled terminals, then analysis can be by standard procedures. It must be remembered however, that in many histological or immunocytochemical procedures the penetration of the reagents into the tissue may be very limited, it is thus important to examine those ultrathin sections that are closest to the surface. In some cases it may even be necessary to angle the tissue during ultrathin sectioning so that the very surface of the tissue is included in the sections.

If the structures under investigation are rare, are rarely stained, or the ultrastructural analysis needs to be related to the three-dimensional or light microscopic morphology of the neuronal structure under investigation, then it is necessary to identify and examine the *same* structures in the electron microscope that were identified in the light microscope. The same is also often the case in multiple labelling studies (see Chapter 11) where a particular event, for instance the close apposition of an anterogradely labelled terminal and a retrogradely labelled cell, is rare for technical reasons. Thus a neurone that is characterized first at the light microscopic level by its morphology (by for instance, Golgi-impregnation see *Protocol 12*, or the intracellular injection of HRP see Chapters 9 and 10), by its projection area (see Chapters 2 and 4), or its chemical characteristics (see Chapters 5 and 7) can then be examined in the electron microscope to characterize its ultrastructure, and its afferent and efferent synaptic connections.

Furthermore, by examination of light microscopically identified neurones in the electron microscope the topography or pattern of afferent synaptic terminals to a particular neurone can be assessed, and *quantitative* aspects of both the input and output can be established. In this way the position of individual neurones and eventually classes of neurones, in the neuronal microcircuitry or networks of a particular area of the brain can be established. The technique by which a structure that is first identified in the light microscope is then examined in the electron microscope, termed 'correlated light and electron microscopy', was pioneered by Blackstad (5, 6) and Smogyi (7, 8) and is described in detail elsewhere (9).

7.1 Correlated light and electron microscopy

Probably the most important step in correlated light and electron microscopy is the detailed records of the structure under investigation at the light microscopic level. In addition to aiding the analysis of the structure in the electron microscope, it is important to make as detailed recordings as possible because once they are sectioned for electron microscopy they are lost. Detailed high magnification photomicrographs and drawings are necessary. It is also valuable to note and record the positions of easily identifiable structures, (e.g. capillaries, neuronal perikarya, etc.) that may be used as 'landmarks' to help locate the neuronal structure under study in the electron microscope. Having decided and recorded those structures that are to be examined in the electron microscope, the coverslip is removed and the tissue re-embedded for ultrathin sectioning (*Protocol 9*).

Once re-embedded the tissue within the block can again be examined in detail in the light microscope and if necessary photographs may be taken, (e.g. see Figure 2A of Bolam *et al.* (10), which was taken from the surface of the block). The block is trimmed to include the area of interest or structures of interest. Rather than using the classical symmetrical trapezium shape for the trimmed block surface, an asymmetrical shape is used to simplify the orientation of the sections in the electron microscope. The distance from the surface of the block to the tissue can be measured by focusing on the surface, and then on a structure in the tissue, and reading off the distance on the microscope vernier. The tissue (or structure of interest) is now approached on an ultramicrotome under manual control, cutting one or two micron sections with regular monitoring in the light microscope. At each examination in the light microscope the size of the block is assessed and trimmed further if necessary to reach optimal size for serial sectioning; the distance of the structure of interest from the surface is also measured. When less than 1 μm from the structure of interest, the ultramicrotome is turned on to automatic, and serial ultrathin sections (silver/grey, approximately 70 nm) are cut. Short series of 50–100 sections are generally cut in one session and are collected on coated single-slot grids (*Protocol 10*). When the sections have been collected, the block is removed from the ultramicrotome chuck and examined again in the light microscope. The location within the block, of the parts of the neuronal structure that have been completely or partly sectioned are noted, and their positions marked on both the drawings and the high magnification micrographs.

After staining the ultrathin sections with lead citrate (*Protocol 11*) they are examined in the electron microscope. The identified structures, (i.e. those examined in the light microscope) are located within the section and examined at high magnification. To localize, or find, the identified structures in the electron microscope, constant comparisons are made between the positions of structures seen in the block in the light microscope (it is useful to have a light microscope adjacent to the electron microscope), the image in the electron microscope, and the high magnification light micrographs. The positions of the identified structures can then be confirmed by their relationships to the 'landmarks' (for instance, unstained neuronal perikarya or blood vessels) in the block and in the light micrographs. Once located, structures are easily examined in serial sections and with careful sectioning on the ultramicrotome, from series to series.

An additional aid to the location of identified structures in the electron microscope are 1 μm sections taken at the beginning or at the end of the series of ultrathin sections (see Section 7.4.3). These sections, suitably counter-stained, are more easily compared than the block surface with the image in the electron microscope. The major problem with 1 μm sections is that structures can no longer be recovered for electron microscopy or can only be done so with great difficulty, thus should only be taken at times when important structures will not be lost.

Records of the observations of the structures examined in the electron microscope should include low and high power light and electron micrographs that include 'landmarks' to demonstrate or 'prove' that the structure examined in the electron microscope is indeed the same structure that had been examined in the light microscope.

8. Single section Golgi-impregnation (11)

Many of the histological procedures designed to stain neurones that are used in experimental neuroanatomy, particularly when preparing for electron microscopy, result in staining of only cell bodies and proximal dendrites. This is a major disadvantage if it is difficult to morphologically characterize a neurone on the basis of the morphology of the cell body and proximal dendrites. It is also a major problem when examining the synaptic input to the neurone since without the distal dendritic tree, both qualitative and quantitative data will be severely limited. One approach to overcome this problem is to Golgi-impregnate the neurones that are stained by the histochemical or immunocytochemical process (11–14). Golgi-impregnated neurones are often stained in their entirety and, following gold-toning, can be examined in the electron microscope (5–8). Although the impregnation of neurones appears to be a random process, staining of sufficient sections eventually results in the impregnation of histochemically stained neurones. A simple and rapid method of impregnation of tissue sections is described that is a modification of the 'single-section-Golgi' procedure of Freund and Somogyi (13).

Protocol 12. Single section Golgi-impregnation (11)

Materials

- 3.5% aqueous potassium dichromate
- 1–2.5% aqueous silver nitrate
- glycerol
- microscope slides and coverslips
- artist's paint brush
- filter paper
- tape (electrician's insulation tape or masking tape)

Method

1. After histological processing and treatment with osmium tetroxide (*Protocol 7*) place the sections in 3.5% aqueous potassium dichromate for 1–3 h, or overnight if convenient, at room temperature.
2. Remove sections, one at a time, and place at one end of a microscope slide. Trim with a razor blade to remove large masses of myelinated axons and ventricles which may hamper diffusion of silver nitrate solution through the section.
3. Remove excess potassium dichromate solution with filter paper and place another slide directly on top of the first. The two slides are held together by gently taping at the opposite end to the sections with the electrician's insulation tape. If the sections are small, then two may be placed side-by-side on a single slide.
4. Place the slide upright in a small beaker that is approximately one third

full of silver nitrate solution. The space between the slides immediately fills with the silver nitrate solution by capillary action.[a] Several slides can be placed in one beaker of silver solution.

5. Monitor progress of the impregnation by examination with a microscope taking care to protect the microscope and lenses from the silver nitrate solution.
6. On completion of impregnation, usually 6–24 h, remove the sections by cutting the edge of the tape that holds the slides together, separating the slides with a razor blade. Lift off the section with an artist's paint brush dipped in glycerol. Place each section between coverslips.

[a] If the silver solution flows over the surface of the section crystals of silver chromate will be formed that will hinder impregnation and obscure any impregnated cells. Remove the section from the slide, briefly rinse in water, and put back into the potassium dichromate solution.

For electron microscopic analysis of Golgi-impregnated neurones it is necessary to carry out a de-impregnation of the neurones to remove the electron dense silver chromate precipitate that fills the cytoplasm of impregnated structures. De-impregnation is carried out by reacting with gold chloride (gold-toning) which results in the deposition of metallic gold within the impregnated neurones. The gold deposit is less dense and allows the visualization of histochemical markers within the neurones at the light level, and allows more detailed ultrastructural analysis of the identified cells and their synaptic inputs (15–17).

Protocol 13. Gold-toning of Golgi-impregnated structures

Materials

- fibre optic lamp (15 V 150 W bulb supplied by Schott)
- cool air blower
- 0.07% $NaHAuCl_4 \cdot 2H_2O$ containing 0.25% glycerol
- 0.2% oxalic acid
- 1% sodium thiosulphate

Method

1. Illuminate sections whilst still sandwiched between two coverslips in glycerol for 30 min using a fibre optic illuminating device containing a 15 V, 150 W bulb focused into an 8 mm circle at full strength. Throughout the illumination the sections are cooled by cold air blowing from a hair dryer.
2. Store sections at 4°C until gold-toning is to be carried out. Remove

Protocol 13. *Continued*

sections from the coverslip by gently separating them with a razor blade, picking them up with a fine paint brush soaked in glycerol, and place in glass vials.

3. Incubate for 15–30 min in 0.07% aqueous solution of $NaHAuCl_4 \cdot 2H_2O$ containing 0.25% glycerol at 0°C with occasional shaking.[a]
4. Wash sections for 3 × 2 min in distilled water, 2 min in 0.2% oxalic acid, and then 3 × 2 min in distilled water.
5. Wash for 3 × 15 min in 1% sodium thiosulphate at room temperature.
6. Rinse briefly in distilled water, dehydrate, and embed in electron microscopy resin according to *Protocol 9*.

[a] The longer the time in the gold solution the heavier is the gold-toning. Select optimal time on each run by incubating test sections.

References

1. Pearse, A. G. E. (1980). *Histochemistry Theoretical and Applied.* Churchill Livingstone, Edinburgh.
2. Glauert, A. M. (1975). *Fixation, Dehydration and Embedding of Biological Specimens.* North Holland Publishing Company, Amsterdam.
3. Sabatini, D. D., Bensch, K., and Barrnett, R. J. (1963). *J. Cell Biol.,* **17,** 19.
4. Reynolds, E. S. (1963). *J. Cell Biol.,* **17,** 208.
5. Blackstad, T. W. (1965). *Z. Zellforsch.,* **67,** 819.
6. Blackstad, T. W. (1975). *Brain Res.,* **95,** 191.
7. Somogyi, P. (1977). *Brain Res.,* **136,** 345.
8. Somogyi, P. (1978). *Neurosci.,* **3,** 167.
9. Bolam, J. P. and Ingham, C. A. (1990). In *Handbook of Chemical Neuroanatomy* (ed. A. Björklund, T. Hökfelt, F. G., Wouterlood, and A. N. van den Pol), Vol. 8, pp. 125–98. Elsevier Science Publishers, Amsterdam.
10. Bolam, J. P., Somogyi, P., Totterdell, S., and Smith, A. D. (1981). *Neurosci.,* **6,** 2141.
11. Izzo, P., Graybiel, A. M., and Bolam, J. P. (1987). *Neurosci.,* **20,** 577.
12. Somogyi, P., Hodgson, A. J., and Smith, A. D. (1979). *Neurosci.,* **4,** 1805.
13. Freund, T. F. and Somogyi, P. (1983). *Neurosci.,* **9,** 463.
14. Gabbott, P. L. and Somogyi, J. (1984). *J. Neurosci. Methods,* **11,** 221.
15. Fairén, A., Peters, A., and Saldanha, J. (1977). *J. Neurocytol.,* **6,** 311.
16. Fairén, A., DeFelipe, J., and Martinez-Ruiz, R. (1981). *11th Int. Cong. Anat.,* 291.
17. Somogyi, P., Freund, T. F., Halasz, N., and Kisvarday, Z. F. (1981). *Brain Res.,* **225,** 431.

Appendix: Tyrode's solution

1. Add to 950 ml distilled water in the following order:
   - 8.0 g NaCl
   - 0.2 g KCl
   - 1 ml of 26.5% $CaCl_2 \cdot 2H_2O$ (the calcium may be omitted)
   - 1 ml of 5% $NaH_2PO_4 \cdot 2H_2O$
   - 1 g $NaHCO_3$
   - 1 g glucose (if solution is made up in advance this should be added on the day of use)
2. make up to 1000 ml with distilled water
3. gas the solution with a mixture consisting of 95% O_2 and 5% CO_2 prior to use.

2

Retrograde tracers for light and electron microscopy

IDA J. LLEWELLYN-SMITH, PAUL PILOWSKY, and JANE B. MINSON

1. Introduction

Retrograde neuronal tract tracing is used to establish where neurones send their axons, and is based on the ability of axons to take up substances from the extracellular fluid and transport them back to cell bodies. Retrograde tracing was introduced to the field of neuroanatomy just over twenty years ago (1, 2). Since then, retrograde tracers have become invaluable tools for the study of nerve pathways in the central and peripheral nervous systems. Initially, horseradish peroxidase (HRP) was the only retrograde tracer available to neuroanatomists. However, in the late 1970s and in the 1980s, a number of new tracers were developed, including fluorescent molecules and fluorescent latex microspheres, HRP conjugated to lectins or toxins, gold-labelled tracers, cholera toxin B subunit (which is detected immunocytochemically), and most recently, viruses. These developments have lead to an explosion in the number of retrograde tracing studies, since there is now a retrograde tracer suitable for virtually any kind of study that the neuroanatomist can imagine. This chapter deals with non-viral retrograde tracers that can be used for both light and electron microscopic studies on neuronal connectivity, i.e. HRP-based tracers, colloidal gold-labelled tracers, and unconjugated cholera toxin B subunit.

2. HRP-based tracers

The most widely used members of this family of tracers are HRP, wheatgerm agglutinin (WGA) conjugated to HRP (WGA-HRP), and cholera toxin B subunit (CTB) conjugated to HRP (CTB-HRP).

HRP is taken up non-specifically by the axons, dendrites, and cell bodies of neurones through pinocytotic vesicles that are constantly sampling the extracellular environment. In contrast, WGA-HRP and CTB-HRP are taken up by way of their lectin (WGA) or toxin (CTB), which bind specifically to different molecules in neuronal plasma membranes. These specific uptake mechanisms make WGA-HRP and CTB-HRP more sensitive retrograde tracers than free HRP (3, 4). Consequently, WGA-HRP and CTB-HRP are generally preferred to HRP for tracing studies within the central nervous system. However, HRP is still commonly used for retrograde tracing from nerve trunks.

After uptake into axons, HRP, WGA-HRP, and CTB-HRP are carried by fast axonal transport to neuronal cell bodies. HRP and WGA-HRP localize in the lysosomes of neuronal somata and proximal dendrites (*Figure 1A–E*). In contrast, CTB-HRP is not confined to lysosomes but can be detected throughout the neuronal cytoplasm, including distal dendrites (see 5, 6 and *Figure 2*), and often yields a Golgi-like image of the neurones that have taken it up. HRP-based tracers can be detected for only a few days after they have reached nerve cell bodies, since the HRP is progressively degraded by proteolytic enzymes that are present in lysosomes.

2.1 Application of HRP-based tracers

HRP and HRP-based tracers are usually used in solution. The tracers discussed in Section 2 are generally supplied in lyophilized form and are reconstituted by the addition of distilled water. HRP (Sigma Type VI or Boehringer Mannheim; *Table 1*) is usually employed at concentrations of 5% to 40%; WGA-HRP, at 0.5% to 4%; and CTB-HRP, at 1%. Sometimes dimethyl sulphoxide (DMSO; 2–10%) is added to the tracer solution. Being highly lipid soluble, DMSO is thought to promote uptake of tracer by nerve fibres. Crystals of HRP can be applied to cut nerve trunks (see Section 2.1.3).

2.1.1 Pressure injection

Many methods have been devised for pressure injection of tracers into the brain or spinal cord (7). The simplest is to use glass tubing with a narrow internal diameter and a fine tip (5–50 μm). Pressure is applied through a length of tubing attached to the glass, and the movement of the meniscus of the tracer solution is monitored through a dissecting or operating microscope with a calibrated graticule in one eyepiece. In the central nervous system, volumes as small as 15 nl can be injected, giving injection sites as small as 300–400 μm in diameter (8), although larger injection sites 1.5–2.0 mm are more usual (9).

HRP-based tracers can also be pressure injected into peripheral nerve trunks or ganglia. The tip of a glass pipette is inserted into the nerve or ganglion by hand while an assistant performs the injection. Alternatively, the nerve can be stabilized with a loop of cotton, and the pipette inserted with an electrode holder. Special care must be taken to avoid drying of the nerve or spillage of tracer that may result in artefactual labelling, particularly when CTB-HRP is used.

2.1.2 Iontophoresis

For very small injection sites, (e.g. 200–300 μm or less in diameter), use iontophoresis from glass electrodes with fine tip diameters (10 μm or less). The electrode is filled with a small amount of tracer, typically 2–5 μl. Connection of the electrode to the current source is through a fine silver wire inserted into the tracer solution. Injections are made by passing an appropriate current, using a duty cycle of 5–10 sec on and 5–10 sec off, to minimize electrode blockage. For most tracing agents, (e.g. HRP, WGA-HRP, CTB) dissolved in physiological solutions, a positive current of 2–15 μA will be optimal, although effective injections have been reported with currents as small as 0.1–0.5 μA for 5–20 min (10, 11). The electrode is connected to the '+' socket of the current source, and a silver wire inserted into the back muscles is connected to the '−' socket. A common reason for injection failure is the use of current sources with low compliance. An electrode with a resistance of 25 MΩ will require a compliance of 250 V to produce 10 μA. We recommend the Midgard CS4, which has a compliance of 2000 V. This means that currents of 5–10 μA can easily be passed through high resistance electrodes. Standard stimulators used for electrophysiology will generally be unsuitable.

2.1.3 Application to cut nerves

Solutions or crystals of HRP-based tracers can be applied directly to the cut ends of nerve trunks. Nerves should be exposed to the tracer for as long as is practicable (usually at least one hour), and then the tracer should be removed to prevent artefactual uptake by adjacent structures. When the tracer is applied in a sealed cuff (12) artefactual labelling is less of a problem.

2.2 Fixation

It is generally agreed that high formaldehyde concentrations reduce the enzyme activity of HRP and should be avoided (13). We find that the inclusion of even 1% formaldehyde in fixative reduces the detectability of HRP-based tracers in the spinal cord. For studies with HRP-based tracers, we routinely perfuse with 2.5% glutaraldehyde, 0.5% formaldehyde in 0.1 M sodium phosphate buffer, pH 7.4 (Chapter 1, *Protocol 2* and *Safety note 1*, p. 5). For more information on perfusion, post-fixation, and section preparation, refer to Chapter 1.

2.3 Detecting HRP-based tracers

Neurones retrogradely labelled with HRP-based tracers are visualized by peroxidase reactions, in which a soluble chromogen is oxidized to a detectable reaction product through the activity of HRP on its substrate, hydrogen peroxide. A variety of chromogens are available, which give reaction products that differ in form, (e.g. crystalline versus amorphous), colour, and

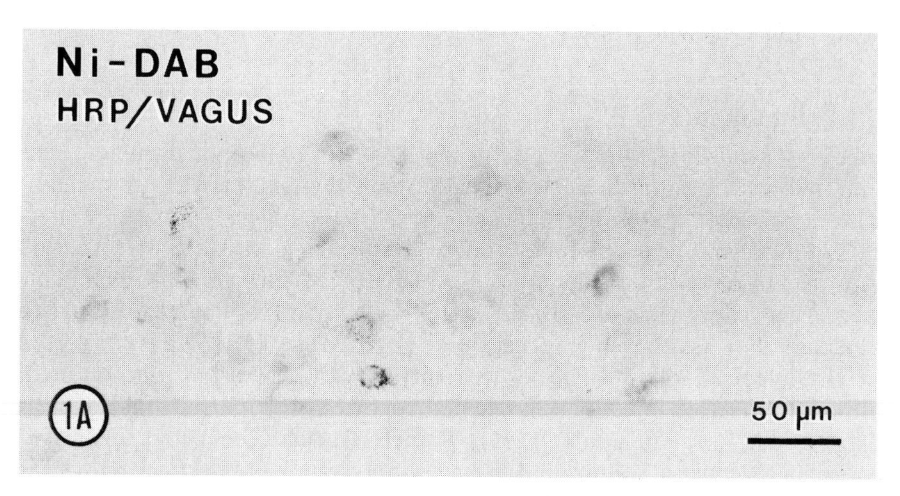
Ni-DAB
HRP/VAGUS
1A
50 μm

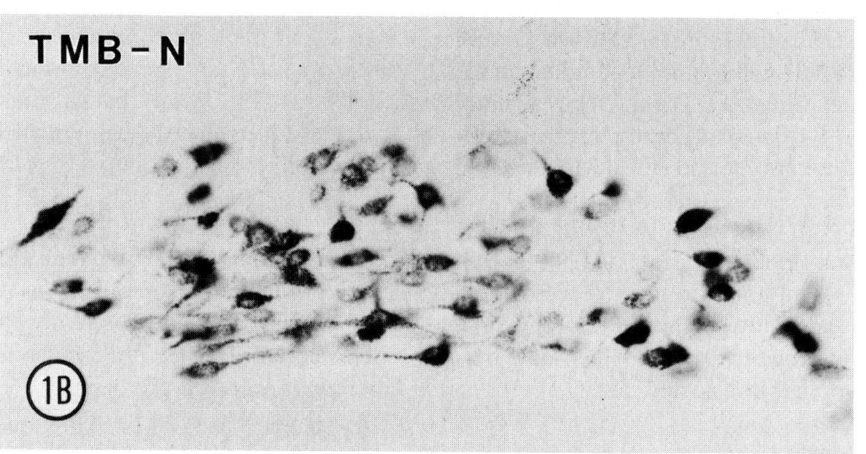
TMB-N
1B

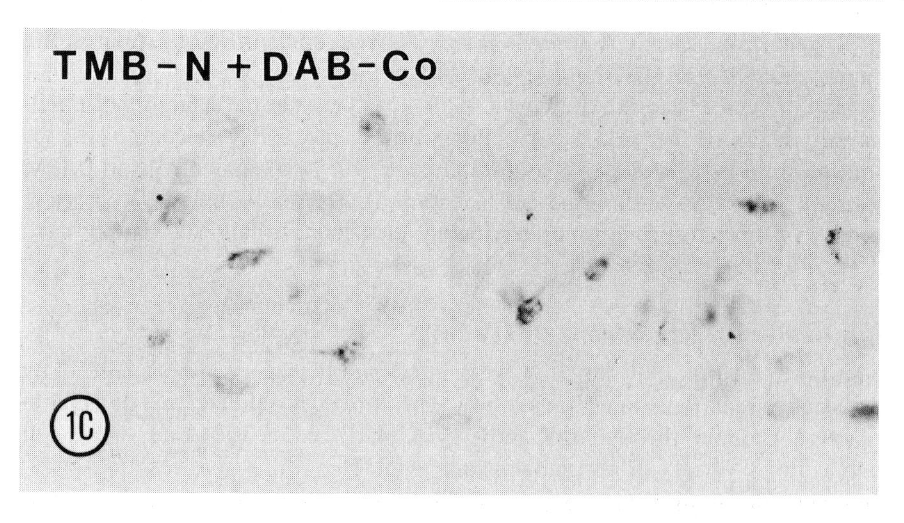
TMB-N + DAB-Co
1C

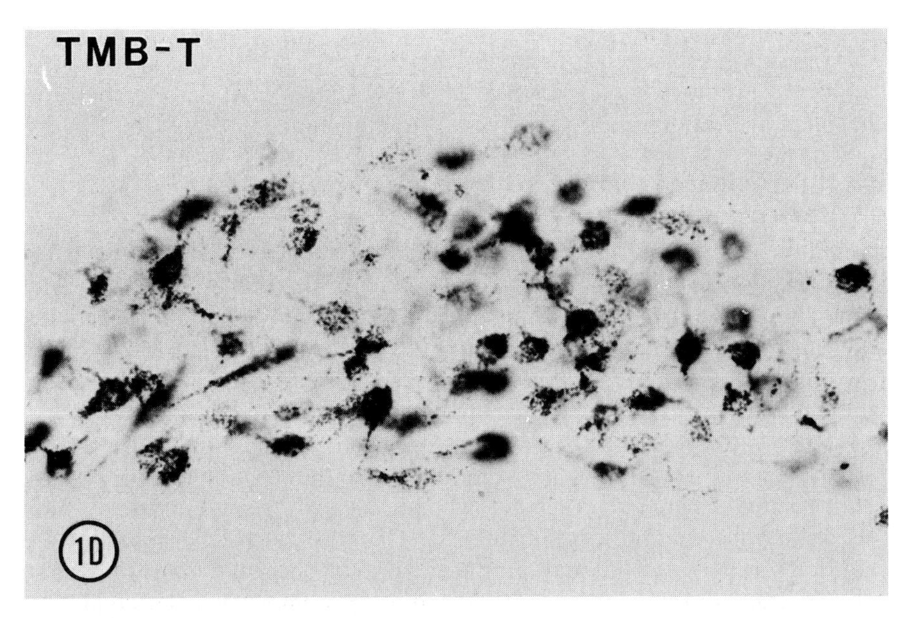

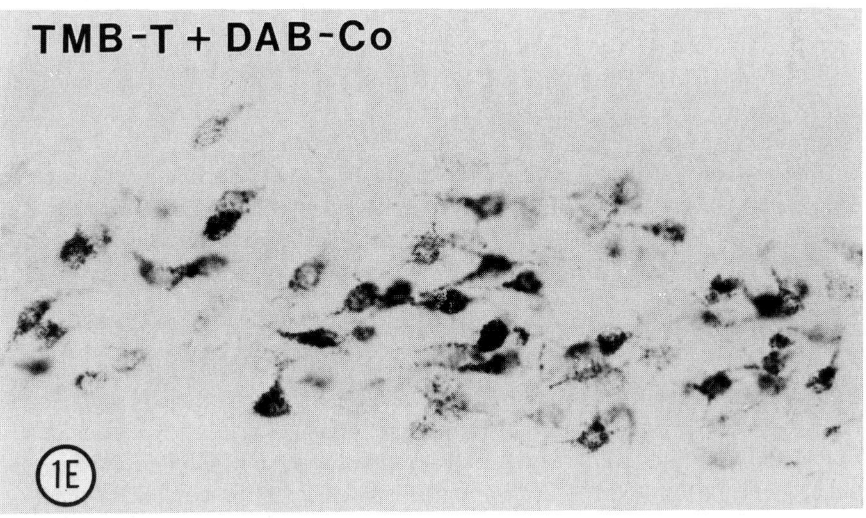

Figure 1. *HRP-based tracers. Comparisons of the sensitivity of peroxidase reactions for detecting retrogradely-transported HRP.* Serial transverse sections through the dorsal motor nucleus of the vagus near the obex, rat. Sigma HRP (10% Type VI in 10% DMSO/distilled water) injected into the cervical vagus nerve. Fixative, 2.5% glutaraldehyde, 0.5% formaldehyde. The injection yielded retrogradely labelled neurones in the dorsal motor nucleus but no anterogradely labelled terminals in the nucleus tractus solitarius. The nickel-DAB reacted section (Ni-DAB; A) shows the fewest retrogradely labelled neurones. The TMB-nitroprusside(TMB-N) reacted section (B) shows the most retrogradely labelled neurones, but most neurones lose their label as a result of treatment with DAB, $CoCl_2$ and H_2O_2 (TMB-N + DAB-Co; C). The TMB-tungstate(TMB-T) reacted section (D) also contains many retrogradely labelled neurones. More neurones from TMB-T reacted sections retain their label through treatment with DAB, $CoCl_2$ and H_2O_2 (TMB-T + DAB-Co; E) than from TMB-N reacted sections (compare E with C).

stability. Chromogens vary in their ability to detect HRP so the choice of chromogen determines the sensitivity of the reaction.

2.3.1 Peroxidase reactions with diaminobenzidine as chromogen

Diaminobenzidine (DAB) was the first chromogen used for detecting retrogradely-transported HRP (1, 2). Peroxidase reactions can be done with DAB alone but are not recommended because of their poor sensitivity. Intensification with either imidazole (14, 15) or heavy metals, such as nickel (see below) or cobalt, or both, increases the sensitivity of the reaction, yielding a larger number and/or more intensely labelled neurones.

We use glucose oxidase to generate hydrogen peroxide in DAB reactions rather than adding hydrogen peroxide directly to the reaction mix because we achieve a better signal to noise ratio. The pre-incubation solution and reaction mix in the following protocol include NH_4Cl and D-glucose because they are required for glucose oxidase to produce hydrogen peroxide. Glucose oxidase solution (Sigma) retains its activity for up to 18 months when stored at 4°C.

Protocol 1 documents our nickel-intensified DAB reaction. In general, metal-intensified DAB reactions produce black reaction products by light microscopy (LM). Unintensified DAB and imidazole-DAB reactions give amber-brown reaction products by LM. See Llewellyn-Smith *et al.* (15) for a description of imidazole-DAB reactions.

Precautions. DAB is a potential carcinogen. Gloves should be worn when handling it. DAB and all DAB-contaminated glassware and disposable items should be inactivated with chlorine bleach (see *Safety note 3* in Chapter 5, p. 119).

i. Nickel-intensified DAB reactions

Appearance.

By LM, black reaction product (*Figure 1A*). At the electron microscope level, nickel-DAB reactions, like other DAB reactions, increase the electron density of lysosomes that contain retrogradely-transported HRP; HRP reaction product also may be found in the Golgi apparatus (*Figure 3B*). Since all DAB reaction products look the same in the electron microscope, cells labelled with one type of DAB reaction cannot be distinguished from cells labelled with another type of DAB reaction at the ultrastructural level.

Sensitivity.

More sensitive than unintensified DAB or imidazole-DAB but less sensitive than tetramethylbenzidine reactions (see *Figure 1*). We have found that when neurones contain little HRP-based retrograde tracer, nickel-intensified DAB reactions yield more labelled cells than imidazole-intensified DAB reactions. However, if the level of tracer is high, nickel-DAB reactions and imidazole-DAB reaction give similar results.

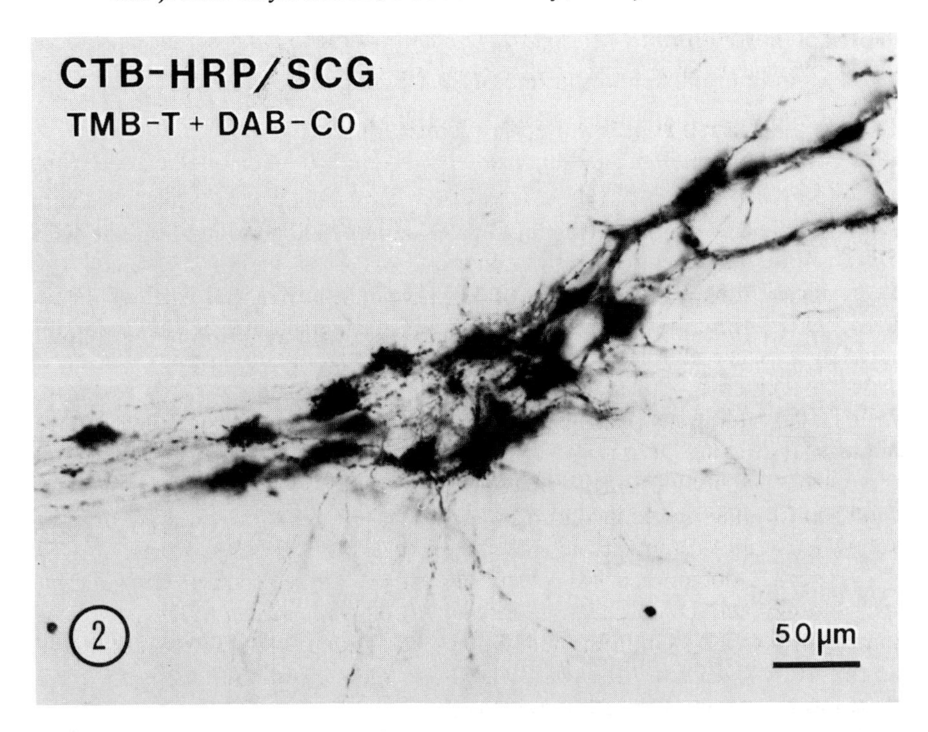

Figure 2. *HRP-based tracers. Retrograde tracing with CTB-HRP.* Transverse section of spinal cord segment T2, rat. List CTB-HRP (1% in 10% DMSO/distilled water) injected into the superior cervical ganglion (SCG). Fixative, 2.5% glutaraldehyde, 0.5% formaldehyde. TMB-tungstate reaction stabilized with DAB, $CoCl_2$ and H_2O_2 (TMB-T + DAB-Co). Many nerve processes are labelled in addition to the cell bodies of sympathetic preganglionic neurones.

Stability.
Nickel-DAB reaction product is extremely stable, being unaffected by exposure to any of the buffers or organic solvents commonly used for histology, histochemistry, immunocytochemistry, or electron microscopy.

Artefacts.
Any cells with high levels of endogenous hydrogen peroxidase, such as red blood cells and pericytes around blood vessels, are revealed.

Protocol 1. Nickel-intensified DAB reaction

Stock solutions

- 1 g nickel ammonium sulphate [$(NH_4)_2SO_4 \cdot NiSO_4 \cdot 6H_2O$] dissolved in 100 ml distilled water

Protocol 1. *Continued*

- 0.2 M sodium phosphate buffer, pH 7.4 (Chapter 1, *Protocol 1*)
- 0.4 g ammonium chloride [NH_4Cl] in 100 ml distilled water
- 20 g D-glucose + 50 mg sodium azide [NaN_3] in 100 ml distilled water (store at 4°C)
- glucose oxidase solution (Sigma G-6891, about 1000 units/ml, store at 4°C)

1. Wash sections 2 × 10 min in 0.1 M phosphate buffer, pH 7.4.
2. Pre-incubate for 10 min at room temperature with agitation in the following solution that has been made up immediately before use:
   - 1 × 10 mg DAB tablet (Sigma D-5905) dissolved in 10 ml of 0.2 M phosphate buffer[a]
   - 200 μl ammonium chloride stock solution
   - 200 μl glucose stock solution
   - 8.8 ml distilled water
   - 800 μl nickel ammonium sulphate stock solution

   Add the nickel ammonium sulphate last, slowly and dropwise; filter the pre-incubation solution before use.
3. Remove pre-incubation solution and replace with reaction mix containing 10 ml pre-incubation solution and 10 μl glucose oxidase solution. Prepare immediately before adding to sections.
4. React for up to 45 min at room temperature with agitation.
5. Remove reaction mix and wash sections in several changes of 0.1 M phosphate buffer, pH 7.4.

Sections can be dried on to chrome alum–gelatin treated slides (Chapter 1, *Protocols 5* and *6*) and histologically stained for LM, or they can be processed for EM (see Chapter 1). They can also be used for LM or EM pre-embedding or post-embedding immunocytochemistry (see Chapters 5 and 6).

[a] Alternatively, pre-weigh DAB (Sigma D-5637) in 10 mg lots; store dry and tightly covered at −15°C or store aliquots of a 5 mg/ml solution frozen.

2.3.2 Peroxidase reactions with tetramethylbenzidine as chromogen

Mesulam (16) introduced the use of tetramethylbenzidine (TMB) with sodium nitroprusside stabilization as a highly sensitive method for the detection of retrogradely-transported HRP. Since Mesulam's method produces a crystalline reaction product that is highly soluble, researchers have used other stabilizing agents, notably ammonium heptamolybdate (17) and ammo-

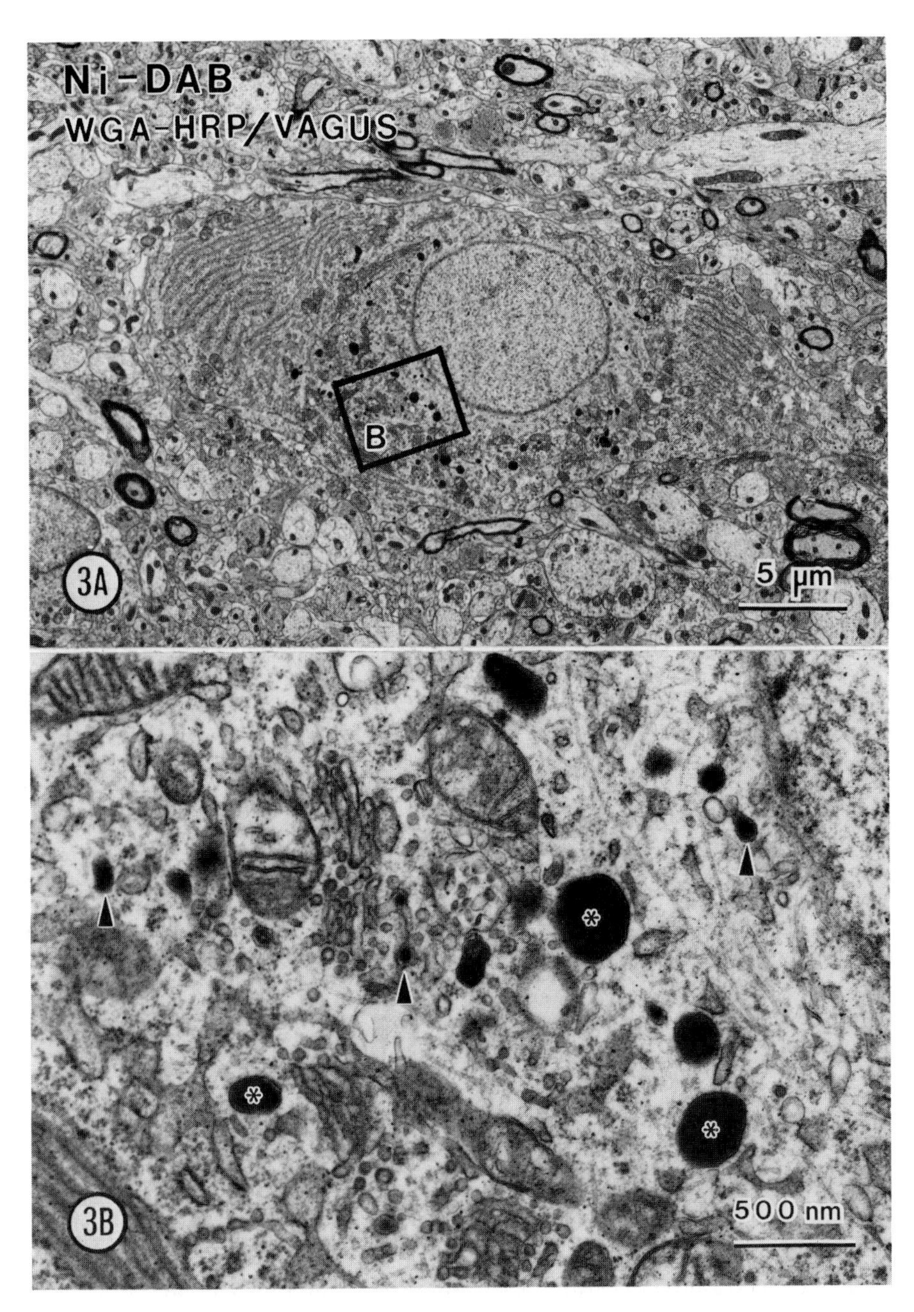

Figure 3. *HRP-based tracers. Ultrastructure of a neurone containing HRP detected with a nickel-intensified DAB reaction (Ni-DAB).* Dorsal motor nucleus of the vagus, rat. Sigma WGA-HRP (4% in 10% DMSO/distilled water) injected into the cervical vagus nerve. Fixative, 2.5% glutaraldehyde, 0.5% formaldehyde. (A) Low magnification micrograph. (B) High magnification micrograph of the area in box B in (A). Lysosomes (asterisks) contain electron-dense reaction product, indicating the presence of WGA-HRP, as do some vesicular and tubular elements of the Golgi apparatus (arrowheads).

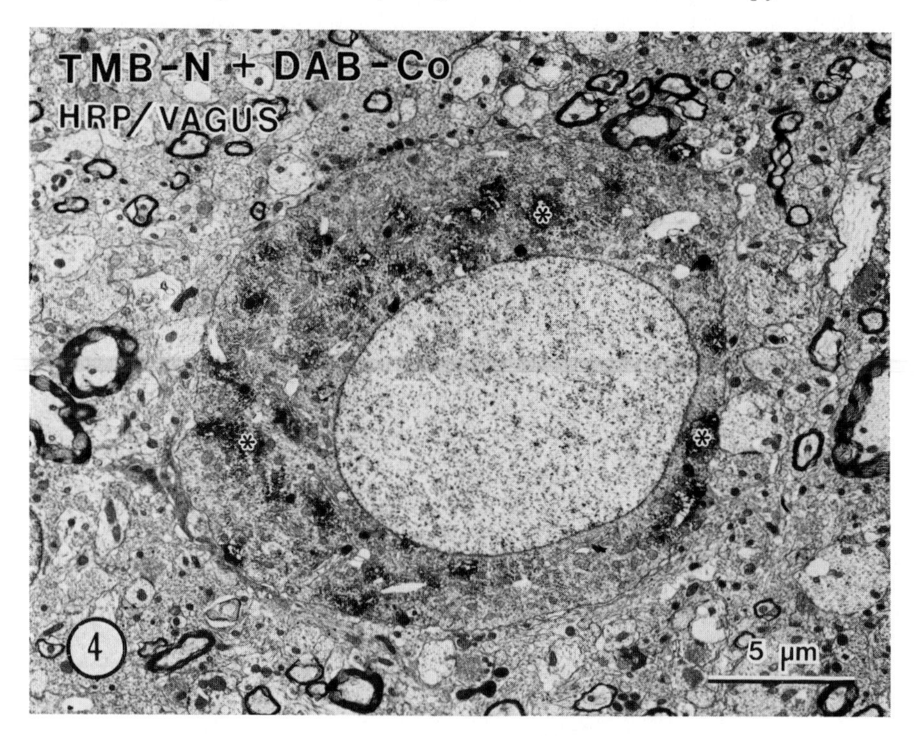

Figure 4. *HRP-based tracers. Ultrastructure of a neurone containg HRP detected with a TMB-nitroprusside reaction and stabilized with DAB, $CoCl_2$ and H_2O_2 (TMB-N + DAB-Co).* Dorsal motor nucleus of the vagus, rat. Sigma HRP (10% Type VI in 10% DMSO/distilled water) into the cervical vagus nerve. Fixative, 2.5% glutaraldehyde, 0.5% formaldehyde. The stabilized TMB-N reaction product (asterisks) appears mainly as semi-crystalline electron-dense deposits, mainly associated with the Golgi apparatus.

nium paratungstate (18), to try to increase the stability of the TMB crystals. Two TMB methods that we have successfully used for LM and EM tracing in combination with immunocytochemistry are described here; a nitroprusside-stabilized reaction (*Protocol 2*) and tungstate-stabilized reaction (*Protocol 3*).

i. Nitroprusside-stabilized TMB reactions

Appearance.

In the light microscope, dark blue crystals (*Figure 1B*). For EM, TMB-nitroprusside (TMB-N) reaction product must be stabilized because it is highly soluble. The TMB-N reaction product stabilized with DAB, $CoCl_2$ and H_2O_2 is black by LM and semi-crystalline by EM (*Figure 1C, Figure 4*).

Sensitivity.

The TMB-N reaction is the most sensitive peroxidase reaction for detecting retrogradely-transported HRP or HRP conjugates. It is considerably more

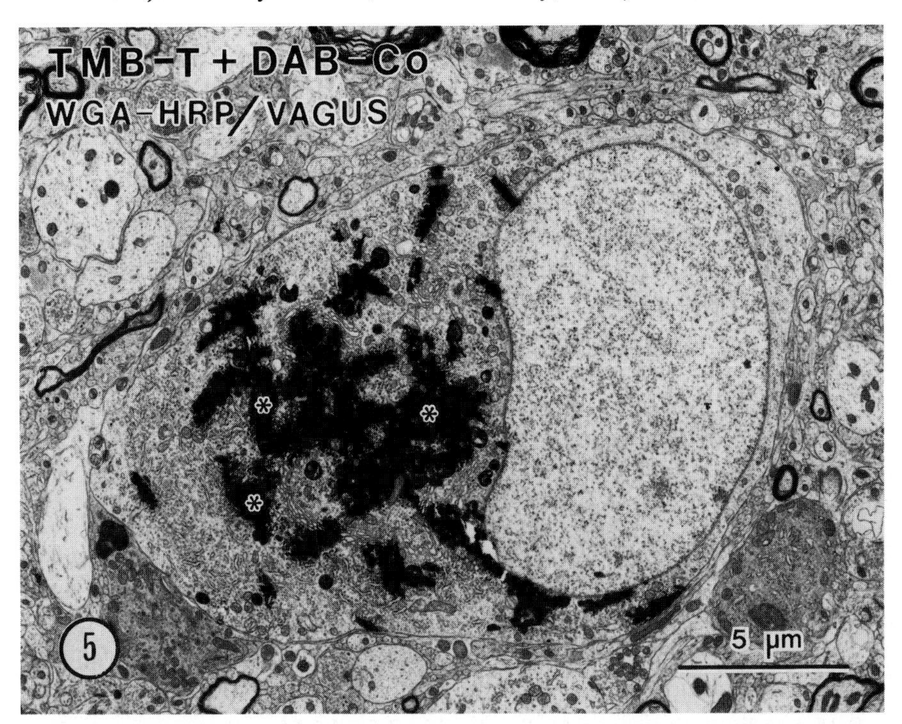

Figure 5. *HRP-based tracers. Ultrastructure of neurone containing WGA-HRP detected with a TMB-tungstate reaction and stabilized with DAB, $CoCl_2$, and H_2O_2 (TMB-T + DAB-Co).* Dorsal motor nucleus of the vagus, rat. Sigma WGA-HRP (4% in 10% DMSO/distilled water) injected into the cervical vagus nerve. Fixative, 2.5% glutaraldehyde, 0.5% formaldehyde. Neurone from the same animal as in *Figure 3*. Stabilized TMB-T reaction product (asterisks) appears as electron-dense crystals.

sensitive than DAB reactions (see *Figure 1*) and slightly more sensitive than TMB-tungstate reactions (see below). However, stabilization of TMB-N reaction product with DAB, $CoCl_2$, and H_2O_2 (DAB-Co; see 19) for EM or immunocytochemistry often results in significant loss of reaction product (see below and *Figures 1B* and *1C*).

Stability.

TMB-N reaction product dissolves readily in buffers and organic solvents. Many TMB-N crystals can be lost during DAB-Co stabilization (compare *Figures 1B* and *1C*) because they are soluble in 10 mM acetate buffer, pH 3.3, the stabilization buffer. The extent of loss seems to depend on the pre-stabilization level of TMB-N crystals in nerve cell bodies. If labelled neurones contain only a few small crystals, all are usually lost during DAB-Co treatment; moderately labelled cells lose most of their crystals, and heavily labelled cells lose many.

Artefacts,

Over-reaction produces needle-like crystals that extend beyond the boundaries of the labelled neurones. Detects endogenous hydrogen peroxidase in pericytes and red blood cells, which often show needle-like crystals.

Safety note 1. Although TMB is non-carcinogenic, nitroprusside can cause poisoning because it contains cyanide. Wear gloves for nitroprusside-stabilized TMB reactions.

Protocol 2. Nitroprusside-stabilized TMB reaction (TMB-N reaction), (adapted from McIlhinney *et al.* (20), very similar to the original Mesulam method (16))

Stock solutions

- 0.1 g tetramethylbenzidine free base (Sigma, T-2885) dissolved in 50 ml of analytical reagent grade absolute ethanol (TMB stock solution is light-sensitive; it lasts for about 2 months if stored in a dark bottle at 4°C)
- 1 M sodium acetate buffer, pH 3.3 (190 ml 1 M acetic acid + 10 ml 1 M sodium acetate)
- 0.15 g sodium nitroprusside dissolved in 7.5 ml 1 M sodium acetate buffer, pH 3.3 + 139 ml distilled water (light-sensitive solution; store in a dark bottle and use within 2 h of preparation)
- analytical reagent grade hydrogen peroxide (approximately 30% solution of H_2O_2, store at 4°C, discard after 6 months)

Method

1. Pre-incubate in the following solution prepared immediately before use:
   - 30 ml of nitroprusside stock solution
   - 375 μl TMB stock solution

   Incubate for 15–20 min at room temperature in the dark on a shaker.
2. Remove pre-incubation solution and replace with reaction mix made up immediately before use from:
   - 30 ml of nitroprusside stock solution
   - 375 μl TMB stock solution
   - 100 μl of 0.3% hydrogen peroxide (100 μl of stock solution in 10 ml of distilled water) made up immediately before use
3. React at room temperature in the dark on a shaker. React sections for 2 × 8 min. The second reaction is done in freshly prepared reaction mixture. The progress of the reaction can be monitored with a dissecting micro-

scope. If the reaction proceeds too rapidly (i.e. if retrogradely labelled cells are visible within 1–2 min), it can be slowed down by carrying out the reaction on ice. For immediate viewing, wash sections for a few seconds in ice-cold nitroprusside stock solution, mount rapidly on chrom alum–gelatin treated slides, air-dry, dehydrate quickly in xylene, and apply coverslip (see Chapter 1, *Protocols* 5 and 6). For EM or immunocytochemistry, wash sections for a few seconds in ice-cold 0.01 M sodium acetate buffer, pH 3.3, and then stabilize sections with DAB-Co (similar but not identical to stabilization procedure in *Protocol 3*; see 20 for details).

---

ii. *Tungstate-stabilized TMB reactions*

Appearance.

By LM, rectangular peacock-blue crystals (*Figure 1D*). The TMB-tungstate (TMB-T) reaction product must be stabilized with a mixture of DAB, $CoCl_2$, and H_2O_2 (DAB-Co) for EM or immunocytochemistry (see below), turning the TMB-T crystals black. In the electron microscope DAB-Co-stabilized TMB-T reaction product appears as electron-dense crystals (*Figure 5*).

Sensitivity.

Much more sensitive than DAB reactions but marginally less sensitive than TMB-N reactions. However, TMB-T crystals are much more effectively preserved by DAB-Co stabilization than TMB-N crystals (compare *Figures 1D* and *1E* with *Figures 1B* and *1C*).

Stability.

TMB-T reaction product is much more stable than TMB-N reaction product, being insoluble in organic solvents and compatible with thionin staining. However, TMB-T crystals do disappear during treatment with osmium (18) and dissolve slowly in buffer. Consequently, if TMB-T reacted sections are to be used for EM or immunocytochemistry, the TMB-T reaction product needs to be stabilized with DAB-Co.

Artefacts.

Over-reaction produces large rectangular crystals that extend beyond the boundaries of the retrogradely labelled neurones. Detects endogenous hydrogen peroxidase in pericytes and red blood cells, which often show large rectangular crystals.

Protocol 3. Tungstate-stabilized TMB reaction (TMB-T reaction, 18)

Stock solutions

- 0.1 g tetramethylbenzidine free base (Sigma) dissolved in 50 ml of analytical reagent grade absolute ethanol (see *Protocol 2*)

Protocol 3. *Continued*

- 1 g ammonium paratungstate (ICN Biomedicals) in 100 ml distilled water (store at room temperature *not* 4°C; discard after 1 week; takes several hours to dissolve at room temperature with stirring)
- 0.1 M sodium phosphate buffer, pH 6.0 (43.8 ml of 0.2 M NaH_2PO_4 + 6.2 ml of 0.2 M Na_2HPO_4 + 50 ml of distilled water)
- analytical reagent grade hydrogen peroxide (see *Protocol 2*)
- 1 g cobalt chloride ($CoCl_2$) in 100 ml distilled water

Method

1. Pre-incubate sections in the following solution that has been made up immediately before use:
   - 10 ml 0.1 M sodium phosphate buffer, pH 6.0
   - 500 μl ammonium paratungstate stock solution
   - 250 μl TMB stock solution

   Incubate for 10–30 min at room temperature on a shaker.
2. Remove pre-incubation solution and replace with reaction mixture made up from 10 ml pre-incubation solution and 100 μl of 0.3% hydrogen peroxide, which has been made up immediately before use.
3. React at room temperature on a shaker. Monitor progress of the reaction with a dissecting microscope. We use reaction times of 5–15 min. If the reaction proceeds too rapidly (i.e. if retrogradely labelled cells are visible within 1–2 min), carry it out on ice.
4. Remove reaction mixture and wash sections in several changes of 0.1 M phosphate buffer, pH 6.0.
5. For immediate viewing, wash sections in distilled water, air-dry on to chrome alum–gelatin treated slides, dehydrate, and apply coverslip (see Chapter 1, *Protocol 6*).
6. For electron microscopy stabilize the sections as soon as possible with DAB-Co that has been made up immediately before use by mixing:
   - 1 × 10 mg DAB tablet (Sigma) dissolved in 10 ml of 0.1 M sodium phosphate buffer, pH 6.0 (or see footnote *a*, *Protocol 1*)
   - 200 μl cobalt chloride stock solution, added slowly dropwise
   - 200 μl of 0.3% hydrogen peroxide, which has been made up immediately before use

   Filter the stabilization immediately before adding the hydrogen peroxide and incubate the sections for 7–10 min at room temperature with agitation.
7. Remove reaction mixture and wash sections in several changes of 0.1 M phosphate buffer, pH 6.0.

8. For EM or immunocytochemistry, wash stabilized sections several times in the appropriate buffer (see Chapter 1, *Protocols 7* and *8* for preparation for electron microscopy and Chapter 6 for immunocytochemistry). For immediate viewing, wash sections in distilled water, air-dry on to chrome alum–gelatin treated slides, dehydrate, and apply coverslip (Chapter 1, *Protocol 6*).

2.3.3 Which peroxidase reaction to use

TMB reactions are the most sensitive way of demonstrating retrogradely-transported HRP (for example, *Figure 1*). Of the two TMB reactions described here, TMB-N reactions are slightly more sensitive than TMB-T reactions but, because of its extreme solubility, the TMB-N reaction product is easily lost unless the reacted sections are mounted quickly and under optimum conditions. TMB-N crystals also disappear during DAB-Co stabilization, which is supposed to prevent the crystals from dissolving. After stabilization, the number and labelling intensity of neurones reacted with TMB-N can be reduced to the level seen after a DAB reaction (*Figure 1A–C*). In contrast, TMB-T crystals are much less soluble, surviving several hours of exposure to water, buffers, organic solvents, and even thionin staining without significant loss. However, TMB-T crystals do disappear in osmium tetroxide and slowly dissolve in buffer, so that stabilization with DAB-Co is necessary for EM or immunocytochemistry. Although there can be some loss of TMB-T crystals during stabilization, it is not nearly as extensive as when TMB-N reaction product is stabilized (compare *Figure 1B* and *C* with *Figure 1D* and *E*). In view of these considerations, we routinely use TMB-T reactions, since the slight loss in sensitivity is more than compensated for by the significantly decreased solubility of the reaction product.

The use of DAB as a chromogen in peroxidase reactions has at least two disadvantages for retrograde tracing studies. First, DAB reactions are the least sensitive for detecting retrogradely-transported HRP or HRP-conjugates. Fewer labelled neurones are usually found after DAB reactions, even with intensification, than after TMB reactions (see, for example, *Figure 1*). Second, although retrogradely labelled neurones revealed with DAB are obvious when tissue is processed for LM, this is not always true in tissue processed for EM. Retrogradely-transported HRP is localized mainly in lysosomes and DAB reaction product shows its presence ultrastructurally by increasing lysosomal electron density (see *Figure 3*). Unfortunately, neurones that are *not* retrogradely labelled also contain lysosomes and it is sometimes difficult to distinguish between neurones with HRP-labelled lysosomes and neurones with unlabelled lysosomes. These considerations argue against using DAB as a chromogen for visualizing HRP-based retrograde tracers.

3. Colloidal gold-labelled retrograde tracers

Several gold-labelled tracers have been introduced over the past five years. These include WGA-gold (21, 22), WGA-HRP-gold (23), WGA-apo-HRP-gold (24), and CTB-gold (25). Retrograde labelling has been successfully achieved after injections of gold-labelled tracers into the brain, spinal cord, ganglia, and nerve trunks but not from dipping cut nerves into tracer. These findings indicate that axon terminals and fibres of passage take up gold-labelled tracers but not cut or damaged axons. Lack of transport from cut nerve fibres may be caused by the limited diffusion of gold particles up damaged fibres; gold-labelled tracers may never reach active uptake sites above the damaged part of the axon.

Neurones appear to transport all gold-labelled tracers in similar ways. The tracers are taken up by way of their lectins or toxins, which bind specifically to different 'receptor' molecules in the axonal plasma membrane. After internalization, the gold-labelled tracers are carried by fast axonal transport and can be detected in nerve cell bodies at similar survival times as for HRP-based tracers. Once the gold particles have been transported to the neuronal cell body, they lodge in lysosomes in somata and proximal dendrites, where they remain permanently. However, the lectins and toxins appear to be stripped from their colloidal gold particles and may be transported to other non-lysosomal locations. Menetrey (23) demonstrated terminals anterogradely labelled with HRP from neurones that had retrogradely-transported WGA-HRP-gold, and we have detected CTB-immunoreactivity throughout the somata and dendrites of neurones retrogradely labelled with CTB-gold (15).

3.1 Preparation of colloidal gold-labelled retrograde tracers

3.1.1 Preparation or purchase of colloidal gold particles

Several methods are available for making colloidal gold particles (26). We use the method of Slot and Geuze (27) to make 7 nm and 15 nm gold particles, and the method of Frens (28) for 20 nm gold particles. It is advisable to measure the mean diameter of the colloidal gold particles on electron micrographs of particles spread on poly-L-lysine-, butvar-, or formvar-coated mesh grids (26) (see Chapter 1, *Protocol 10* for coating grids). In our experience, the size of the gold particle can influence the size of the injection site (25; see Section 3.2).

Several companies sell colloidal gold particles of defined sizes in the form of sols that can be used for the preparation of gold-based tracers (see *Table 1*).

3.1.2 Preparation or purchase of gold-labelled retrograde tracers

Protein molecules combine with colloidal gold particles through complex electrostatic interactions rather than through direct chemical bonding. This electrostatic binding means that the adsorbed proteins retain their biological activity in protein–gold complexes. Consequently, lectins and toxins adsorbed to gold particles can still bind to the appropriate molecules in neuronal membranes.

(a) *Cholera Toxin B-Gold.* The method of Horisberger and Rosset (29) has been used to link CTB to colloidal gold particles of any size. Refer to Llewellyn-Smith *et al.* (15, 25) for instructions. Use CTB purchased from List as a starting material. CTB conjugated to 7 nm gold particles can now be purchased in lyophilized form from Gilt Products (*Table 1*).

(b) *Wheatgerm agglutinin-apo-HRP-Gold.* For instructions on how to prepare WGA-apo-HRP-gold, refer to Basbaum and Menetrey (24) or Menetrey and Basbaum (30). Unconjugated WGA-apo-HRP is available from Sigma (*Table 1*).

(c) *Wheatgerm agglutinin-gold.* Methods for preparation of WGA-gold can be found in Seeley and Field (21) and Morilak *et al.* (22). Unconjugated WGA can be bought from Sigma (*Table 1*). WGA adsorbed to 10 nm particles of colloidal gold is available from E-Y Laboratories and from Sigma (*Table 1*).

3.2 Applications of gold-labelled retrograde tracers

Gold-labelled retrograde tracers are pressure injected into the brain, spinal cord, ganglia, or nerve trunks (see Section 2.1.1). Menetrey and Basbaum (30) indicate that they have been unsuccessful at applying WGA-apo-HRP-gold by iontophoresis.

Gold-labelled tracers give well defined injection sites that are small compared to the injection sites obtained after pressure injection of either HRP-based tracers or CTB. We have found with CTB-gold, that the size of the gold particle in the tracer will determine the size of the injection site, if similar volumes of gold conjugate are injected (25). We obtained bigger injection sites with CTB-7 nm gold than with CTB-20 nm gold.

3.3 Fixation

Unlike HRP-based tracers, gold-labelled tracers are unaffected by fixation conditions. We have successfully localized gold-labelled tracers in tissue perfused with a wide variety of fixatives from 4% formaldehyde to 5% glutaraldehyde (see Chapter 1 for preparation of fixatives and perfusion). Gold-labelled tracers can be visualized in vibrating microtome, paraffin, frozen, or plastic-embedded sections.

3.4 Detection of gold-labelled retrograde tracers

Retrogradely-transported gold-labelled tracers are detected for LM by silver intensification (*Figure 6*). Silver intensification is basically a photographic

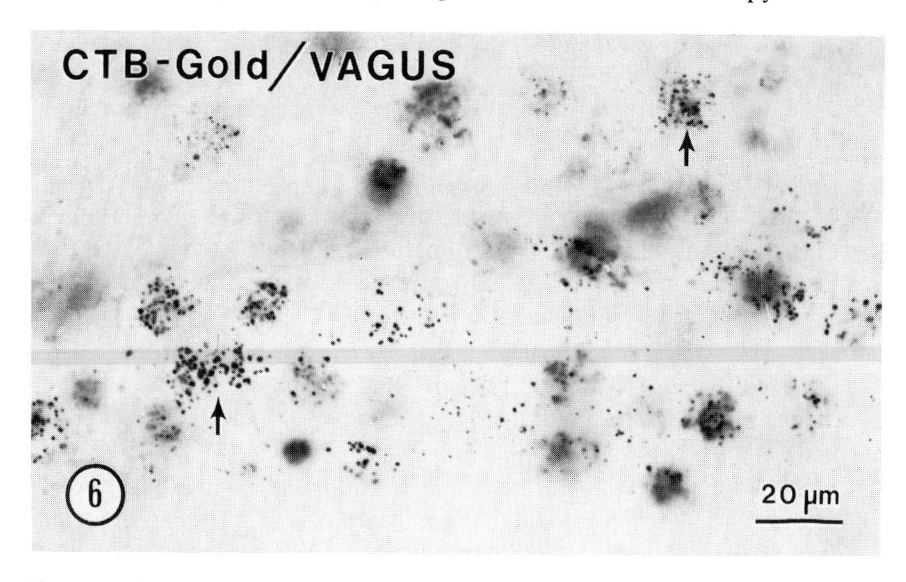

Figure 6. *Gold-labelled tracers. Retrograde tracing with CTB-gold.* Transverse section through the dorsal motor nucleus of the vagus near the obex rat. Gilt Products CTB-7 nm gold injected into the cervical vagus nerve. Fixative, 2.5% glutaraldehyde, 0.5% formaldehyde. Silver-intensification (Amersham kit) with gold-toning. Many vagal motor neurones, some of which are indicated by arrowheads, contain black puncta due the presence of silver-intensified CTB-gold. Many retrogradely labelled neurones are out of the plane of focus of the micrograph.

process, in which growing shells of metallic silver are deposited over the colloidal gold particles. When the silver shells become large enough, the retrograde tracer can be seen by LM.

We routinely silver intensify sections with commercial kits because they are easy to use, reliable, relatively insensitive to light, relatively inexpensive, and give less background than most published recipes. We have had success with both the Silver Enhancer kit from Sigma and the IntenSE kits from Amersham. Other silver intensification kits are also available (*Table 1*). Retrogradely-transported gold tracers can also be revealed using published silver intensification methods, most of which are based on the technique of Danscher (31–33). For a more detailed discussion of these methods and their use, see Scopsi (34) and Hacker (35).

In addition to silver intensification, we often gold-tone our sections for LM. By bright field microscopy, silver intensified and gold-toned sections often contain more retrogradely labelled neurones with heavier deposits than sections that have only been silver-intensified. Gold-toning is essential for EM sections because untreated silver deposits disappear during osmication. Gold-toning does not significantly affect either ultrastructure (*Figure 7*) or subsequent immunocytochemistry for neurotransmitter-related markers (15, 25).

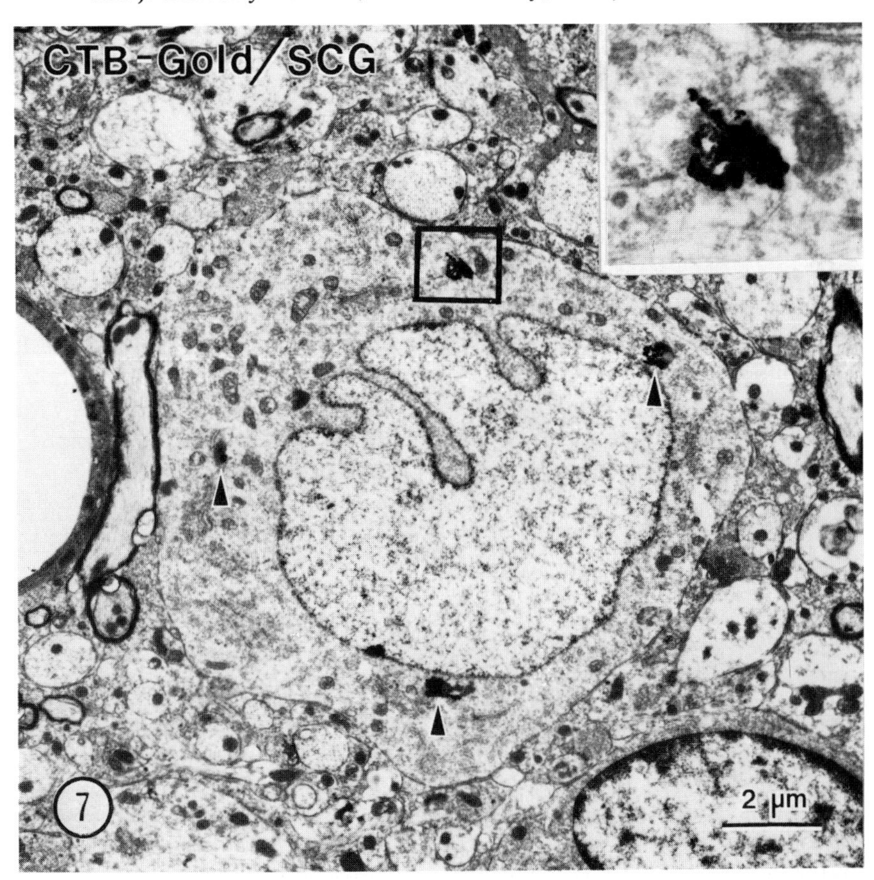

Figure 7. *Gold-labelled tracers. Ultrastructure of a neurone containing retrogradely transported CTB-gold.* Intermediolateral cell column of spinal segment T2, rat. Gilt Products CTB-7 nm gold injeced into the superior cervical ganglion (SCG). Fixative, 1% glutaraldehyde, 1% formaldehyde. Silver-intensified, gold-toned particles of CTB-gold (arrowheads) occur in lysosomes in the cell body of the sympathetic preganglionic neurone. The gold particle in the box is shown at higher magnification in the inset.

Although gold-labelled tracers can be seen at the electron microscopic level without silver intensification, we usually do silver intensify sections for EM. We find silver intensification advantageous for EM because we can select individual retrogradely labelled neurones by LM for subsequent study by EM, and because silver-intensified gold particles are much easier to detect at low magnification with the electron microscope than unintensified particles.

Protocol 4 is used for detecting gold particles in free-floating vibrating microtome sections of fixed nervous tissue. Gold-labelled tracers can also be visualized in slide-mounted sections.

Protocol 4. Detection of gold-labelled retrograde tracers with two commercial silver intensification kits

A. *Silver intensification*

1. Cut sections on a Vibratome or other vibrating microtome *into distilled water.*[a] (We use 50 μm thick sections for LM and 70 μm thick sections for EM) (see Chapter 1, *Protocol 4*).)
2. *Optional.* Wash sections in 50% ethanol in distilled water on a shaker at room temperature.[b] Wash sections for LM for 30–45 min. For EM, wash sections fixed with 0.1% glutaraldehyde or less for 10 min; wash sections fixed with 1% or more glutaraldehyde for 30 min; wash sections fixed with 2.5% glutaraldehyde for 45 min. Transfer sections from 50% ethanol to distilled water. Swirl them vigorously so that they sink.
3. Wash sections in distilled water. If the sections *have* been exposed to 50% ethanol, wash them 2 × 10 min. If the sections *have not* been exposed to 50% ethanol, wash them 3 × 30 min.[c]
4. Immediately before use, prepare the silver intensification solution according to the manufacturer's instructions.
5. Silver-intensify the sections. With the Sigma kit, incubate sections 3 × 5 min. With the Amersham kit, incubate sections 2 × 20 min. Make up fresh silver intensification solution immediately before each incubation. Decrease or increase the development steps in time or number if sections have a high background of silver particles over their surfaces, or if the silver deposits in the retrogradely labelled neurones are small and faint.

B. *Gold-toning (optional)*

1. Wash sections 3 × 10 min in distilled water.
2. Incubate sections for 10 min in the dark in 0.05% (w/v) gold chloride [$HAuCl_4 \cdot 3H_2O$] in distilled water.
3. Wash sections 3 × 10 min in the dark in distilled water.
4. Incubate sections for 2 min in the dark at 4°C in 0.2% (w/v) oxalic acid [$(COOH)_2 \cdot 2H_2O$] in distilled water.
5. Wash sections 3 × 5 min in the dark in distilled water.

C. *Fixation*

1. Fix sections for 5 min in 2.5% (w/v) sodium thiosulphate [$Na_2S_2O_3 \cdot 5H_2O$] in distilled water.
2. Wash sections for a few minutes in two changes of distilled water, or in distilled water followed by buffer or phosphate-buffered saline.

Sections can be mounted on chrome alum–gelatin treated slides (see Chapter 1, *Protocol 5*) and histologically stained. They can also be used for post-embedding immunocytochemistry (see Chapter 6) or for light or electron microscopic pre-embedding immunocytochemistry with peroxidase or fluorescence detection systems (see Chapters 5 and 11).

[a] Since phosphate ions in the silver intensification solution can cause it to precipitate, avoid the use of phosphate buffer until after fixation.
[b] We have shown that ethanol treatment allows antibodies to penetrate completely through vibrating microtome sections without significantly destroying ultrastructure (36, 37). If sections for immunocytochemistry have been washed in ethanol before silver intensification, detergent treatment with Triton X-100 is unnecessary. Ethanol treatment also helps to decrease background labelling during silver enhancement.
[c] If it is desirable to limit exposure of the sections to hypo-osmotic solutions and the Amersham kit has been used, sections can be washed 3 × 20 min in citrate-acetate buffer, pH 5.5 (50 ml 0.2 M citric acid and 50 ml 0.2 M ammonium acetate, pH adjusted to 5.5 with 25% ammonia solution) rather than distilled water. Citrate-acetate buffer speeds up the silver intensification reaction with the Sigma kit to unacceptably rapid rates.

3.5 Which gold-labelled tracer to use?

Both CTB-gold and WGA-apo-HRP-gold have been widely used for retrograde tracing in the central nervous system. We have successfully used both for tracing from sympathetic ganglia to the spinal cord, and from injections into the cervical vagus nerve, but not from cut nerve trunks. Hence, either tracer is recommended for tracing studies as long as they can be applied by pressure injection. WGA-apo-HRP-gold is used in preference to WGA-HRP-gold. Unlike WGA-HRP, WGA-apo-HRP has no enzyme activity so WGA-apo-HRP-gold can be used in combination with peroxidase-based immunocytochemistry. We cannot recommend WGA-gold since we have found WGA-gold prepared according to the method of Seeley and Field (21) to be unstable in the presence of physiological saline and achieved poorer results with this tracer than with CTB-gold or WGA-apo-HRP-gold.

4. Unconjugated cholera toxin B subunit

Immunocytochemically detected CTB was introduced for retrograde tracing in the mid-1980s (38–40). Its major advantage is that it labels not only somata and proximal dendrites but also distal dendrites and axons, often producing a Golgi-like image of the labelled neurones (*Figure 8*).

4.1 Application of cholera toxin B subunit

Cholera toxin B subunit can be either pressure injected or applied iontophoretically. A 1% solution of unconjugated CTB (List, *Table 1*) is generally used. A dye such as Evans blue can be added to the CTB for injection into nerves or ganglia so that the progress of the injection can be monitored. With

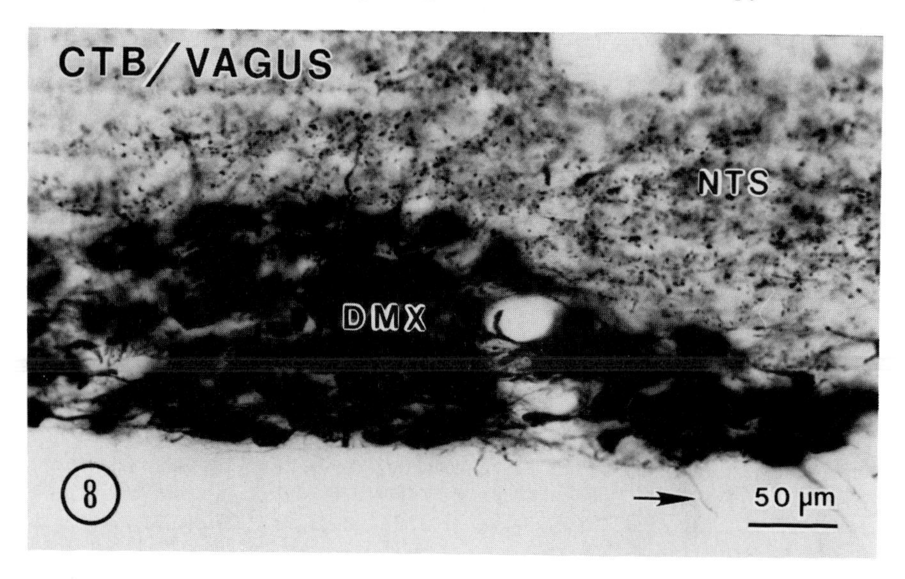

Figure 8. *Retrograde tracing with unconjugated CTB.* Transverse section through the dorsal motor nucleus of the vagus (DMX) near the obex, rat. List CTB (1%) injected into the cervical vagus nerve. Immunocytochemical detection with a nickel-DAB reaction. Fixative, 4% formaldehyde, 0.05% glutaraldehyde, 0.2% picric acid. The somata and processes of vagal motor neurones are heavily immunoreactive for the retrogradely-transported CTB. Anterogradely labelled fibers, also immunoreactive for CTB, are present in the adjacent nucleus tractus solitarius (NTS). Arrow, CTB-immunoreactive process of a vagal motor neurone.

application by pressure, injection sites within the central nervous system can be quite large. However, iontophoretic application of CTB gives small, well-localized injection sites with little associated cellular damage. Refer to Luppi *et al.* (41) and Section 2.1.2 for details on iontophoresis of tracers. CTB is a very sensitive tracer so spillage or inaccurate placement of injectate should be avoided to minimize artefactual labelling.

4.2 Fixation

CTB-immunoreactivity is sensitive to fixation (15, 38, 41). We have found that CTB-immunoreactivity is affected both by glutaraldehyde concentration and by exposure time to glutaraldehyde (15). Rat sympathetic preganglionic neurones retrogradely labelled with CTB are well revealed after perfusion with 4% formaldehyde and post-fixation for one to several days, or with 4% formaldehyde and 0.05–1% glutaraldehyde as long as post-fixation is decreased to only a few hours. If exposure to glutaraldehyde is increased, CTB-immunoreactivity becomes increasingly restricted to the Golgi apparatus in cell bodies and proximal dendrites (*Figure 9*).

Fixation parameters for demonstrating CTB-immunoreactivity should be

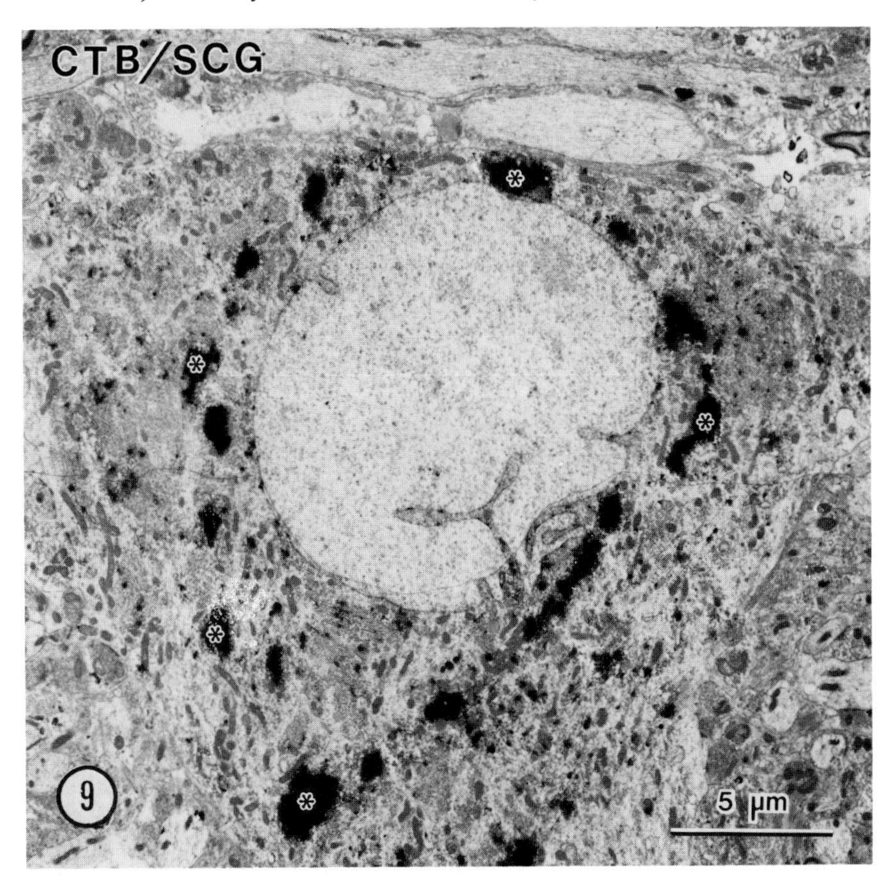

Figure 9. *Ultrastructure of a neurone containing retrogradely-transported CTB.* Intermediolateral cell column of spinal segment T2, rabbit. List CTB (1%) injected into the superior cervical ganglion (SCG). Immunocytochemical detection with a nickel-DAB reaction. Fixative, 4% formaldehyde, 0.5% glutaraldehyde, 0.2% picric acid. Large deposits of CTB-immunoreactivity occur in the Golgi apparatus (asterisks); smaller deposits are present throughout the neuronal cytoplasm.

chosen on the basis of how the tissue will be subsequently processed. If the tissue is to be used for LM studies on the projection patterns of neurones, or if other glutaraldehyde-sensitive antigens are to be localized in conjunction with CTB, 4% formaldehyde or fixatives containing only 0.05% glutaraldehyde should be used. For other applications, it is advisable to test the effects on CTB-immunoreactivity of different fixatives and post-fixation times. We have successfully localized CTB-immunoreactivity in sympathetic preganglionic neurones after perfusion with 2.5% glutaraldehyde and very brief post-fixation, but this regime may be too severe for visualizing retrogradely-transported CTB in other areas of the central nervous system (see Chapter 1, *Protocols 2* and *3* for preparation of fixative and perfusion fixation).

4.3 Detection of retrogradely-transported cholera toxin B subunit

Retrogradely-transported CTB is detected with goat anti-CTB antibodies (List, *Table 1*). CTB-labelled neurones can be revealed for either LM or EM with *Protocol 5*. Staining is carried out on free-floating Vibratome sections. We use 50 μm sections for LM and 70 μm for EM.

Protocol 5. Immunocytochemical detection of retrogradely-transported CTB (see Chapter 5 for more details on immunocytochemistry, see also Chapter 4, *Protocol 2*)

1. To improve antibody penetration, wash vibrating microtome sections in 50% ethanol in distilled water *immediately* after they are cut, using similar wash times as under step **2** of *Protocol 4*.
2. Swirl sections quickly in 0.1 M sodium phosphate buffer, pH 7.4, until they sink. Wash in another quick change of 0.1 M sodium phosphate buffer, pH 7.4.
3. Pre-incubate sections for at least 30 min in 10% normal horse serum (NHS) in 10 mM Tris, 0.05% merthiolate (Thimerosal; Sigma), 10 mM sodium phosphate buffer, pH 7.4, (TPBS).
4. Place sections in anti-CTB antiserum[a] (List) diluted with TPBS containing 10% NHS. Incubate LM sections at room temperature for at least 24 h; EM sections, for 2–4 days. Incubations should be carried out in sealed containers or in a humid chamber on a slowly rotating shaker.
5. Wash sections 3 × 10 min for LM, or 3 × 30 min for EM in TPBS.
6. Incubate sections in 1:200 dilution of biotinylated donkey anti-sheep IgG[b] (Sigma) in TPBS containing 1% NHS. Incubations are carried out at room temperature overnight for LM or 24 h for EM as in step **4**.
7. Wash sections as in step **5**.
8. Incubate sections as in step **4** in a 1:1000 or 1:1500 dilution of ExtrAvidin–HRP (Sigma), Avidin–HRP (Sigma), or ABC Reagent (Vector Laboratories) in TPBS at room temperature for at least 4 h for LM, or 16–24 h for EM.
9. Wash sections as in step **5**.
10. Do a peroxidase reaction with DAB (see *Protocol 1* and reference 15), or benzidine dihydrochloride (see Chapter 5, *Protocol 11* and reference 15) to reveal the retrogradely-transported CTB.

Sections for LM can be dried on to chrome alum–gelatin treated slides, dehydrated, and coverslip applied (Chapter 1, *Protocol 6*). They can also be used for LM or EM pre-embedding immunocytochemistry (see Chapter 5), or embedded in resin for LM or EM (Chapter 1, *Protocols 7* and *8*) post-embedding immunocytochemistry (see Chapter 6).

[a] Determine the optimal dilution of anti-CTB antiserum (to give the maximum number of retrogradely-labelled neurones with the minimal amount of non-specific background staining) by titration. As a guide, with a nickel-intensified diaminobenzidine reaction, we use a 1:25 000–1:200 000 dilution, depending on fixation conditions.
[b] Anti-sheep IgG binds avidly to goat IgG as well as sheep IgG.

5. Which retrograde tracer to use?

Defining a neuronal pathway. Immunocytochemically detected CTB would probably be the best choice for this type of study. The advantages of CTB are:

(a) it is comparatively cheap ($0.66US/μl of 1% CTB plus a few cents for anti-CTB),
(b) it is readily detectable in neurones for several weeks after injection,
(c) it gives very reproducible results with fixatives containing little or no glutaraldehyde and, most importantly,
(d) it demonstrates beautifully the proximal and distal dendrites and even the axons of retrogradely labelled neurones.

This last feature means that CTB is also ideal for studying the morphology of retrogradely labelled neurones by LM and EM. The major disadvantage of CTB is that immunocytochemical detection requires several days.

CTB-HRP or WGA-HRP are reasonable alternatives to CTB for defining a nerve pathway, now that a reliable variant of the highly sensitive TMB reaction (TMB-tungstate) is available. CTB-HRP is more expensive than CTB ($5.00US/μl of 1% solution) but also gives excellent labelling of cell bodies, dendrites, and often axons. WGA-HRP, like HRP, is localized in lysosomes and so labels only somata and proximal dendrites, but this may not be a problem if neuronal morphology is not of interest. A disadvantage of CTB-HRP and WGA-HRP is that retrogradely-transported HRP can be detected for only a few days after it has reached nerve cell bodies. Furthermore, we find that the retrograde labelling seen with CTB-HRP and WGA-HRP is much more variable than that seen with CTB detected immunocytochemically.

Determining the neurotransmitter content of retrogradely labelled neurones. Gold-labelled tracers are ideal for LM or EM studies. Since CTB-gold and WGA-apo-HRP-gold are insensitive to fixation conditions, they can be combined with immunocytochemistry for any neuronal antigen. Gold-labelled tracers also persist in neurones for many months, giving the investigator time

Table 1. Suppliers

Supplier	Address	Product (catalogue number)
Amersham	Check for local office/agent	IntenSE Kits (RPN 491, RPN 492)
BioClin	P.O. Box 129 Cardiff CF4 4YU UK Fax: 44-222-752645	Gold sols—5,10,15,20,40 nm particle sizes (GC-gold particle size)
BioRad	Check for local office/agent	Gold sols—5,10,15,20 nm particles sizes, 100 ml (A2700–A2703 in increasing size)
Boehringer Mannheim	Check for local office/agent	Peroxidase from horseradish (814-393 for 10 mg)
Energy Beam Sciences	P.O. Box 468 11 Bowles Road Agawam, MA 01001 USA Fax: 1-413-789-2786	BioSite gold sols—1,2,5,10,15,20,30,40,50,80 nm particle sizes (BC-sol-gold particle size)
E-Y Laboratories	107 North Amphlett Blvd. San Mateo, CA 94401 USA Fax: 1-415-342-2648	Gold sols—3,5,10,15,20,30,40 nm particle sizes (G-gold particle size) Silver intensification kit (SET10) WGA-10 nm gold (GP2101)
Gilt Products	Department of Medicine Flinders Medical Centre Bedford Park, SA 5042 Australia Fax: 61-8-204-5268	CTB-7 nm gold

ICN Biomedicals, Inc.	Check for local office/agent	Ammonium para-tungstate (204104)
List Biological Laboratories	501-B Vandell Way Campbell, CA 95008-6967 USA Fax: 1-408-866-6364	CTB (Choleragenoid) (103) Goat anti-choleragenoid (703) CTB-HRP (105)
Pelco	P.O. Box 492477 Redding CA, 96049-2477 USA Fax: 1-916-243-3761	BioCell gold sols—1,2,5,10,15,20,30,40 nm gold particle sizes, 100 ml (15 700-1 to 707-1, in increasing particle size) Silver intensification kits (15718)
Sigma Chemical Company	Check for local office/agent	Avidin–HRP (A3151) Biotinylated donkey anti-sheep IgG (B-7390) 3,3′-diaminobenzidine tetrahydrochloride—powder (D-5637) 3,3′-diaminobenzidine tetrahydrochloride—10 mg tablets (D-5905) ExtrAvidin–HRP (E-2886) Glucose oxidase solution, type VS in acetate buffer (G-6891) Horseradish peroxidase—Type VI (P-8375) Silver Enhancer kit (SE-100) Thimerosal (T-5125) Tetramethylbenzidine free base (T-2885) WGA (L-9640) WGA-gold (L-1994) WGA-apo-HRP (L-0390)
Vector Laboratories	Check for local office/agent	ABC reagent—standard kit (PK400) ABC reagent—Elite standard kit (PK6100)

to do other long, or short-term experimental manipulations before animals are sacrificed. HRP or WGA-HRP can be used for LM studies if a nickel-DAB reaction is used to detect the HRP (black) and an unintensified DAB or imidazole-DAB reaction is used to detect the transmitter or enzyme (brown). However, the sensitivity of HRP-based tracers to formaldehyde and their short survival time in retrogradely labelled neurones makes them less flexible than gold-labelled tracers for these types of studies.

Determining the neurotransmitter content of synapses on to retrogradely labelled neurones. For these experiments, the choice of tracer should be determined by the expected density of synaptic input to the retrogradely labelled neurones. If the density of input is likely to be low, CTB or CTB-HRP should be used, as these tracers reveal retrogradely labelled neurones to the maximal extent. CTB should be used if the markers to be detected are glutaraldehyde-sensitive, (e.g. serotonin); CTB-HRP if the markers prefer high glutaraldehyde, (e.g. GABA). Gold-labelled tracers can also be used, as long as synapses are numerous and occur on cell bodies and proximal dendrites, so that gold particles are likely to be visualized in the same or adjacent sections as labelled synapses. HRP and WGA-HRP are less desirable because they label only cell bodies and proximal dendrites, and are sensitive to fixation parameters.

Acknowledgements

This work was supported by the National Health and Medical Research Council of Australia, the National Heart Foundation of Australia, the National SIDS Council of Australia, and the Flinders Medical Centre Research Foundation. We would like to thank Prof John Chalmers for many fruitful discussions. Adrian Wright, Margaret McLaren, Claudine Frisby, and Rachael Coffey provided expert technical assistance.

References

1. Kristensson, K. and Olsson, Y. (1971). *Brain Res.,* **29,** 363.
2. LaVail, J. H. and LaVail, M. M. (1972). *Science,* **17,** 1416.
3. Gonatas, N. K., Harper, C., Mizutani, T., and Gonatas, J. O. (1979). *J. Histochem. Cytochem.,* **27,** 728.
4. Trojanowski, J. Q., Gonatas, J. O., and Gonatas, N. K. (1982). *Brain Res.,* **231,** 33.
5. Ju, G., Liu, S., and Tao, J. (1986). *Neurosci.,* **19,** 803.
6. Bacon, S. J. and Smith, A. D. (1988). *J. Autonom. Nerv. Syst.,* **24,** 97.
7. Amaral, D. G. and Price, J. L. (1983). *J. Neurosci. Methods,* **9,** 35.
8. Chan, S. H. H., Chan, J. Y. H., and Ong, B. T. (1986). *Neurosci. Letts.,* **71,** 277.
9. Dampney, R. A. L., Czachurski, J., Dembowsky, K., Goodchild, A. K., and Seller, H. (1987). *J. Autonom. Nerv. Syst.,* **20,** 73.

10. Cederbaum, J. M. and Aghajanian, G. K. (1978). *J. Comp. Neurol.,* **178,** 1.
11. Aston-Jones, G., Ennis, M., Pieribone, V. A., Nickell, W. T., and Shipley, M. T. (1986). *Science,* **234,** 734.
12. Velley, L., Milner, T. A., Chan, J., Morrison, S. F., and Pickel, V. M. (1991). *Brain Res.,* **550,** 298.
13. Malmgren, L. and Olsson, Y. (1978). *Brain Res.,* **148,** 279.
14. Straus, W. (1982). *J. Histochem. Cytochem.,* **30,** 491.
15. Llewellyn-Smith, I. J., Minson, J. B., and Pilowsky, P. (1992). In *Methods in Neurosciences* (ed. P. M. Conn), Vol. 8, 'Neurotoxins', pp. 180–201. Academic Press, New York.
16. Mesulam, M.-M. (1978). *J. Histochem. Cytochem.,* **26,** 106.
17. Olucha, F., Martinez-Garcia, F., and Lopez-Garcia, C. (1985). *J. Neurosci. Methods,* **13,** 131.
18. Weinberg, R. J. and van Eyck, S. L. (1991). *J. Histochem. Cytochem.,* **39,** 1143.
19. Rye, D. B., Saper, C. B., and Wainer, B. H. (1984). *J. Histochem. Cytochem.,* **32,** 1145.
20. McIlhinney, R. A. J., Bacon, S. J., and Smith, A. D. (1988). *J. Neurosci. Methods,* **22,** 189.
21. Seeley, P. J. and Field, P. M. (1988). *Brain Res.,* **449,** 177.
22. Morilak, D. A., Somogyi, P., McIlhinney, J., and Chalmers, J. (1989). *Neurosci.,* **31,** 187.
23. Menetrey, D. (1985). *Histochemistry,* **83,** 391.
24. Basbaum, A. I. and Menetrey, D. (1987). *J. Comp. Neurol.,* **261,** 306.
25. Llewellyn-Smith, I. J., Minson, J. B., Wright, A. P., and Hodgson, A. J. (1990). *J. Comp. Neurol.,* **294,** 179.
26. Handley, D. A. (1989). In *Colloidal Gold. Principles, Methods and Applications* (ed. M. A. Hayat), Vol. 1, pp. 13–32. Academic Press, New York.
27. Slot, J. W. and Geuze, H. J. (1985). *Eur. J. Cell Biol.,* **38,** 87.
28. Frens, G. (1973). *Nature,* **241,** 20.
29. Horisberger, M. and Rosset, J. (1977). *J. Histochem. Cytochem.,* **25,** 295.
30. Menetrey, D. and Basbaum, A. I. (1989). In *Colloidal Gold. Principles, Methods and Applications* (ed. M. A. Hayat), Vol. 2, pp. 203–26. Academic Press, New York.
31. Danscher, G. (1981). *Histochemistry,* **71,** 1.
32. Danscher, G. (1981). *Histochemistry,* **71,** 77.
33. Danscher, G. (1981). *Histochemistry,* **71,** 81.
34. Scopsi, L. (1989). In *Colloidal Gold. Principles, Methods and Applications* (ed. M. A. Hayat), Vol. 1, pp. 251–95. Academic Press, New York.
35. Hacker, G. W. (1989). In *Colloidal Gold. Principles, Methods and Applications* (ed. M. A. Hayat), Vol. 1, pp. 297–321. Academic Press, New York.
36. Llewellyn-Smith, I. J., Minson, J. B., Morilak, D. A., Oliver, J. R., and Chalmers, J. P. (1990). *Neurosci. Letts.,* **108,** 243.
37. Llewellyn-Smith, I. J., Minson, J. B., Pilowsky, P. M., and Chalmers, J. P. (1991). *Clin. Exp. Physiol. Pharmacol.,* **18,** 111.
38. Horikawa, K. and Powell, E. W. (1986). *J. Neurosci. Methods,* **17,** 287.
39. Luppi, P.-H., Sakai, K., Salvert, D., Fort, P., and Jouvet, M. (1987). *Brain Res.,* **402,** 339.
40. Ericson, H. and Blomqvist, A. (1988). *J. Neurosci. Methods,* **24,** 225.
41. Luppi, P.-H., Fort, P., and Jouvet, M. (1990). *Brain Res.,* **534,** 209.

3

Anterograde tracing with PHA-L and biocytin at the electron microscopic level

YOLAND SMITH

1. Introduction

The neuronal circuitry of the mammalian brain is an extremely complex meshwork of highly ordered interconnections between billions of neurones. In order to be able to analyse and understand the organization of the circuitry of the central nervous system (CNS) it is essential to label a particular population of axonal structures to differentiate them from the unlabelled elements and study their connections.

In the middle of the last century Waller demonstrated that axons of neurones degenerate if they are severed from their parent cell bodies (Wallerian degeneration). Twenty years later Von Gudden showed in young animals that many neurones were degenerated following lesion of their axonal projections. These major discoveries served as a basis for the development of various retrograde and anterograde degeneration methods that have been used for nearly a century in attempts to determine the projection sites of particular population of cells (1). However, despite the fact that these techniques have led to major findings about the neuronal circuity in the mammalian CNS, the lack of sensitivity and the problems in the interpretation of data were the two major drawbacks of these methods. For these reasons, numerous connections remained unknown until the recent introduction of more sensitive tract-tracing methods. These new tracing techniques are based on physiological properties rather than on pathological changes of the neurones following experimental lesions. The demonstration that the perikaryon is the major site of protein synthesis in the neurone, and that these proteins once synthesized are transported along the axonal projections led in the late sixties, to the development of the autoradiographic method to trace connections in the peripheral and central nervous system (see 2–4 for reviews). A few years later, Kristensson and Olson (5) demonstrated that large protein molecules such as horseradish peroxidase (HRP) or bovine serum albumin (BSA) can be transported retrogradely from the periphery to the central nervous system. Subsequently, analogous retrograde transport of HRP was demonstrated within the CNS from the retina to the isthmo-optic nucleus (6). During the 1970s, efforts were directed at improving the uptake and transport of the enzyme as well as the sensitivity of the histochemical procedure to reveal the tracer. A major advance in this direction occurred when Gonatas and his colleagues (7) demonstrated that the conjugation of HRP with the lectin wheatgerm agglutinin (WGA) significantly improves the sensitivity of this method in the tracing of connections in the CNS (see 8 and Chapter 2).

Although the above-mentioned techniques, with all the modifications added over the years, represent a major step forward over the early degeneration methods, these tracers do not offer the possibility of visualizing the population of labelled neurones in their full extent, including the axonal segment and the terminal specializations. In this regard, Gerfen and Sawchenko discovered in 1984 that the kidney bean lectin, *Phaseolus vulgaris*–leucoagglutinin (PHA-L), fulfils most of the criteria for the ideal anterograde tracer (9). Recently, biocytin (biotinylated lysine) was introduced as a neuronal tracer that leads to anterograde labelling of axons and terminals with morphological details as great as those visualized with PHA-L (10–12).

The purpose of this chapter is to examine the advantages, limitations, and technical pitfalls of PHA-L and biocytin as anterograde tracers in the mammalian central nervous system. This chapter is intended for those starting to use these methods although it should also be useful to the more experienced worker. Detailed protocols for the use of PHA-L and biocytin alone, or in combination with other histochemical methods (see Chapter 11; see also Chapter 9, *Protocol 9*) are given. Because of the space limitation, particular emphasis will be given to the application and localization of the tracers at electron microscopic level. The reader who requires information about the use and the localization of these tracers at the light microscopic level only are referred to recent extensive reviews prepared by Gerfen and his colleagues (13), or Groenewegen and Wouterlood (14).

2. *Phaseolus vulgaris*–leucoagglutinin

The introduction of PHA-L as an anterograde tracer in the central nervous system represents one of the major advances in neuroanatomical techniques over the past ten years (9). Since the original report (9) showing the high level of specificity and sensitivity of PHA-L as an anterograde tracer, the lectin has been extensively used to study the organization of various neuronal systems at both light and electron microscopic levels. The use of PHA-L is now well established as a highly sensitive anterograde tracing technique that reveals details of axonal projections that could not be visualized with other anterograde tracing methods. In addition to its superiority over other techniques as an anterograde tracer, PHA-L offers a wide spectrum of possibilities in chemoanatomical research. The present section will briefly summarize the major characteristics of PHA-L and discuss the usefulness, but also the disadvantages of the technique (see *Table 1*).

2.1 Isolation of PHA-L

The phytohaemagglutinin (PHA) extracted from the red kidney bean, *P. vulgaris* is a mixture of several proteins that is best known for its capacity to agglutinate human erythrocytes and leucocytes (9). In 1964, Nordman and his colleagues, using serological methods, demonstrated that PHA contains a pure leucoagglutinin and an erythroagglutinin that has the capacity to produce mixed leukocyte–erythrocyte agglutinate at high concentrations (15). Three years later, the same group isolated two glycoprotein components from PHA which stimulated mitosis in lymphocytes but differed from each other in that one component had predominantly erythroagglutinating activity, whereas the other had leucoagglutinating activity (16). Two categories of subunits have since been characterized (M. wt 33 000 Daltons) from lectin extracts; a leucoagglutinating subunit (L) and an erythroagglutinating subunit (E). In 1977, Leavitt and co-workers demonstrated that PHA consists of five isolectins that have approximately the same amino acid composition and the same molecular weight (M. wt 115 000 Daltons). Each of these isolectins consists of a unique tetrameric combination of subunits (17).

Although the commercially available preparation of PHA-L (Vector Lab.) contains a significant proportion of E subunits, it is very likely that these subunits are not detected in labelled axon terminals, since Gerfen and Sawchenko (9) have shown that PHA-E is not taken up and transported by neurones when injected under the experimental conditions described in *Protocol 1*.

2.2 Administration of PHA-L

The most widely used method of administration of PHA-L in the central nervous system is iontophoresis (9). However, a few authors have reported that conventional pressure injections of PHA-L result in significant anterograde labelling (18). Pilot experiments in our laboratory revealed that injections of 100–150 nl of 2.5% PHA-L solution into the monkey striatum using a 1 μl Hamilton microsyringe result, at the injection site, in a diffuse area of labelling surrounded by a few heavily stained neurones. However, the density of anterogradely labelled elements following such injections is much lower than obtained after iontophoretic delivery of the tracer in the same region. Therefore, despite the fact that pressure injections are much easier and quicker to perform, we are in agreement with Gerfen and Sawchenko (9), that iontophoresis is the optimal method to deliver PHA-L. The parameters for iontophoretic injections of PHA-L are given in *Protocol 1* as is information about the post-injection survival time.

Protocol 1. Preparation and administration of PHA-L

Materials

- current source device (Model CS-3 from Transkinetics systems, Inc.)
- electrode puller
- glass capillaries (o.d. 1.0 mm, i.d. 0.5 mm; A-M Systems Inc.)
- silver wire (200 μm × 7.6 m; A-M Systems Inc.)
- stereotaxic frame with micromanipulator and electrode holder (David Kopf)
- peristaltic pump

Solutions

- PHA-L (Vector Laboratories)
- phosphate buffer (PB; 0.01 M, pH 8.0) and phosphate-buffered saline (PBS; 0.01 M, pH 7.4) (Chapter 1, *Protocol 1*)
- saline (0.9% NaCl in distilled water)
- fixative (1–4% paraformaldehyde and 0.1–5% glutaraldehyde in phosphate buffer 0.1 M, pH 7.4) (Chapter 1, *Protocol 2*)

Method

1. Dissolve PHA-L in PB (0.01 M, pH 8.0) as a 2.5% solution.[a]
2. Prepare glass micropipettes (tip diameters ranging from 10–40 μm) with an electrode puller.
3. Attach a micropipette to an electrode holder fixed to a micromanipulator of a stereotaxic frame.
4. Connect a small plastic tube (inner diameter of 1 mm) to the pipette and attach to a 1 ml syringe. Lower the tip of the micropipette into the PHA-L solution. Backfill the pipette by slowly pulling the plunger of the syringe.
5. Insert the silver wire into the pipette until it reaches the PHA-L solution.
6. Anaesthetize animal, place in stereotaxic frame and using appropriate stereotaxic coordinates, position the tip of the pipette in the target region of the brain.
7. Connect the wire to the positive terminal of the current source device. The negative terminal is used to ground the animal via a connection with any part of the animal's body.
8. Deliver the tracer by means of a 5–7 μA positive current pulsed for 20 min using a 7 sec on/7 sec off cycle.[b]

9. Allow the animal to survive for 7–12 days.[c]
10. Perfuse–fix the animal (Chapter 1, *Protocol 3*) with a mixture of paraformaldehyde and glutaraldehyde in phosphate buffer (Chapter 1, *Protocol 2*).
11. Dissect the brain from the skull. Cut in 5 mm-thick blocks and store in PBS at 4°C until sectioning.

[a] Once dissolved the PHA-L solution can be stored in 20 μl aliquots at −20°C for many months.
[b] Although PHA-L has been delivered using conventional pressure injections (18), it has been shown that the morphological characteristics of labelled neuronal elements at both the injection site and the termination areas are visualized with much greater detail when the tracer is delivered iontophoretically (9).
[c] It has recently been shown that the appearance of PHA-L immunoreactivity in labelled neurones at the injection site, and in the anterogradely labelled axons and terminals in the termination areas do not vary over a period ranging from a few days to 4.5 weeks (19).

2.3 Uptake of PHA-L

Once injected, PHA-L is taken up predominantly by neuronal perikarya and dendrites as well as astrocytes, in the vicinity of the site of delivery. Although the exact mechanism of uptake of PHA-L still remains to be determined, the pattern of intracellular labelling and the long survival time before the tracer is degraded suggests that it is different from the mechanism by which other lectins such as WGA are incorporated (13). In fact, it has been shown that in contrast to other tracers, the iontophoretically delivered PHA-L is not incorporated by endocytosis and does not enter the lysosomal system. Gerfen and his colleagues have recently suggested two possibilities by which PHA-L may be incorporated into neuronal structures (13). One possibility is that during the iontophoretic injection of the tracer, the membranes of neurones are temporarily opened and the tracer gains access to the cell (13). The second hypothesis is based on the fact that iontophoretic delivery of PHA-L might disrupt the association between astrocytes and dendrites opening a site of entry for the tracer to the intracellular compartment (13). Obviously, future experiments are still needed to clearly understand the exact mechanism by which PHA-L gains access to neuronal structures. So far there is no evidence that specific populations of neurones fail to transport PHA-L.

The appearance and the size of PHA-L injection sites are dependent, at least in part, on the cellular architecture of the area of delivery. In structures where the cells are densely packed, (e.g. striatum, subthalamic nucleus), iontophoretic injections of PHA-L lead to injection sites of approximately 400–600 μm in diameter with a darkly labelled central core, whereas similar injections in an area where the cells are loosely arranged, (e.g. globus pallidus) result in a more diffuse injection site having a diameter twice as large (*Figure 1A*). The pattern of labelling at the injection site is often the same, i.e. a central core containing densely labelled neuronal and glial processes surrounded by neurones that appear to be completely filled with the lectin. Although direct evidence is still lacking, it seems likely that the labelled axon terminals that emerge from a PHA-L injection site arise from the population of neurones that are filled with the lectin (9). Occasionally, a few intensely-labelled cells are found outside the confines of the injection site proper. The extension of dendrites from these neurones into the injection area probably accounts for this labelling (9).

2.4 Anterograde transport of PHA-L

The axonal transport of PHA-L is a relatively slow process that occurs at a rate of 5–6 mm/day in the anterograde direction (9). Therefore, in most of the neuronal systems that have been investigated with this method, optimal anterograde labelling was obtained seven to ten days after the injection. However, it appears that even after four to five weeks post-injection survival, the labelling at the injection site and the termination areas is not significantly changed (19). After this period the tracer gradually disappears from the perikarya, dendrites, and axonal structures. Post-injection survival times of less than four weeks are therefore recommended after intracerebral injections of PHA-L. The quality of the anterograde labelling of axon terminals obtained with PHA-L is not dependent on the neuronal system under investigation. In general, the PHA-L labelled structures can be visualized in great morphological detail from the injection site to the termination areas including the axonal segment (*Figure 1B*). The morphology of PHA-L labelled terminals can be studied in much greater detail in both light and electron microscopes than terminals labelled with either WGA-HRP or tritiated amino acids (*Figure 1C*). The high level of resolution offered by the PHA-L method allows one to follow single axons through brain sections and analyse their pattern of terminal arborization. It is thus highly recommended to use the PHA-L method in experiments where the pattern of arborization of the anterogradely labelled elements need to be analysed in detail. However, in experiments where large targets must be injected, the WGA-HRP and the autoradiographic methods should be considered.

Protocol 2. Localization of injected and transported PHA-L

Materials

- rotating agitator
- vibrating microtome
- glass vials (20 ml)

Solutions

- phosphate-buffered saline (0.01 M, pH 7.4) (Chapter 1, *Protocol 1*)

- Tris-HCl buffer (0.05 M, pH 7.6)
- sodium borohydride (1% solution in PBS)

Reagents for immunohistochemical reaction

- rabbit anti-PHA-L (Dakopatts)
- biotinylated goat anti-rabbit IgG (Vector Laboratories)
- avidin–biotin–peroxidase complex (ABC, Vector Laboratories)
- normal goat serum (NGS; Vector Laboratories)
- Triton X-100 (Sigma Chemical Company)
- bovine serum albumin (BSA) (Sigma Chemical Company)
- 3,3′-diaminobenzidine tetrahydrochloride (DAB, Sigma Chemical Company) (see *Safety note 3*, Chapter 5, p. 119)
- imidazole (BDH Chemicals)
- hydrogen peroxide (Sigma Chemical Company)

Method (see Chapter 5 for further details on immunocytochemistry, see also Chapter 9, *Protocol 9*)

1. Cut brain areas containing the injection sites and the transport sites at 50–70 μm on a vibrating microtome (Chapter 1, *Protocol 4*).
2. Collect the sections in PBS.
3. Treat the sections for 20 min with sodium borohydride (1% solution in PBS) (Chapter 5, *Protocol 6*).
4. Wash the sections several times in PBS.
5. Separate sections that are to be processed for electron microscopy from those that are to be prepared for light microscopy.
6. Freeze-thaw in liquid nitrogen the sections for electron microscopy (Chapter 5, *Protocol 4*). For sections that are prepared for light microscopy, add 0.3% Triton X-100 to the antisera and the ABC solutions.
7. Incubate the sections for 48 h at 4°C in rabbit anti-PHA-L IgG (1:1000 dilution in PBS) including 1% NGS.
8. Wash the sections three times (for a total of 45 min) in PBS.
9. Incubate the sections for 12 h at 4°C in biotinylated goat anti-rabbit IgG (1:200 dilution in PBS) including 1% NGS.
10. Wash the sections three times (for a total of 45 min) in PBS.
11. Incubate the sections for 12 h at 4°C in ABC (1:100 dilution in PBS) including 1% BSA.
12. Wash the sections two times (10 min each) in PBS, and then two times (10 min each) in Tris-HCl buffer (0.05 M, pH 7.6).

Protocol 2. *Continued*

13. Reveal PHA-L immunoreactivity using diaminobenzidine as the chromogen in the peroxidase reaction, by incubation for 10–12 min in Tris-HCl buffer (0.05 M, pH 7.6; 20 ml) containing:
- 0.025% DAB (5 mg)
- 0.01 M imidazole (200 μl of a 1.0 M stock solution)
- 0.006% of hydrogen peroxide (400 μl of a 0.3% stock solution)

14. Stop the reaction by extensive washings in PBS (5 × 5 min).

15. Post-fix the sections for electron microscopy in osmium tetroxide (Chapter 1, *Protocol 7*), dehydrate, and embed in an electron microscope resin on microscope slides (Chapter 1, *Protocol 8*).

16. Mount on to gelatin-coated slides, dehydrate, and apply coverslips to the sections that have been processed for light microscopy (Chapter 1, *Protocols 5* and *6*).

2.5 Is PHA-L transported by fibres of passage?

In their original report, Gerfen and Sawchenko (9) suggested that PHA-L is not taken up by fibres of passage traversing the injected area; at least when it is delivered iontophoretically using pipettes with a small tip diameter. Experiments in our laboratory and in others (19) have confirmed this observation. After iontophoretic injections of PHA-L into the striatum that involved fibres of the internal capsule, no anterogradely labelled elements were found in the thalamus or the cerebral cortex which are known to send their axons through the internal capsule. On the other hand, a few authors have reported that after injections of PHA-L centred in fibre bundles, (e.g. spinal trigeminal tract, dorsal column, trapezoid body, and inferior cerebral peduncle), a small number of labelled axons emerging from the injection sites can be visualized over relatively long distances into the brain (20, 21). Therefore, it is important to keep this possibility in mind but under normal experimental conditions, this problem should not complicate the interpretation of the results (14).

2.6 Is PHA-L transported retrogradely?

Although it is predominantly transported in the anterograde direction, various reports suggest that in some situations PHA-L is also transported in the retrograde direction. The appearance of retrogradely-transported PHA-L in neuronal structures is either granular or homogeneous. In the cases where the labelling is granular, it is confined to the perikaryon and proximal dendrites of the labelled cells. However, when the labelling is homogeneous, it entirely fills the retrogradely labelled cell in a Golgi-like manner. In our experience, the granular retrograde labelling is more commonly found than the Golgi-like labelling. The reason for a particular type of retrograde labelling to prevail in a specific neuronal system is not known, although it appears that the Golgi-like retrograde labelling is found more frequently in cells that arborize profusely into the injected areas. A typical example of such a system is the striatopallidal projection. A single iontophoretic injection of PHA-L into the pallidal complex of rats and monkeys invariably leads to Golgi-like retrograde labelling of medium-sized spiny cells into the striatum. On the other hand, after injections of PHA-L into the striatum, only very few perikarya in the substantia nigra compacta contain granules of retrogradely-transported PHA-L and none display Golgi-like labelling. In our experience, it seems that in some neuronal systems, (e.g. striatopallidal projection) the retrograde transport of PHA-L is unavoidable while in other systems, (e.g. nigrostriatal projection) the number of retrogradely labelled cells can be significantly reduced if PHA-L is injected according to the standard experimental protocol (*Protocol 1*). The reason why some neuronal systems transport PHA-L in the retrograde direction more efficiently than others remains to be determined.

2.7 Localization of PHA-L labelled elements in the electron microscope

In the electron microscope, the PHA-L labelled axon terminals are recognized by the presence of immunoperoxidase reaction product attached to the inner surface of the cell membrane and the outer surface of cytoplasmic organelles (*Figure 1C*). The texture of the reaction product depends on the nature of the chromogen that has been used (see Chapter 5). For example, the use of DAB leads to an amorphous reaction product that is often homogeneously distributed inside the labelled structures whereas benzidine dihydrochloride (BDHC) forms crystals that are evenly distributed throughout the labelled elements (Chapter 5). One of the major advantages of using PHA-L at the electron microscopic level is the possibility of investigating in much more detail, the ultrastructural characteristics and the synaptic relationships between the PHA-L labelled varicosities and their post-synaptic targets. However, the localization of PHA-L in the electron microscope is technically more complicated than the localization in the light microscope because additional technical demands need to be satisfied. One of the major technical problems that investigators need to overcome when using the PHA-L method at the electron microscopic level, is to find a compromise between good preservation of ultrastructural details and the localization of PHA-L labelled elements deep within the section. These two demands are difficult to reconcile because they are mutually exclusive; good ultrastructural preservation needs strong fixation, whereas weaker fixation is better for the penetration of the antibody into the tissue. Therefore, it is important to find a method by which the PHA-L antibody can penetrate through strongly fixed tissue without damaging too much the membranes of neural elements. One of the most commonly used detergents to improve penetration of antibody through brain tissue is Triton X-100. However, because it dissolves membranes and results in poor preservation of ultrastructural details it is not recommended to use Triton X-100 on tissue that must be examined in the electron microscope. Although various approaches have been suggested (14), we routinely use in our laboratory a single section freeze-thawing method to enable the PHA-L antibody to reach the antigen located deep within brain sections (see Chapter 5, *Protocol 4*). In our experience this method allows the PHA-L antibody to penetrate at least the first 10–15 μm on both sides of brain sections that have been fixed with solutions containing as much as 3% glutaraldehyde.

Another problem that may occur when PHA-L labelled elements are examined in the electron microscope is the scarcity of labelled structures visualized in single ultrathin sections. In order to avoid ultrathin sectioning and examination of areas that do not contain immunoreactive structures, it is advisable to analyse carefully the areas of interest in the light microscope first, and then select part of the structures rich in immunoreactive elements for electron microscopic analysis (see Chapter 1 for more details). A detailed experimental protocol for the localization of PHA-L in the electron microscope is given in *Protocol 2*. Further information can also be found in recent reviews by Gerfen and his colleagues (13) or by Groenewegen and Wouterlood (14).

2.8 Combination of PHA-L with other tract-tracing methods and immunohistochemical techniques

Because it is localized by means of immunohistochemical procedures, the PHA-L method can easily be combined with other techniques to address additional problems concerning the chemo-anatomical organization of neuronal circuits in the central nervous system. So far, most of the combined approaches that have been introduced have been used at the light microscopic level only (13, 14). However, recent developments suggest that the use of PHA-L can also be combined with other tract-tracing methods and immunohistochemical procedures at electron microscopic level. In Chapter 11 detailed protocols for the use of these combined techniques are provided (see also references 13, 14, 22).

3. Biocytin

Biocytin (biotinyl–lysine) was recently introduced as an intracellular marker of neurones following electrophysiological recordings (23) (see also Chapter 10). Furthermore, a few reports suggested that biocytin can also be used as a powerful anterograde tracer in the mammalian central nervous system (10, 11). We have recently used biocytin to trace various neuronal pathways in rat and monkey brains (12, 24, 25). In light of the findings obtained in these studies the major characteristics of biocytin and the advantages and limitations of this method, in comparison to the PHA-L technique, will be described (*Table 1*).

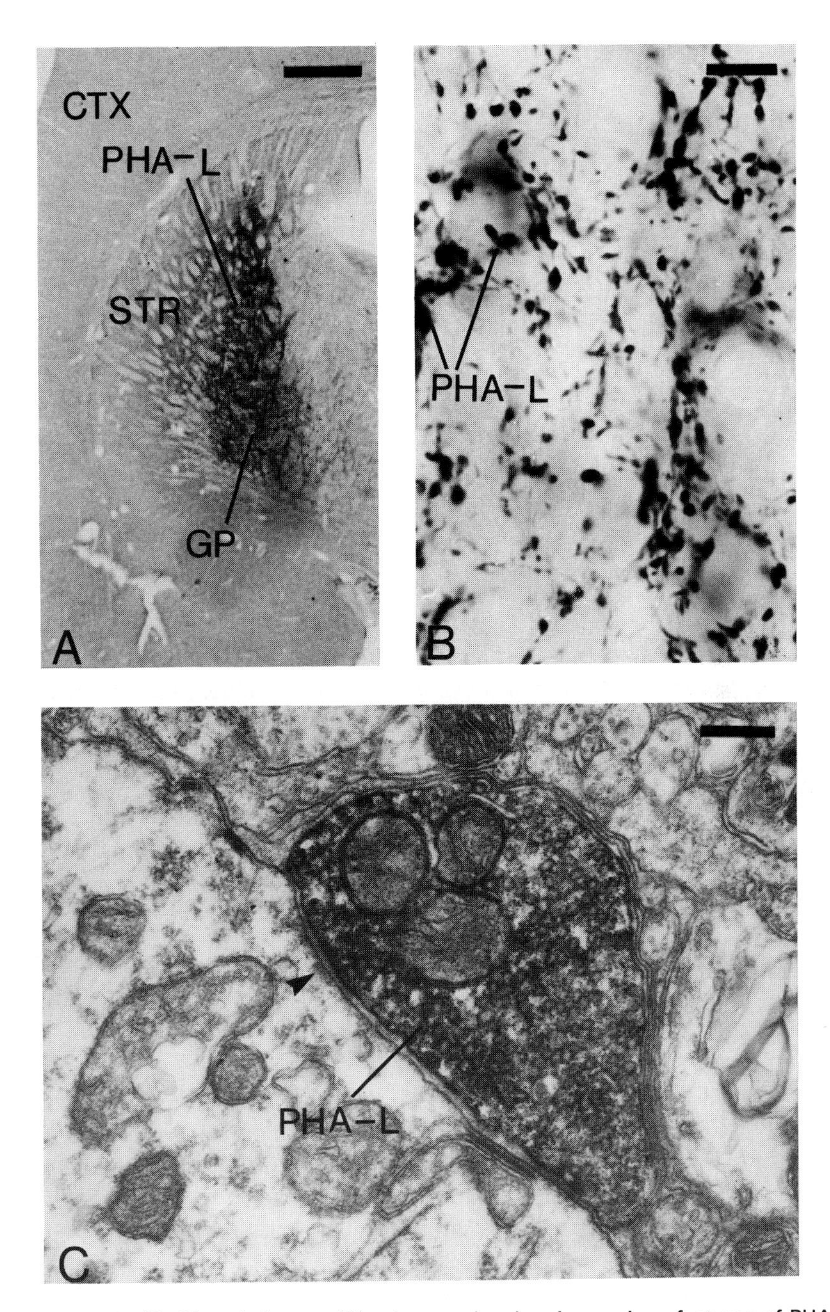

Figure 1. Light (A–B) and electron (C) micrographs showing various features of PHA-L labelling in the subthalamic nucleus after injection in the globus pallidus (GP) of the rat. (A) depicts the extent of the PHA-L injection site in the GP. (B) shows a rich plexus of PHA-L labelled varicosities in the subthalamic nucleus after injections in the GP. (C) illustrates a PHA-L immunoreactive pallidosubthalamic terminal that forms a symmetric synapse (arrowhead) with a perikaryon. CTX, cortex; STR, striatum. Scale markers: (A) 0.5 mm, (B) 10 μm, (C) 0.1 μm.

3.1 Biochemical characteristics of biocytin

Biocytin is a low molecular weight complex of biotin combined with the E-amino group of lysine that was first isolated from yeast by Wright and his colleagues (26). It is now well established that biocytin occurs in traces in eukaryotic organisms. Although the exact role of this complex is not fully understood, biochemical evidence suggests that it may serve as an intermediate carrier of carbon dioxide during carboxylation reactions mediating gluconeogenesis, synthesis of fatty acids, and amino acid oxidation (27, 28). Biocytin is highly soluble in aqueous solutions and the biotin moiety retains a high binding affinity for avidin. This latter characteristic was used to develop histochemical approaches to localize the tracer in fixed tissue using markers, (e.g. peroxidase and fluorescent molecules) conjugated with molecules of avidin.

3.2 Uptake of biocytin and pattern of neuronal labelling at the injection site

The exact way by which biocytin is taken up from the extracellular space into intracellular compartments still remains to be determined. The appearance of biocytin injection sites is similar to PHA-L injections, i.e. a central core where neuronal elements and glial cells are completely filled with the tracer, surrounded by a zone containing labelled neurones that display a Golgi-like staining. It is thus possible to analyse at both light and electron microscopic levels the morphological characteristics and synaptic inputs of neurones that have taken up the tracer, and most likely give rise to the anterograde labelling in the termination areas (12). As is the case for PHA-L, the size of biocytin injection site is highly dependent on the cytoarchitecture of the target; in areas where the cells are tightly packed, (e.g. striatum) the extent of single biocytin injections is much more restricted than in areas where the cells are more loosely organized, (e.g. cerebral cortex). Another similarity between biocytin and PHA-L at the level of the injection sites is that both tracers are taken up by neuronal elements confined to the very close vicinity of the site of delivery even when large volumes (<400 nl) of biocytin are administered. Therefore, it seems that over a certain limit (200–300 nl), the size of biocytin injection sites is not directly proportional to the volume of tracer that is injected. For this reason, it is essential to make multiple penetrations when large areas need to be injected.

Protocol 3. Preparation and administration of biocytin

Materials

- the materials required for the injection of PHA-L are also necessary for the delivery of biocytin (see *Protocol 1*)

- a 10 μl Hamilton microsyringe with a glass micropipette (tip 20–60 μm) glued to the needle
- a syringe holder on a stereotaxic frame (David Kopf)

Solutions

- biocytin (5% solution in Tris-HCl buffer 0.05 M, pH 7.6; Sigma Chemical Company)
- PBS (0.01 M, pH 7.4) (Chapter 1, *Protocol 1*)
- Tris-HCl buffer (0.05 M, pH 7.6)
- saline (0.9% NaCl in distilled water)
- fixative (1–4% paraformaldehyde and 0.5–2.5% glutaraldehyde in phosphate buffer 0.1 M, pH 7.4) (Chapter 1, *Protocol 2*)

Method

1. Dissolve biocytin in Tris-HCl buffer (0.05 M, pH 7.6) as a 5% solution.[a]
2. Fill a 10 μl Hamilton microsyringe, with a micropipette attached to the tip, with the biocytin solution.[b]
3. Anaesthetize the animal, place in stereotaxic frame, and position the tip of the syringe in the target brain region according to stereotaxic coordinates.
4. Deliver between 0.25–0.40 μl of biocytin/site. This can be delivered by steps of 0.1 μl over a period of 10–15 min.[c]
5. Wait 5–10 min and withdraw the syringe slowly from the brain.
6. Allow the animal to survive between 24–36 h.
7. Perfuse–fix the animal (Chapter 1, *Protocol 3*) with a mixture of paraformaldehyde and at least 0.1% glutaraldehyde (Chapter 1, *Protocol 2*).
8. Dissect the brain from the skull. Cut in 5 mm-thick blocks, and store in PBS until sectioning.

[a] Once dissolved the tracer can be stored in 20 μl aliquots at −20°C for many months. Repeated freeze-thawing may inactivate the tracer.

[b] Biocytin can also be delivered iontophoretically using parameters similar to those described in *Protocol 1* for the administration of PHA-L.

[c] If large areas need to be injected it is recommended to deliver the tracer at many adjacent sites since there is no linear relationship between the size of the biocytin injections and the volume of tracer delivered.

3.3 Anterograde transport of biocytin and examination of labelled terminals

Once injected, biocytin is taken up very rapidly by neuronal elements and transported predominantly in the anterograde direction. The exact speed at which biocytin is transported has not been determined precisely but it has been shown that in the rat, some neuronal connections, (e.g. corticostriatal pathway) can be labelled as quickly as four to eight hours after the injection (11). However, in our experience it seems that the optimal survival time after biocytin injections in the rat and monkey central nervous system ranges between 24 and 48 hours. Pilot experiments are recommended to determine the optimal post-injection survival period for each neuronal pathways under investigation. This step is critical since biocytin is degraded very rapidly once it has been delivered and taken up by neuronal elements (see below).

The biocytin-labelled axon terminals can be visualized with a high level of resolution in both light and electron microscopes. In the light microscope, a detailed morphological analysis of anterogradely labelled axons and terminals can be performed. Individual biocytin-labelled fibres can be followed over long distances through the sections, and can be seen to give rise to many axonal swellings that sometimes are apposed to the surface of unlabelled dendritic shafts and perikarya in the termination areas (*Figure 2A*). Examination of the anterogradely labelled axonal swellings in the electron microscope reveals that these varicosities are axon terminals packed with vesicles and mitochondria that often form synaptic contact with their targets (*Figure 2B*). In the cases where DAB is used to localize the peroxidase bound to biocytin (*Protocol 4*), the electron-dense reaction product is floccular, homogeneously distributed, and associated with the internal surface of plasma membranes. The form and distribution of the reaction product is very similar to that seen following immunoperoxidase reactions. The labelled terminals can be easily differentiated from the unlabelled structures because of their dark staining that stands out from the unstained neuropil.

Protocol 4. Localization of injected and transported biocytin

Materials

- the materials needed to localize biocytin are the same as for PHA-L (*Protocol 2*)

Solutions

- the solutions needed are the same as those used for the localization of PHA-L (*Protocol 2*)

Reagents for the histochemical reaction

- avidin–biotin–peroxidase complex (ABC, Vector Laboratories)
- bovine serum albumin (Sigma Chemical Company)
- Triton X-100 (Sigma Chemical Company)

- 3,3′-diaminobenzidine tetrahydrochloride (DAB, Sigma Chemical Company) (see *Safety note 3*, Chapter 5, p. 119)
- imidazole (BDH Chemicals)
- hydrogen peroxide (Sigma Chemical Company)

Method

1. Follow steps **1–6** in *Protocol 2*.
2. Incubate the sections for 24 h at room temperature in ABC (1:100 dilution in PBS) including 1% BSA.
3. Wash the sections two times in PBS (10 min each) and two times (10 min each) in Tris-HCl buffer (0.05 M, pH 7.6).
4. Perform peroxidase reaction using DAB as the chromogen as described in step **13,** *Protocol 2*.
5. Stop the reaction by several washes in PBS (5 × 5 min).
6. Post-fix in osmium tetroxide (Chapter 1, *Protocol 7*), dehydrate, and embed in resin the sections prepared for electron microscopy (Chapter 1, *Protocol 8*).
7. Mount on gelatin-coated slides, dehydrate, and apply coverslips to the sections processed for light microscopy (Chapter 1, *Protocols 5* and *6*).

3.4 Retrograde transport of biocytin

Although it is preferentially taken up by neuronal perikarya and transported in the anterograde direction, biocytin is occasionally transported retrogradely. As is the case with PHA-L, the retrograde transport of biocytin occurs more frequently in some neuronal systems, (e.g. thalamocortical and striatonigral projections) than in others, (e.g. nigrostriatal). In our experience it seems that biocytin is transported retrogradely when large volumes of tracer are delivered at multiple adjacent sites into the target (10). However, it is worth noting that even in such cases, the retrograde labelling produced following injections of biocytin is far less marked than that occurring after injections of retrograde tracer such as WGA-HRP. The retrogradely labelled cells are often extensively filled with the tracer giving them a Golgi-like appearance.

3.5 Transport of biocytin along fibres of passage

The fibres of passage coursing through the injection sites do not seem to take up and transport biocytin, at least in the striatum. After multiple intrastriatal pressure injections of biocytin, the fibre bundles of the internal capsule remained unlabelled. Furthermore, these injections resulted only in terminal labelling in the targets of striatal cells, i.e. the substantia nigra and the pallidal complex; no labelling was found in the thalamus or the cerebral cortex which

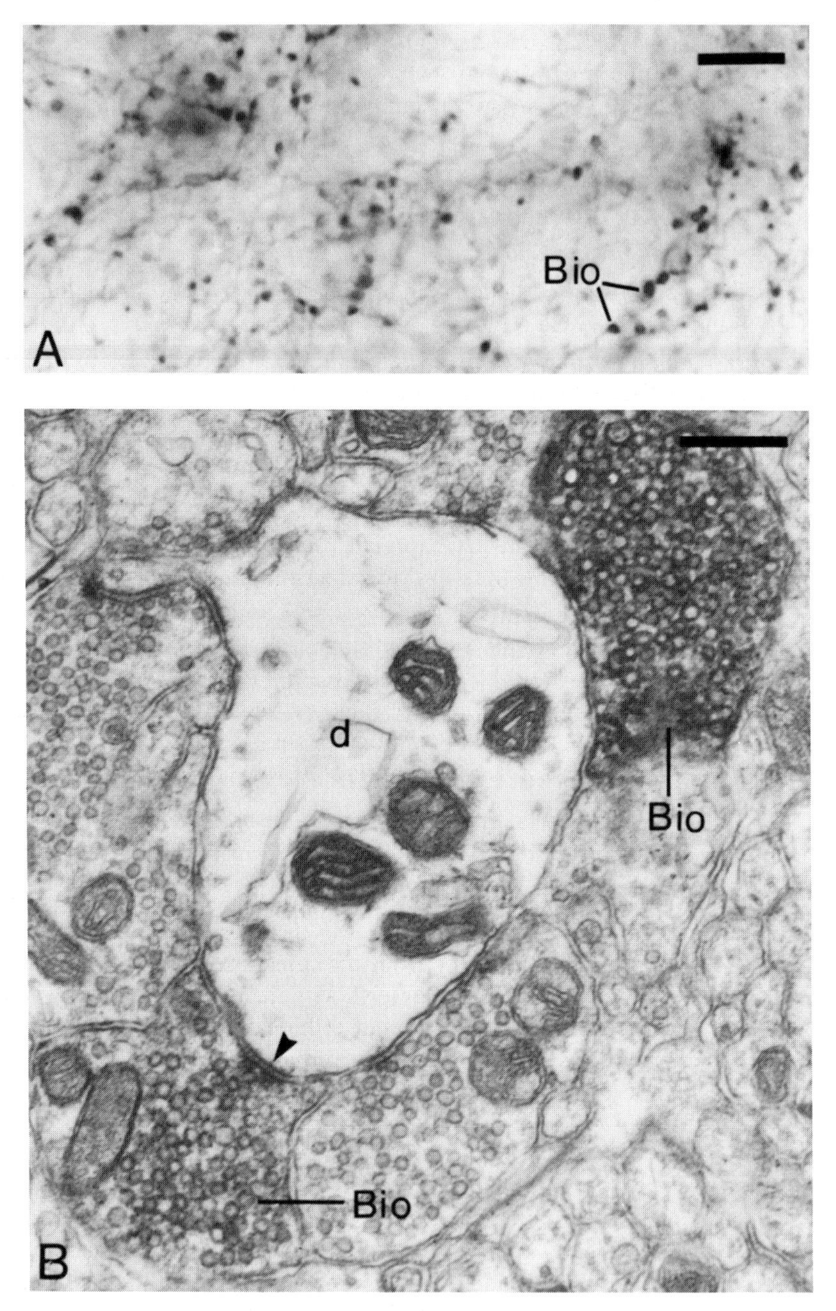

Figure 2. Light (A) and electron (B) micrographs showing examples of anterogradely labelled terminals (Bio) in the substantia nigra after injection of biocytin in the striatum of the rat. In (B), one of the labelled terminals forms a symmetric synapse (arrowhead) with the dendritic shaft (d). Scale markers: (A) 10 μm, (B) 0.5 μm.

are known to send their axons through the internal capsule (12). A slight transport of biocytin along fibres of passage has been reported in rats when the tracer was delivered by pressure using large tip needle injections (10, 11).

4. Advantages and limitations of biocytin in comparison to PHA-L

The PHA-L and biocytin anterograde transport methods offer to neuro-anatomists the possibility of visualizing anterogradely labelled terminals with great morphological detail in both light and electron microscopes. Despite the fact that biocytin has not been used extensively as an anterograde tracer, the results that have been obtained in our laboratory and in others (10, 11) suggest that it offers some advantages over PHA-L. It is well established that PHA-L must be delivered iontophoretically to get optimal anterograde labelling (see above). Although iontophoresis is the best approach to get well-defined small injection sites, it is very time consuming when large areas, (e.g. striatum, cerebral cortex, etc.) need to be injected, since a single PHA-L injection takes at least 20 to 30 minutes to be completed. Thus, when numerous injection sites are needed it may easily take a full day to complete the experiment. In contrast, biocytin is much easier and less time-consuming to deliver, since it can be applied by pressure over a period of 5 to 10 minutes per injection. Furthermore, it is worth noting that the morphological details displayed by biocytin-labelled elements at both the site of delivery and the termination areas are as great as those displayed by PHA-L immunoreactive structures.

A major difference between PHA-L and biocytin is the speed of transport in the anterograde direction. A post-injection survival time of 7 to 12 days is necessary for an optimal anterograde labelling with PHA-L. However, in our experience it appears that a period of 12 to 48 hours is long enough for biocytin to be transported effectively from the injection site to the termination areas. It has been reported that some short neuronal connections in the brainstem can even be labelled four hours after biocytin injections (11). This relatively short survival period significantly reduces the time necessary to complete a series of experiments. However, the major disadvantage of biocytin is the fact that it is degraded very rapidly after injection into CNS. With post-injection survivals longer than 48 hours, the density of biocytin-labelled structures is significantly reduced. In contrast, PHA-L is much more stable and can be visualized even after 4 to 5 weeks post-injection survival periods.

The histochemical reaction to localize biocytin is less costly and much quicker to perform than the immunohistochemical reaction to localize PHA-L. In addition, the fact that no antibodies are needed to localize biocytin offers a wider spectrum of possibilities for combination with other immunohistochemical techniques (see Chapter 11, and Chapter 9, *Protocol 9*), since antibodies raised in any species can be used to localize the second antigen.

Another difference between biocytin and PHA-L is that a certain percentage of glutaraldehyde (at least 0.1%) must be included in the fixative to retain biocytin in the tissue. This is not the case with PHA-L which can be localized in tissue that has been perfused with fixative containing either paraformaldehyde only, or a mixture of paraformaldehyde and glutaraldehyde. The presence of a high concentration of glutaraldehyde is not compatible with the immunohistochemical localization of certain neurotransmitter-related substances. For this reason, in cases where the anterograde tracer is combined with immunohistochemical procedures (see Chapter 11), PHA-L must be used when the second antigen does not tolerate glutaraldehyde. However, experiments in our laboratory have revealed that biocytin can be combined with the immunohistochemical localization of enzymes such as tyrosine hydroxylase and choline acetyltransferase without significant loss of immunoreactivity (see Chapter 11).

Table 1. Comparison between PHA-L and biocytin anterograde labelling techniques

	PHA-L	**Biocytin**
Preparation	2.5% solution in PB (0.01 M, pH 8.0)	5% solution in Tris-HCl buffer (0.05 M, pH 7.6)
Administration	Iontophoresis, 7μA, 7 sec on/ 7 sec off	Iontophoresis (7 μA, 7 sec on, 7 sec off) or pressure (0.3 μl/ site)
Survival period	7–14 days	12–48 hours
Perfuse–fixation	2–4% paraformaldehyde and 0.1–1% glutaraldehyde	2–4% paraformaldehyde and 0.1–1% glutaraldehyde
Localization	Immunohistochemistry; ABC or peroxidase anti-peroxidase methods	Histochemistry; ABC method

References

1. de Olmos, J. S., Ebbesson, S. O. E., and Heimer, L. (1981). In *Neuroanatomical Tract-tracing Methods* (ed. L. Heimer and M. J. Robards), pp. 117–70. Plenum Press, New York.
2. Cowan, W. M., Gottlieb, D. I., Hendrickson, A. E., Price, J. L., and Woolsey, T. A. (1972). *Brain Res.,* **37,** 21.
3. Edwards, S. B. and Hendrickson, A. E. (1981). In *Neuroanatomical Tract-tracing Methods* (ed. L. Heimer and M. J. Robards), pp. 171–205. Plenum Press, New York.
4. Jones, E. G. and Hartman, B. K. (1978). *Ann. Rev. Neurosci.,* **1,** 215.
5. Kristensson, K. and Olsson, Y. (1971). *Brain Res.,* **29,** 363.
6. LaVail, J. H. and LaVail, M. M. (1972). *Science,* **176,** 1416.

7. Gonatas, N. K., Harper, C., Mizutani, T., and Gonatas, J. O. (1979). *J. Histochem. Cytochem.*, **27**, 728.
8. Mesulam, M.-M. (1982). In *Tracing Neural Connections with Horseradish Peroxidase* (ed. M.-M. Mesulam), pp. 1–151. John Wiley and Sons Ltd., Chichester.
9. Gerfen, C. R. and Sawchenko, P. E. (1984). *Brain Res.*, **290**, 219.
10. King, M. A., Louis, P. M., Hunter, B. E., and Walker, D. W. (1989). *Brain Res.*, **497**, 361.
11. Izzo, P. N. (1991). *J. Neurosci. Methods*, **36**, 155.
12. Smith, Y. and Bolam, J. P. (1991). *Neurosci.*, **44**, 45.
13. Gerfen, C. R., Sawchenko, P. E., and Carlsen, J. (1989). In *Neuroanatomical Tract-Tracing Methods 2, Recent Progress* (ed. L. Heimer and L. Z. Zaborszky), pp. 19–47. Plenum Press, New York.
14. Groenewegen, H. J. and Wouterlood, F. G. (1990). In *Handbook of Chemical Neuroanatomy: Analysis of Neuronal Microcircuits and Synaptic Interactions* (ed. A. Björklund, T., Hökfelt, F. G., Wouterlood, and A. N. van den Pol), Vol. 8, pp. 7–124. Elsevier Science Publishers, Amsterdam.
15. Nordman, C. T., de la Chapelle, A., and Gräsbeck, R. (1964). *Acta med. scand.*, Suppl. **412**, 49.
16. Weber, T., Nordman, C. T., and Gräsbeck, R. (1967). *Scand. J. Haematol.*, **4**, 77.
17. Leavitt, R. D., Felsted, R. L., and Bachur, N. R. (1977). *J. Biol. Chem.*, **252**, 2961.
18. Russchen, F. T., Amaral, D. G., and Price, J. L. (1985). *J. Comp. Neurol.*, **242**, 1.
19. Wouterlood, F. G., Goede, P. H., and Groenewegen, H. J. (1900). *J. Chem. Neuroanat.*, **3**, 11.
20. Cliffer, K. D. and Giesler Jr, G. J. (1988). *Brain Res.*, **458**, 185.
21. Schofield, B. R. (1990). *J. Neurosci. Methods*, **35**, 47.
22. Bolam, J. P. and Ingham, C. A. (1990). In *Handbook of Chemical Neuroanatomy: Analysis of Neuronal Microcircuits and Synaptic Interactions* (ed. A. Björklund, T. Hökfelt, F. G., Wouterlood, and A. N. van den Pol), Vol. 8, pp. 125–98. Elsevier Science Publishers, Amsterdam.
23. Horikawa, K. and Armstrong, W. E. (1988). *J. Neurosci. Methods*, **25**, 1.
24. Bolam, J. P. and Smith, Y. (1990). *Brain Res.*, **529**, 57.
25. Lapper, S. R., Smith, Y., Sadikot, A. F., Parent, A., and Bolam, J. P. (1992). *Brain Res.*, **580**, 215.
26. Wright, L. D., Cresson, E. L., Liebert, K. V., and Skeggs, H. R. (1952). *J. Am. Chem. Soc.*, **74**, 2004.
27. Dreyfus, P. M. (1985). In *Handbook of Neurochemistry* (ed. A. Lajtha), p. 773. Plenum Press, New York.
28. Friedrich, W. (1988). *Biotin from Vitamins.* Walter de Gruyter, Berlin.

4

Transneuronal mapping of neural circuits with alpha herpesviruses

PETER L. STRICK and J. PATRICK CARD

1. Introduction

The use of alpha herpesviruses for defining functionally interconnected populations of neurones has generated considerable interest in recent years (1). Two of the most attractive aspects of using viruses for circuit definition are the fact that they pass transneuronally and replicate in synaptically linked populations of neurones. Thus, the virus is transported through a multi-synaptic pathway and the signal, (i.e. intracellular concentration of virus) progressively increases with time (*Figures 1* and *2*). These two attributes are clearly superior to those offered by other neuronal tracers which have been shown to pass transneuronally. Wheatgerm agglutinin horseradish peroxidase (WGA-HRP) and the C fragment of tetanus toxin (cTT) are both known to cross synapses, but they do so in such limited amounts that it is at times difficult to identify synaptic transfer with confidence. For these reasons, there has been a dramatic increase in the number of studies which have utilized herpesviruses to characterize functionally distinct populations of neurones.

The neurotropic properties of herpesviruses are well known, and the fundamental mechanisms which underlie neuro-invasiveness and virulence have been the subject of intense analysis (2, 3). The utility of using herpesviruses to identify functional circuits is based upon the assumption that virus replicates within synaptically linked populations of neurones, and that neuronal infection is the product of trans-synaptic passage of virus rather than lytic release of virions into the extracellular space. Although this conclusion is supported by numerous studies which have shown projection-specific patterns of neuronal infectivity (4–27), the precise route of viral spread in the nervous system remains to be established. Consequently, it is clear that optimal results and appropriate interpretation of the pattern of viral transport is dependent upon critical consideration of the strain of virus employed, the route of injection, the temporal aspects of transport, and a clear understanding of the fundamental principals which direct viral uptake, replication, and transport in the nervous system.

Our objective in writing this chapter is to provide a critical overview of the above issues and how they can be effectively addressed to optimize the use of alpha herpesviruses in mapping multi-synaptic circuits. The primary emphasis has been placed upon the practical application of the method and the interpretation of the resulting data. The literature citations are not meant to be inclusive, but have been selected to illustrate issues which are most important in the design and interpretation of experimental results.

2. Considerations in designing viral studies

2.1 Safety

Alpha herpesviruses are classified as biohazardous agents and specific safety regulations are imposed upon their use. The human herpesvirus strains pose obvious dangers to investigators, but *all* alpha herpesvirus strains must be used in accordance with biosafety level II (BSL II) restrictions. These regulations are detailed in Health and Human Services publication number 88-8395 entitled *Biosafety in Microbiological and Biomedical Laboratories*. The following list highlights the most important issues that should be considered in designing viral studies, but it is not meant to be exhaustive. Some institutions impose further restrictions upon use of virus and it is the responsibility of each investigator to seek out this information from the Biosafety Officer at their institution.

(a) *Laboratory*. Most institutions require a separate laboratory equipped with a biosafety hood. Restricted access and biohazard signs (indicating BSL II restrictions are in force) should be placed on the door and the door should be locked during the course of each study. *Anyone* (especially animal resources personnel and custodial staff) who might require access to the room should be made aware of the nature of the experiments and the regulations imposed upon their conduct. The name and phone number of the person(s) to be contacted in the event of an emergency should be clearly indicated on the door.

(b) *Personnel*. A baseline serum titer should be obtained for all personnel working with HSV prior to the onset of experiments.

(c) *Animal housing*. Once an animal has received an injection of virus it is considered to be 'infected' and should be separated from the remainder of the animal population. With rodents we accomplish this by isolating animals in the BSL II laboratory throughout the course of the study. Commercially available housing units for rodents provide the best solution for laboratories that will be using this method on a routine basis. These units can accommodate multiple cages and are ventilated into the biosafety hood ductwork. Alternatively, individual cages can be housed in the biosafety hood or equipped with dust covers and kept on the benchtop of the BSL II lab. Larger animals and primates pose different problems. Infected primates should be housed separately and stored in a squeeze cage which is carefully labelled to identify it for Animal Care personnel. The room housing an infected animal also should be labelled. Infected primates, like any other animal, should be sedated prior to any manipulation. Virus injected into the brain generally remains confined to the nervous system, minimizing the risks of blood-borne or secretion-borne contamination. Despite this, the cage and excretions of infected primates should be treated as contaminated materials. Only the pans of a primate cage containing an infected animal should be cleaned. This cleaning should be done in a manner which avoids the production of aerosols. The excretions should be double bagged, labelled as biohazardous, and incinerated. At the end of the experiment, cages should be decontaminated by autoclaving.

(d) *Virus storage and access*. Virus should be stored at −70°C in a freezer compartment solely designated for virus storage. Under optimal circumstances the freezer should be located in the BSL II laboratory. If this is not an option the freezer and/or the room housing it should be locked and labelled with a biohazard sign. The temperature at which aliquots of virus are stored should be carefully monitored. We freeze virus in small aliquots and discard unused portions after each experiment. Repeated thawing and freezing of virus dramatically reduces the titer and should be avoided. Stocks which have been exposed to increased temperature (−40°C or higher) as a result of freezer malfunction should be discarded. If it is necessary to transport the virus to the surgical suite, it should be transported on dry ice in a sealed container labelled with a biohazard tag.

(e) *Experimental precautions*. BSL II regulations mandate that laboratory coats should be worn throughout the course of each experiment. In addition, we wear gloves and goggles whenever handling virus or an infected animal. These protective garments should be removed and left in the BSL II laboratory upon completion of the experiments. Hypodermic needles and syringes should only be used for parenteral injection and aspiration of fluids from experimental animals and diaphragm bottles. Only needle-locking syringes or disposable syringe needle units, (i.e. the needle is integral to the syringe) should be used for the injection or aspiration of infectious fluids. *Extreme caution should be used when handling contaminated needles and syringes to avoid autoinoculation* and the generation of aerosols during use and disposal. Needles should not be bent, sheared, replaced in the sheath or guard, or removed from the syringe following use. Rather, they should be promptly placed in a puncture-resistant container and decontaminated before they are discarded.

(f) *Animal surgery*. All animals should be deeply anaesthetized prior to any manipulation and surgical procedures should be performed using sterile techniques. If the procedure involves primates, it should be conducted in a sterile operating room.

(g) *Decontamination procedures.* Work surfaces and instruments exposed to the virus should be decontaminated with a quaternary ammonium disinfectant or 5% chlorox after spills and upon completion of each experiment.

(h) *Waste disposal.* All excess virus and contaminated waste should be inactivated and disposed of appropriately at all stages of each experiment. Excess virus should be inactivated with 5% chlorox or 70% ethanol and collected in a biosafety waste container for incineration. Solid waste, (i.e. surgical gauze and dressings) should be decontaminated and disposed of in the same manner. Experiments should be terminated by perfusing infected animals with buffered aldehyde solutions (see below). This inactivates the virus within the animals and preserves the tissue for subsequent viral localization. Nevertheless, the animal carcass should be considered biohazardous waste and disposed of by incineration.

2.2 Virus strain

Differences in the strain of virus can have profound effect upon the uptake and subsequent transport of virus through neural circuits. This is vividly illustrated in our recent analyses of the infectivity of central visual circuits by different strains of pseudorabies virus (PRV) (5, 6). Following intra-ocular injection of wild type PRV (Becker strain; 28) the virus ultimately infected all central visual circuits in two temporarily separated waves (*Figure 3A*). The first wave of infection occurred at 48 hours post-inoculation and targeted neurones in the dorsal lateral geniculate nucleus and tectum. This was followed by a second wave of infection at 72 hours that involved retinorecipient neurones of circadian centres (suprachiasmatic nuclei and intergeniculate leaflets). This pattern of neuronal infectivity was markedly different from that which resulted from identical administration of an attenuated strain of the same virus (Bartha; 29). The attenuated strain never infected neurones susceptible to the first wave of wild type infection (even at post-inoculation intervals extending to 125 hours), but was quite efficient in infecting neurones in circadian centres within a temporal framework that was essentially identical to that resulting from wild type injection (*Figure 3B*). Subsequently we found that the differing ability of these two closely related strains to infect visual circuity is related to differences in the complement of glycoproteins found in the viral envelope (6). The genome of the attenuated strain of virus exhibits prominent deletions which eliminate the genes for two glycoproteins and substantially reduces the concentration of a third glycoprotein in the viral envelope (30). Our findings indicate that one of these gene deletions is responsible for the inability of the attenuated strain to infect the subset of visual circuitry involved in the first wave of infectivity. Thus, it is clear that

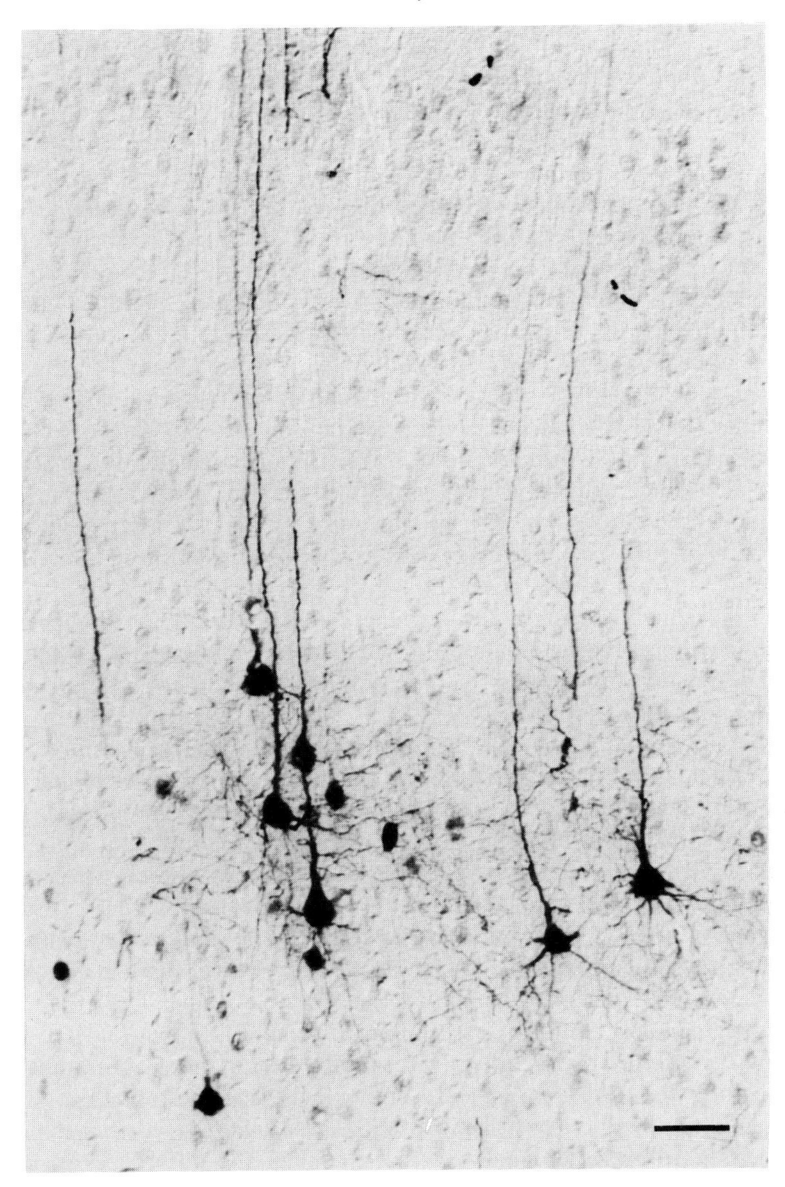

Figure 1. Neurones in the perirhinal cortex of the rat infected by transneuronal passage of the Bartha strain of pseudorabies virus from medial prefrontal cortex of the adult rat. The post-inoculation interval was 36 hours, and the virus was detected by the avidin–biotin immunoperoxidase procedure (*Protocol 1*) using a rabbit polyclonal antiserum generated against acetone inactivated wild type virus. Note the dense immunoreactivity filling the cell nucleus and cytoplasm and large portions of the dendritic tree (scale bar = 100 μm.) (From a study by J. P. Card, L. W. Enquist, and P. Levitt that is currently in preparation.)

the pattern of neuronal infection achieved with any strain of virus should be closely compared to the circuitry revealed by classical neuronal tract tracers and, if possible, verified with another strain of virus.

We have seen equally dramatic differences in the transport of two different strains of *Herpes simplex* virus (HSV-1) after their injection into the 'arm' area of the primary motor cortex of cebus monkeys (27). One strain, HSV-1 (H129), was transported transneuronally in the *anterograde* direction (*Figure 2*). It infected 'second order' neurones at sites known to receive input from the arm area of the primary motor cortex, (e.g. putamen, pontine nuclei). In addition, 'third order' neurones were labelled in the cerebellar cortex (granule and Golgi-cells) and in the globus pallidus (largely the external segment). In contrast, the other strain, HSV-1 (McIntyre-B), was transported transneuronally in the *retrograde* direction. It infected neurones at sites known to project to the arm area of the primary motor cortex, (e.g. ventrolateral thalamus). In addition, 'second' order neurones were labelled in the deep cerebellar nuclei (dentate and interpositus) and in the globus pallidus (internal segment). McLean *et al.* (16) also have observed largely retrograde transneuronal transport of this strain after its injection into several different sites of the rat central nervous system. Taken together, these observations suggest that strain differences have an important impact not only on which neurones become infected, but also on the direction of transneuronal transport within infected neurones.

Virulence is also a major consideration in selecting the strain of virus. Virulence can be defined both in terms of the post-inoculation survival of the animal and the lytic effects of viral infection upon neurones in the brain. Both of these aspects of viral infectivity are extremely important in defining the extent of a circuit, (i.e. the number of cells involved) and the specificity of viral transport. There is considerable evidence that strains of HSV-1 vary in their neurovirulence. For example, Dix *et al.* (31) compared the ability of 23 different strains of HSV-1 to induce acute neurological disease in BALB/c mice after either peripheral or intracerebral inoculation. They found that strains segregated into three classes of neurovirulence: those that were highly virulent by both peripheral and intracerebral routes of inoculation, those that were highly virulent by intracerebral routes only, and those that were highly attenuated by both routes of inoculation. The *in vivo* growth curves for the three classes of virus did not appear to explain the differences in neurovirulence. Dramatic differences in virulence have also been reported with closely related strains of PRV. In general, wild type strains of virus are most virulent and induce prominent infection of glia in response to lytic release of virus from infected neurones (6, 22). In some instances, the lytic release is contained by reactive astroglia and the circuit specific transport is maintained (6, 7). However, Strack and Loewy (22) reported widespread necrosis that was clearly non-specific following injection of another wild type strain of PRV (K strain). Wild type strains of PRV also produce very prominent infection of

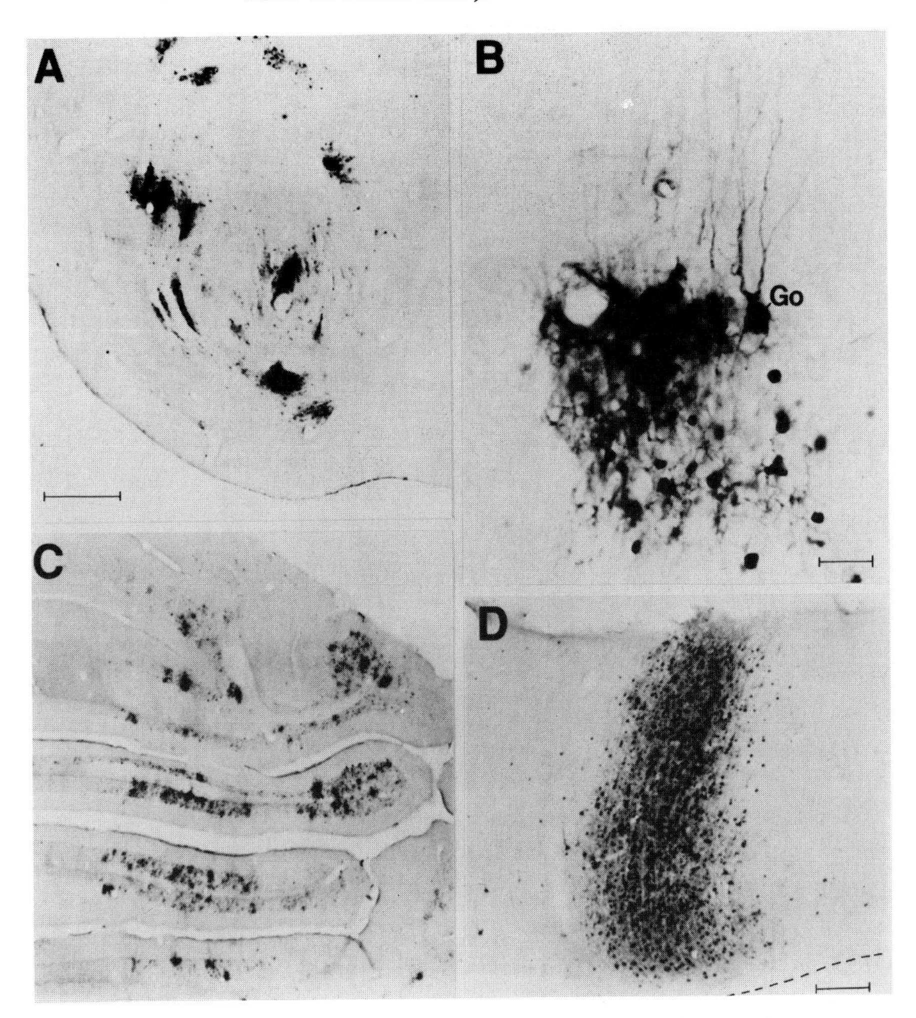

Figure 2. Neurones labelled by transport of HSV-1 (strain H129) from the primary motor cortex of a cebus monkey. (A) Labelled neurones in the pontine nuclei (scale bar = 1 mm). (B) A patch of labelled granule cells and a Golgi-cell (Go) in cerebellar cortex (scale bar = 30 μm). (C) Multiple patches of labelled neurones in the granular layer of cerebellar cortex (scale is same as (A)). (D) A 'column' of labelled neurone in cerebral cortex buried within the dorsal bank of the cingulate sulcus. The dashed line indicates the border between white and grey matter (scale bar = 300 μm). (From Zemanick *et al.* reference 27).

the respiratory system which severely compromises the animal at longer survival intervals (55–65 hours post-inoculation). These undesirable effects can be largely eliminated with the use of attenuated strains of virus. Animals injected with the attenuated strain of PRV known as Bartha are largely unencumbered with the lytic cellular effects of wild type strains, survive

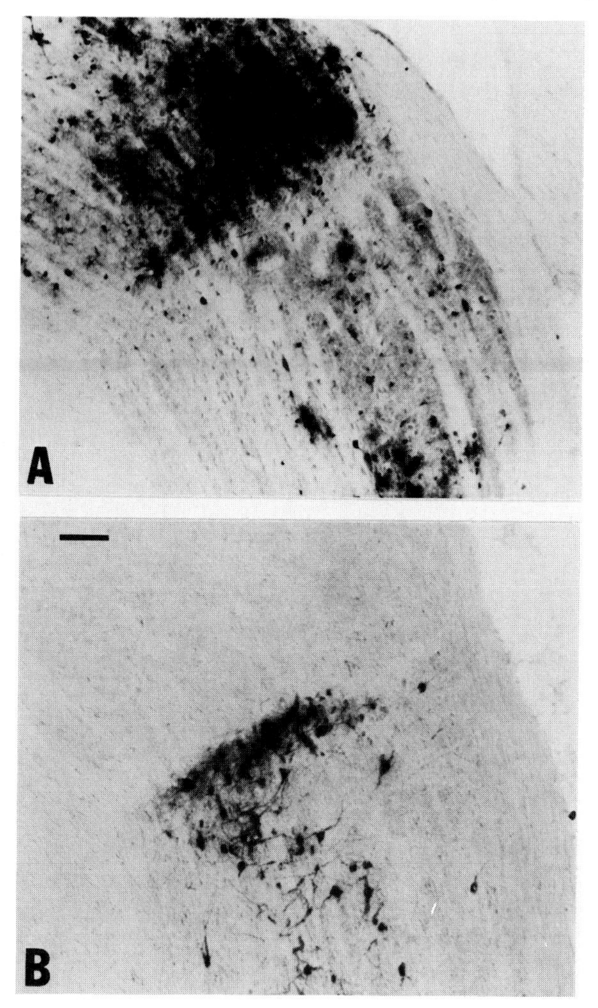

Figure 3. Differential infection of the lateral geniculate complex of the rat by two strains of pseudorabies virus are illustrated. (A) The wild type strain known as Becker infects neurones in all three geniculate subdivisions (dorsal geniculate nucleus, ventral geniculate nucleus, and intergeniculate leaflet) within 55 hours of injection of the virus into the vitreous body of the eye. (B) In contrast, an attenuated strain of PRV known as Bartha only infects neurones in the intergeniculate leaflet, and a subset of those in the ventral geniculate nucleus at survival times extending to 125 hours. Other retinorecipient regions of the brain also exhibit differential patterns of infectivity with these two strains of PRV. (Scale bar = 500 μm.) (From Card *et al.* reference 5.)

longer than animals injected with wild type strains, and do not exhibit the pronounced respiratory pathology that accompanies more virulent strains. As a result, multi-synaptic pathways can be identified more effectively due to the longer survival and reduction of symptoms of the infection.

2.3 Viral infectivity

The infectivity of all alpha herpesviruses are dramatically influenced by titer (concentration) and the method of storage. Titer is measured in plaque-forming units (p.f.u.) and is extremely sensitive to fluctuations in temperature. In our studies with PRV (the wild-type Becker strain and the Bartha attenuated strain), we achieve 100% infectivity with average titers of 5×10^8 p.f.u./ml. Similarly, we have achieved 100% infectivity in our primate experiments using HSV titers of at least 10^8 p.f.u./ml. In contrast, Strack and collaborators (22–24) reported that only 20% of injected animals were infected with the K strain of PRV at a titer of 2×10^5 p.f.u./ml. Differences in the strain of virus and route of injection may have contributed to these differences, but recent unpublished observations from our laboratory indicate that rate of infectivity of PRV is directly tied to the titer of virus. Furthermore, Ugolini and collaborators (24) have demonstrated that titers of HSV-1 lower than 10^7 p.f.u./ml did not lead to infection of hypoglossal motor neurones after injection of the nerve. Thus, if the ultimate goal of the experiment is to infect synaptically linked populations of neurones one should use titers of 10^8 p.f.u./ml or higher to optimize infectivity at the site of injection.

2.4 Route of administration

A clear understanding of the patterns of transport of any strain of virus is very dependent upon careful consideration of the route of administration. The parameters which govern viral transport following intracerebral injection are relatively straightforward and easily evaluated. These do not differ significantly from that which would be considered with the use of conventional neural tracers. In particular, it is necessary to determine the optimal volume and coordinates of injection in order to confine virus to the desired site. In rats, we find that there is very little diffusion of virus from the injection site, even with injection volumes as large as 200 nl. This has also been convincingly demonstrated by peripheral injection of virus into either the stomach or oesophagus. Each of these organs receive direct projections from the brainstem via the vagus nerve (32, 33), but the location of the neurones differs substantially; motor neurones in the nucleus ambiguus innervate the oesophagus, and the stomach receives projections from motor efferents arising from neurones in the dorsal motor vagal nucleus. Consequently, even slight spread of virus from one organ to the other would be easily detected by viral replication in both motor neurone groups in the brainstem. Nevertheless, viral infectivity resulting from injection of the stomach or oesophagus near the gastro-oesophageal junction always infected the appropriate population of motor neurones with no apparent spread of virus to the adjacent organ (7).

Two recent studies further illustrate the importance of carefully considering the route of injection when evaluating patterns of central viral transport after peripheral injection. In our analysis of the transport of PRV through the vagus nerve, we injected the end organ, (i.e. oesophagus or stomach) and demonstrated that viral infectivity in the brainstem was initially evident in motor neurones innervating these organs (7). Infectivity of sensory afferents innervating these organs also occurred, but transganglionic infection of brainstem neurones via these sensory afferents *always* followed infectivity of the motor neurones. This finding contrasted with the pattern of central infection reported by Blessing and collaborators (4) following direct injection of HSV-1 into the vagus nerve. These authors demonstrated that virus injected into the nerve preferentially targeted sensory axons and appeared to spare motor axons. This conclusion was based upon the appearance of infected glia in subnuclei of the nucleus of the solitary tract (NTS) which are innervated by vagal sensory afferents, and the absence of infected motor neurones in the same tissue samples. The differential infectivity of sensory and motor components of the vagus in these investigations could be explained by differences in the strain of virus and/or the route of injection. In considering the route of injection, organ injection exposes virus to both motor and sensory terminals, while nerve injection would seemingly provide greater access of virus to the unmyelinated sensory axons in the nerve. In any event, the differing patterns of infectivity produced by the organ versus nerve inoculation clearly illustrate the importance of considering route of injection in designing experiments.

2.5 Experimental animals

The choice of experimental animal is also critical to the success of viral tracing studies. It has long been known that animals vary in their susceptibility to infection with herpesviruses. Hunt and Melendez (34) provide a succinct summary of this issue: 'In general, for each herpesvirus there exists a host(s) in which the virus exits as a subclinical or latent infection. As examples, Herpesvirus suis is latent in swine and fatal to cattle; Herpesvirus hominis is latent in man and fatal in owl monkeys; and Herpesvirus B is latent in rhesus monkeys and fatal in man'. Susceptibility to infection can vary even within a single species. For example, Lopez (35) demonstrated that different strains of mice varied in their resistance to infection with HSV-1. He found that the C57BL strain was very resistant, the BALB/c and CBA strains were moderately susceptible, and the AKR and A/J strains were quite susceptible to infection following an intra-peritoneal inoculation of one strain of HSV-1. Furthermore, he reported that resistance is a dominant trait governed by two (or more) genes.

The age of an animal at the time of exposure to virus also is an important factor in determining susceptibility to infection. Serious and even fatal infections can occur in the young of a normally resistant reservoir host, (e.g. human infants infected with HSV-1 and piglets infected with PRV). In experimental studies, the C57BL/6 strain of mice is resistant to infection with HSV-1 as adults, but is highly susceptible to infection as newborns (36, 37). Resistance to infection in this mouse strain develops at about 20 days of age. Thus it is clear that the age of the animal and its susceptibility to infection must be carefully considered in designing an experimental analysis.

Among non-human primates, there is enormous variation in the manner that different species respond to HSV. Naturally occurring HSV infections in laboratory primates appear to be infrequent and have been reported for only two species, owl monkeys and gibbons (34, 38, 39). However, as noted above, owl monkeys are highly susceptible to morbidity and mortality caused by HSV infection. In fact, it has been suggested that the LD50 for owl monkeys after intra-vaginal inoculation with wild type HSV is at or near 10 p.f.u. (40). Consequently, it is apparent that successful tracing experiments require the appropriate match between the strain of herpesvirus and the experimental animal. While there is a considerable literature regarding PRV infections in rodents, there are few reliable reports of such infections in laboratory primates (41, 42). Similarly, different strains of PRV produce excellent results for tracing studies in rodents, but have not been used successfully in primates (Hoover and Strick, unpublished observations).

3. Methods of detection

3.1 Immunohistochemistry

Immunohistochemical detection of replicating virus is easily the most straightforward method of defining viral transport in the nervous system. Rabbit polyclonal antisera generated against both human and swine strains of the alpha herpesviruses are readily available (both commercially and through a number of laboratories) and application of the immunohistochemical method is straightforward (*Protocol 1*). In addition, limits of detection are only a consideration at early survival times since continuous replication of virus over time leads to a progressive increase in signal in infected neurones. In most instances, the available polyclonal antisera detect virus within both the nucleus and cytoplasm of infected cells and often reveal a large proportion of their dendritic arborization.

Although the virus can be easily detected with both fluorescence and immunoperoxidase procedures, we prefer the latter method because it creates a permanent record which is not encumbered with the fading problems that occur with fluorescence labelling. However, with few exceptions, co-localization of virus with peptides, neurotransmitters, or other neural tracers is most effectively accomplished with fluorophors (see below). The following immunoperoxidase procedure is based upon the avidin–biotin modification (43) of Sternberger's (44) immunoperoxidase procedure. We have applied it for viral localization in a number of species with equal success.

Protocol 1. Immunohistochemical localization of virus (see also Chapter 5)

1. Perfuse the anaesthetized animal transcardially with paraformaldehyde–lysine–periodate fixative (PLP; 45) preceded by physiological saline, pH 7.4. Best results are achieved when solutions are infused under controlled pressure with a peristaltic pump (see Chapter 1, *Protocol 3* for details of perfuse–fixation).
2. Post-fix the tissues with PLP fixative for 1 h at 4°C. Post-fixation can be extended up to one week with no apparent loss of immunoreactivity.
3. Wash the tissue in 0.1 M sodium phosphate buffer for 1 h at 4°C (see Chapter 1, *Protocol 1*). This can be extended to 24 h without consequence.
4. Cryoprotect the tissue in a 20% phosphate-buffered sucrose solution overnight (or until tissue sinks) at 4°C. A 30% solution should be used for tissue that will be sectioned with a cryostat.
5. Section at 30–40 μm with a freezing microtome; collect sections in 0.1 M sodium phosphate buffer (pH 7.4) and store at 4°C. It is best to process the tissue immediately, but the sections may be stored for two weeks without problems. Add the preservative, sodium azide to the solutions used to store the large number of sections that come from a single primate brain.
6. Incubate tissue in primary antiserum diluted with 0.1 M sodium phosphate buffer containing 1% normal serum (species of origin of the secondary antibody), and 0.3% Triton X-100 detergent (PBGT; the Triton X-100 is omitted when localizing HSV-1). The length of incubation and final dilution is dependent upon the antiserum being used. All incubations should be conducted at 4°C.[a]
7. Bring the tissue to room temperature over 30 min with agitation.
8. Wash tissue in three changes of phosphate buffer over a period of 30 min.
9. Place tissue in biotinylated goat anti-rabbit IgG diluted to 1:200 (5 μl/ml) with PBGT, and incubate for 60–90 min at room temperature with agitation.
10. Wash tissue as in step **8**.
11. Incubate tissue in avidin–biotin–peroxidase complex (ABC) for 90–120 min at room temperature. We use the Vectastain kit (Vector Laboratories) as follows: combine 9 μl of each component (A and B) *90 min prior to use* and bring to a final volume of 1 ml with PBGT just before use.
12. Wash with buffer as in steps **8** and **10**.
13. Make a 'saturated' solution of diaminobenzidine (DAB). Saturated in this context is defined as the amount of DAB that will go into solution

during 5 min of vigorous stirring at room temperature. Use either phosphate buffer (first choice) or 0.1 M Tris-buffered saline, pH 7.6 (see *Safety note 3* in Chapter 5, p. 119).

14. Pre-incubate the tissue in the DAB solution for 10 min with agitation (room temperature).

15. Add 100 μl of 30% stock solution of hydrogen peroxide per 100 ml of DAB and monitor the reaction visually by occasionally removing a section and examining it under the microscope.

16. Terminate the reaction (usually within 2–5 min) by washing with fresh buffer, mount sections on coated slides, dehydrate, and apply coverslips (Chapter 1, *Protocols 5* and *6*).

[a] We use our rabbit polyclonal antisera at a primary dilution of 1:2000 with overnight incubation at 4°C. However, with nickel intensification procedures (46) the antiserum can be used at dilutions as high as 1:8000.

The procedural aspects of *Protocol 1* do not differ significantly from those employed for immunohistochemical localization of most peptides and neurotransmitters in the CNS (see Chapter 5). Successful application of this protocol is primarily dependent upon the *method of sampling* and *knowledge of the literature* relevant to the circuits of interest. With rodents we routinely section the entire neuraxis and collect the tissue sections in six serial wells of buffer. In the initial analysis we localize virus in sections from one well of tissue (a one in six series through the brain) and make a determination of the full extent of viral transport. If analysis of more frequent series of sections is necessary we process other bins of tissue. With this approach it is also possible to use the remaining tissue to localize other antigens in adjacent sections and thereby acquire a substantial amount of information on both the connectivity and chemical content of neurones in the infected circuit.

Knowledge of the connectivity or chemical content of a circuit can also be obtained by co-localization of virus with peptides or neurotransmitters in the same section. This can be accomplished through the use of two different chromogens or with different fluorphors. In either case it is necessary to use antisera generated in different species. We often inject the neural tracer cholera toxin (B subunit) with virus in order to definitively separate first and second order neurones; cholera toxin (CT) will remain trapped within the first order neurone while the virus will pass transneuronally. This approach is particularly valuable when the first and second order neurone populations are in close proximity or share overlapping domains (see Chapter 2 for details of retrograde labelling). *Protocol 2* provides a detailed method for localizing CT and virus in the same section with chromogens of different colour. This method provides a permanent record of the distribution of neurones labelled with the two tracers which is not subject to the fading that would occur if fluorescent tags were used.

Protocol 2. Double labelling immunohistochemical localization

See Chapter 2 for details of retrograde labelling with CT, Chapter 2, *Protocol 5* for alternative method for CT immunohistochemistry, and Chapter 11 for various combined methods.

1. Follow steps **1–5** of *Protocol 1*.
2. Incubate sections in goat anti-cholera toxin antiserum diluted to 1:5000 with 0.1 M phosphate buffer containing 0.3% Triton X-100 and 1% normal horse serum (PBHT) for 24 h at 4°C.
3. Incubate sections in anti-goat IgG diluted to 1:200 with PBHT for 1 h at room temperature.
4. Wash tissue in 0.1 M sodium phosphate buffer: 2 × 15 min.
5. Incubate in peroxidase anti-peroxidase (PAP) complex diluted to 1:500 with PBHT for 1 h at room temperature.
6. Wash tissue in 0.1 M sodium phosphate buffer: 2 × 15 min.
7. React tissue in first substrate (0.04% diaminobenzidine, 0.5% nickel sulphate, 0.01% hydrogen peroxide in 0.2 M sodium acetate buffer, pH 7.0) to produce a blue reaction product.
8. Wash tissue in 0.1 M sodium phosphate buffer: 2 × 15 min.
9. Incubate tissue in the rabbit anti-virus antiserum diluted to 1:2000 with PBHT, for 24 h at 4°C.
10. Process tissue according to same procedures detailed in steps **7–16** in *Protocol 1*.
11. Wash tissue several times in 0.1 M sodium phosphate buffer and mount sections on gelatin-coated slides, dehydrate, and apply coverslips (Chapter 1, *Protocols 5* and *6*).

Double labelling of virus with other antigens in the same tissue section can also be accomplished by using different colour fluorphors. For example, we have localized virus with a fluorocein conjugated secondary antibody (green fluorescence), and other antigens with secondary antibodies conjugated to rhodamine (red fluorescence). The success of this method is obviously dependent upon the use of antisera generated in different species and the appropriate choice of secondary antiserum.

3.2 [^{3}H] thymidine

The tritiated thymidine method has been applied very effectively to localize HSV-1 in the trigeminal complex following eye inoculation (11–13). Thymidine is taken up by dividing neurones and, therefore, cannot be applied to the adult nervous system under normal circumstances because neurones are postmitotic. However, the cascade of cellular events resulting from viral infection includes extensive replication of viral DNA and thymidine is taken up quite avidly under these circumstances. Consequently, it is possible to use autoradiographic localization of tritiated thymidine to identify the location of virally infected neurones.

There are three limitations to the routine application of this method for thorough mapping of a neural circuit. Tissue routinely requires four or more weeks of exposure to photographic emulsion before adequate signal can be detected. This is far longer than the three to four days required for immunohistochemical processing. In addition, the autoradiographic label is confined almost exclusively to the cell nucleus, precluding a full characterization of the morphology of the infected cell. Finally, Margolis and colleagues (11) have noted that the density of silver grains over neurones in advanced stages of infection is reduced and suggest that the autoradiographic method 'may be disadvantageous for identifying neurones in which massive DNA replication has already taken place'. Nevertheless, when used appropriately, this method is a very effective means of detecting viral replication in the nervous system, and is probably superior to immunohistochemistry for detecting cells at early stages of infection when cellular levels of mature virus are low. The following procedure (adapted from 11) has been successfully applied for detection of HSV in the trigeminal and superior cervical ganglia following ocular inoculation.

Protocol 3. [^{3}H] thymidine localization of infected cells

1. Inject animals intra-peritoneally with [^{3}H] thymidine. Best results are achieved by a single injection of 400 μCi two and one half hours prior to sacrifice. Multiple injections over a longer period of time do not enhance the signal and increase the background.
2. Perfuse the anaesthetized animal transcardially with cacodylate-buffered saline solution (pH 7.2) followed by 3% glutaraldehyde in the same buffer (see *Safety note 1*, Chapter 1, p. 5). Best results are achieved when solutions are infused with a peristaltic pump (see Chapter 1, *Protocol 3*).
3. Post-fix the tissues in the primary fixative overnight at 4°C.
4. Dehydrate the tissue in multiple changes of methyl cellulosolve (ethylene glycol monomethyl ether).
5. Embed the tissue in glycol methacrylate.
6. Section tissue at 2–3 μm.
7. Mount sections on glass microscope slides and dip in photographic emulsion.[a]
8. Develop slides after four weeks exposure.
9. Counterstain sections with thionine and apply coverslips.

[a] See Chapter 8, *Protocol 6* for further details of autoradiographic method.

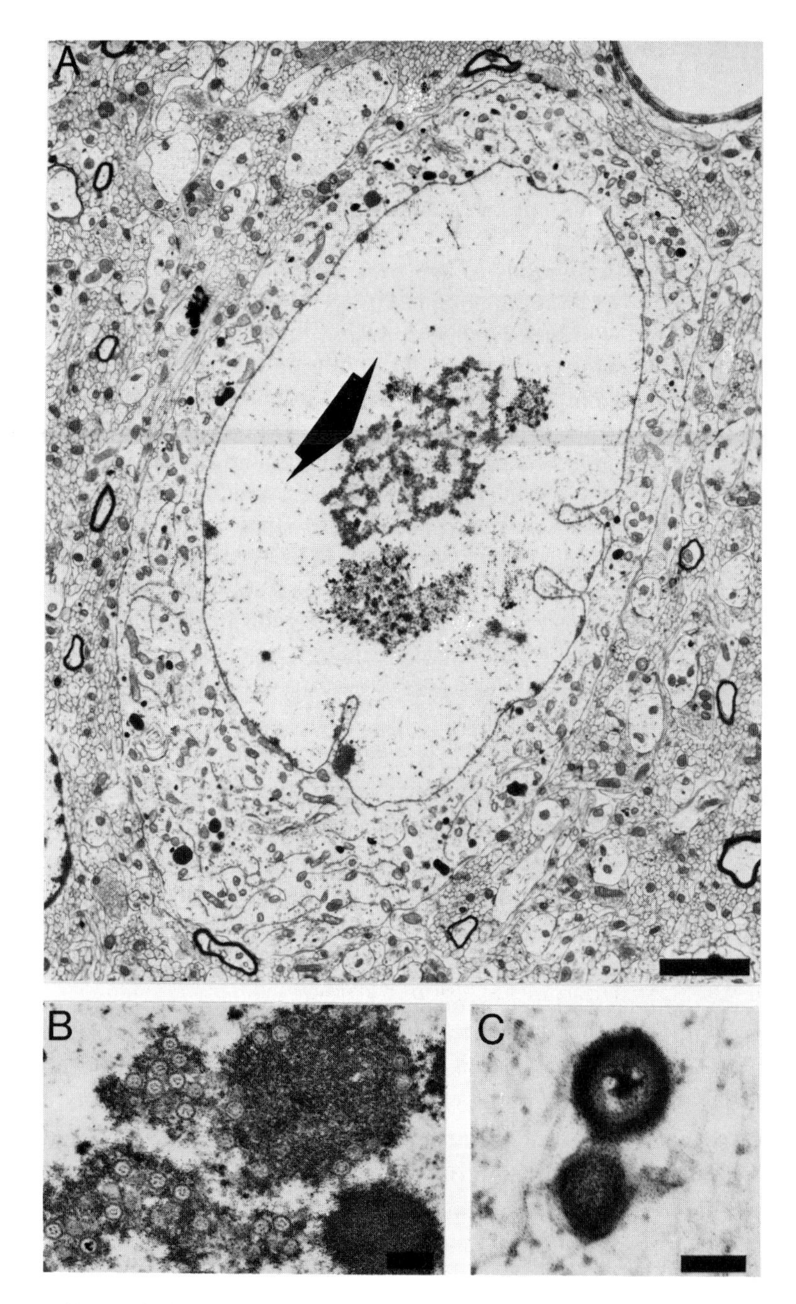

Figure 4. Transmission electron micrographs of virus in a neurone in the dorsal motor vagal nucleus infected by injection pseudorabies virus into the wall of the stomach. Pathological inclusions of the cell nucleus (arrow in (A)) represent replication of the viral capsids (shown at higher magnification in (B)). Capsids acquire a membrane envelope from the Golgi apparatus in the cell cytoplasm to attain the mature conformation shown in (C). This envelope is essential for the virus to leave the parent cell and gain access to other cells. Scale bars = (A) 2 μm, (B) 200 nm, (C) 100 nm.

3.3 Transmission electron microscopy (TEM)

Considerable information on virus uptake, replication, assembly, and transport can be gleaned from ultrastructural analysis of infected tissue (*Figure 4*). However, transmission electron microscopic analysis is most useful in focused analyses of viral replication and transport (8, 9, 11, 15, 47) rather than in the definition of a multisynaptic circuit, Nevertheless, TEM provides an extremely powerful means of examining the specificity of viral transport through circuits previously defined with light microscopic methods and is the method of choice for definitive characterization of the extent of viral pathogenesis.

Successful application of the TEM method (*Protocol 4*) is heavily dependent upon rigorous light microscopic characterization of both the route of viral transport and the temporal aspects of viral replication in the area of interest. Thus, the most fruitful ultrastructural analysis will be based upon a thorough documentation of these parameters using light microscopic immunohistochemical procedures. We generally subject two animals to identical inoculation procedures and process one for light microscopic localization of virus and the other for ultrastructural analysis.

Protocol 4. Ultrastructural localization of virus

See Chapter 1 for the preparation of tissue for electron microscopy.

1. Perfuse anaesthetized animal initially with 30–50 ml physiological saline followed by 1% glutaraldehyde and 0.8% paraformaldehyde in 0.1 M phosphate buffer (pH 7.4), and then 5% glutaraldehyde and 4% paraformaldehyde in the same buffer. (The former buffer is a 1:5 dilution of the latter.) (See Chapter 1, *Protocol 2* for preparation of fixative, and *Protocol 3* for details of perfusion–fixation.)
2. Remove tissue, trim around the area of interest and post-fix overnight at 4°C in 5% glutaraldehyde and 4% paraformaldehyde in 0.1 M phosphate buffer.
3. Wash specimens in several changes of buffer over a period of approximately 30 min to remove all traces of fixative.
4. Section tissue with a vibrating microtome at 50–100 μm (Chapter 1, *Protocol 4*). Best results are achieved by maintaining the vibratome bath at 4°C. Collect sections in buffer.
5. Treat the tissue with osmium tetroxide solution for 1–2 h at room temperature. The solution consists of 1.0% osmium tetroxide, 1.5% potassium ferricyanide (48) in 0.1 M phosphate buffer. (See Chapter 1, *Protocol 7* and *Safety note 3*, p. 13.)
6. Wash the tissue several times in phosphate buffer over a period of 30–45 min.

Protocol 4. *Continued*

7. Dehydrate the sections in serial dilutions of ethanol for 10 min each and two 15 min changes of transitional fluid (either acetone or propylene oxide; see *Safety note 4* in Chapter 1, p. 17). (See Chapter 1, *Protocol 8*.)
8. Infiltrate and embed tissue with plastic resin as follows: epon araldite (EA): transitional fluid (TF) (1:1)—overnight; EA:TF (3:1)—1/2 day; 100% EA—1/2 day; flat-embed sections in 100% resin—overnight at 60°C. The resin consists of:
   - Epon 812 or Polybed 15.5 g
   - Araldite 502 10.7 g
   - DDSA 30.0 g
   - DMP-30 1.6 g

   Alternatively follow the dehydration and embedding procedure described in Chapter 1, *Protocol 8*.
9. Examine tissue in the electron microscope, see Chapter 1.

4. Interpretation of results

4.1 Spread from site of injection

The spread of any tracer from the site of injection has important implications for interpreting the validity of the labelled connection. The neurotrophic properties of alpha herpesviruses effectively limit the spread of virus from the site of injection and thereby contribute to one's ability to define specific connections. This has been convincingly demonstrated following both intracerebral (27) and peripheral (5–7) injections. As noted previously, we were able to demonstrate that injection of PRV into either the oesophagus or stomach always infected the appropriate population of motor neurones, even when the site of inoculation was close to the gastro-oesophageal junction. Other studies involving injection of PRV into the adrenal gland (23), the pancreas (18), the anterior chamber of the eye (14, 22), the pinna of the ear (22), the nares (14) or head, and neck musculature (14, 20, 21) have also demonstrated remarkable specificity and an absence of infectivity that would be expected if virus were diffusing significantly from the site of injection. Nevertheless, careful documentation of the full extent of spread of virus from the site of injection is essential for validating the resulting pattern of infectivity.

4.2 Lytic release and non-specific spread in the CNS

It is important to realize that alpha herpesviruses produce lytic neuronal infections in the CNS. This has obvious implications in evaluating the specificity of viral transport through neural circuits, and has stimulated a critical evaluation of the utility of using viruses for transneuronal tracing. It is obvious that lytic release of virus into the extracellular space would lead to indiscriminate uptake and infectivity of all neurones and processes in the afflicted area. The reproducible, projection-specific organization of circuits identified by viral transport in numerous investigations argue convincingly against non-specific infectivity when the strain of virus is well characterized. In addition, it is becoming increasingly clear that reactive astroglia play a prominent role in restricting the spread of virus from lytic neurones. Our studies have demonstrated that reactive gliosis and invasion of peripheral macrophages into the CNS occurs in response to neuronal infection (19). This response always follows the neuronal infection and is most pronounced in relation to the most seriously afflicted neurones. Ultrastructural analysis indicates that elaboration of these processes effectively isolates the infected cell and thereby restricts non-specific spread of virus from the site of infection. This process is certainly aided by the fact that glia cells exhibit a pronounced affinity for virus (49, 50). Furthermore, Rinaman and collaborators (19) have recently demonstrated that microglia and macrophages also are recruited to areas that contain seriously infected neurones and appear to participate in preventing non-specific spread of virus.

4.3 Temporal aspects of transport

The significance of infection of non-neuronal cells should also be considered within the context of the temporal course of their appearance. As noted previously, the glial response is generally associated with only the most severely compromised neurones. By this point in time the virus has replicated extensively and has already passed transneuronally. Consequently, lytic release of virus from these neurones should have little impact upon the specific transport of virus through synaptically linked populations of cells, especially when one considers the fact that reactive glia are limiting spread of virus from these lytic cells. Nevertheless, one should carefully characterize the full extent of viral infectivity in each case, and the pattern of viral transport in animals subjected to the same experimental paradigm should be carefully compared to determine if the same circuit of neurones is infected.

5. Conclusions

The use of alpha herpesviruses for mapping synaptically linked populations of neurones holds great promise for advancing circuit analysis of the nervous system. The usefulness of this method, and the factors which can complicate its applications, are in large part related to the neurotropic properties of this class of viruses. For this reason, it is absolutely essential that every investigator carefully selects the reagents and considers all of the factors which can have an impact upon the experimental results. We have attempted to provide a thorough overview of the issues which must be considered in designing a study, and conducting it in a safe and efficient manner. Our presentation is based upon the current understanding of the biology of these viruses and their ability to infect the nervous system. However, this is a rapidly expanding field of analysis and one can conservatively predict that continued application of the method and further research into the fundamental mechanisms underlying viral neurotropism and neuro-invasiveness will have a considerable impact on its use in the future.

References

1. Kuypers, H. G. J. M. and Ugolini, G. (1990). *Trends Neurosci.,* **13,** 71.
2. Izumi, K. M. and Stevens, J. G. (1990). *J. Exp. Med.,* **172,** 487.
3. Lominicz, B., Watanabe, S., Ben-Porat, T., and Kaplan, A. S. (1984). *J. Virol.,* **52,** 198.
4. Blessing, W. W., Li, Y.-W., and Wesselingh, S. L. (1991). *Neurosci.,* **42,** 261.
5. Card, J. P., Whealy, M. E., Robbins, A. K., Moore, R. Y., and Enquist, L. W. (1991). *Neuron,* **6,** 957.
6. Card, J. P., Whealy, M. E., Robbins, A. K., and Enquist, L. W. (1992). *J. Virol.,* **66,** 3032.
7. Card, J. P., Rinaman, L., Schwaber, J. S., Miselis, R. R., Whealy, M. E., Robbins, A. K., and Enquist, L. W. (1990). *J. Neurosci.,* **10,** 1974.
8. Dolivo, M., Beretta, E., Bonifas, V., and Foroglou, C. (1978). *Brain Res.,* **140,** 111.
9. Kristensson, K., Vahlne, A., Persson, A., and Lycke, E. (1978). *J. Neurol. Sci.,* **35,** 331.
10. Kristensson, K., Nennesmo, I., Persson, L., and Lycke, E. (1982). *J. Neurol. Sci.,* **54,** 149.
11. LaVail, J. H., Zhan, J., and Margolis, T. P. (1990). *Brain Res.,* **514,** 181.
12. Margolis, T. P., Togni, B., LaVail, J., and Dawson, C. R. (1987). *Curr. Eye Res.,* **6,** 119.
13. Margolis, T. P., LaVail, J. H., Setzer, P. Y., and Dawson, C. D. (1989). *J. Virol.,* **63,** 4756.
14. Martin, X. and Dolivo, M. (1983). *Brain Res.,* **273,** 253.
15. McCracken, R. M. and Clarke, J. K. (1971). *Archiv fur die gesamte Virusforschung,* **34,** 189.
16. McLean, J. H., Shipley, M. T., and Bernstein, D. I. (1989). *Brain Res.,* **22,** 867.
17. Norgren, R. B. Jr. and Lehman, M. N. (1988). *Brain Res.,* **479,** 374.
18. Rinaman, L., Enquist, L. W., and Card, J. P. (1991). *Soc. for Neurosci.* Abstract 456.10, 1148.
19. Rinaman, L., Card, J. P., and Enquist, L. W. (1992). Submitted for publication.
20. Rouiller, E. M., Capt, M., Dolivo, M., and De Ribaupierre, F. (1986). *Neurosci. Lett.,* **72,** 247.
21. Rouiller, E. M., Capt, M., Dolivo, M., and De Ribaupierre, F. (1989). *Brain Res.,* **476,** 21.
22. Strack, A. M. and Loewy, A. D. (1990). *J. Neurosci.,* **10,** 2139.

23. Strack, A. M., Sawyer, W. B., Platt, K. B., and Loewy, A. D. (1989). *Brain Res.,* **491,** 274.
24. Strack, A. M., Sawyer, W. B., Hughes, J. H., Platt, K. B., and Loewy, A. D. (1989). *Brain Res.,* **491,** 156.
25. Ugolini, G., Kuypers, H. G. J. M., and Simmons, A. (1987). *Brain Res.,* **422,** 242.
26. Ugolini, G., Kuypers, H. G. J. M., and Strick, P. L. (1989). *Science,* **243,** 89.
27. Zemanick, M. C., Strick, P. L., and Dix, R. D. (1991). *Proc. Natl Acad. Sci. USA,* **88,** 8048.
28. Becker, C. H. (1967). *Experientia,* **23,** 209.
29. Bartha, A. (1961). *Magy. Allatorv. Lapja,* **16,** 42.
30. Robbins, A. K., Ryan, J. P., Whealy, M. E., and Enquist, L. W. (1989). *J. Virol.,* **63,** 250.
31. Dix, R. D., McKendall, R. R., and Baringer, J. R. (1983). *Immunity,* **40,** 103.
32. Shapiro, R. E. and Miselis, R. R. (1985). *J. Comp. Neurol.,* **238,** 473.
33. Altschuler, S. M., Bao, X., Bieger, D., Hopkins, D. A., and Miselis, R. R. (1989). *J. Comp. Neurol.,* **283,** 248.
34. Hunt, R. D. and Melendez, L. V. (1969). *Laboratory Animal Care,* **19,** 221.
35. Lopez, C. (1975). *Nature* (*Lond.*), **258,** 152.
36. Kohl, S. and Loo, L. S. (1980). *Infect. Immun.,* **30,** 847.
37. Zawatzky, R., Engler, H., and Kirchner, H. (1982). *J. Gen. Virol.,* **60,** 25.
38. Emmons, R. W. and Lennette, E. H. (1970). *Archiv für die gesamte Virusforschung,* **31,** 215.
39. Kalter, S. S. (1988). In *Viral diseases in Laboratory and Captive Animals* (ed. G. Darai), pp. 101–33. Martinus Nijhoff Publishers, Boston.
40. Meignier, B., Jourdier, T. M., Norrild, B., Pereira, L., and Roizman, B. (1987). *J. Infect. Dis.*, **155,** 921.
41. Gustafson, D. P. (1975). In *Diseases of Swine* (ed. H. W. Dunne and A. D. Leman), pp. 391–410. The Iowa State University Press, Ames.
42. Wittmann, G. and Rziha, H.-J. (1989). In *Herpesvirus Diseases of Cattle, Horses and Pigs* (ed. G. Wittmann), pp. 230–333. Kluwer Academic, London.
43. Hsu, S., Raine, L., and Fanger, H. (1981). *J. Histochem. Cytochem.,* **29,** 577.
44. Sternberger, L. A. (1979). In *Immunocytochemistry* (ed. L. A. Sternberger), pp. 104–69. Wiley, New York.
45. McLean, I. W. and Nakane, P. K. (1974). *J. Histochem. Cytochem.,* **22,** 1077.
46. Adams, J. C. (1977). *Neurosci.,* **2,** 141.
47. Lycke, E., Hamark, B., Johansson, M., Krotochwil, A., Lycke, J., and Svennerholm, B. (1988). *Arch. Virol.,* **101,** 87.
48. Langford, L. A. and Coggeshall, R. E. (1980). *Anat. Rec.,* **197,** 297.
49. Vahlne, A., Nystrom, B., Sandberg, M., Hamberger, A., and Lycke, E. (1978). *J. Gen. Virol.,* **40,** 359.
50. Vahlne, A., Svennerholm, B., Sandberg, M., Hamberger, A., and Lycke, E. (1980). *Infect. Immunol.,* **28,** 675.

5

Immunocytochemistry I: pre-embedding staining

S. TOTTERDELL, C. A. INGHAM, and J. P. BOLAM

1. Introduction

Immunocytochemistry is a technique which has become widely used in experimental neuroanatomy. It enables one to morphologically characterize neurones containing a specific chemical moiety, and since the major means of communication between neurones in the nervous system is by chemical transmission, immunocytochemistry represents one of the most powerful techniques available to the experimental neuroanatomist in the study of the nervous system. The approach relies on the fact that an antibody directed against a specific substance will bind avidly to that substance. With antibodies directed against neurotransmitters or an enzyme related to the neurotransmitter it is possible to morphologically characterize those neurones expressing the transmitter (or enzyme), to analyse their afferent synaptic input, and by analysis of terminals that are immunostained, to analyse their synaptic output. Furthermore, immunocytochemistry can be used to detect *exogenous* substances, for instance the anterograde axonal tracers *Phaseolus vulgaris*–leucoagglutinin (PHA-L) (1) (see Chapter 3). The combination of immunocytochemistry for endogenous or exogenous substances with other techniques has added further dimensions to the study of the nervous system (see Chapter 11).

The term 'pre-embedding' refers to the stage at which the tissue is in during its preparation for light or electron microscopy. Pre-embedding immunocytochemistry is carried out on the tissue before it is embedded in a light microscopic mounting medium or electron microscopic resin. This contrasts with post-embedding immunocytochemistry which is carried out on material that has been embedded in an electron microscopic resin (see Chapter 6).

The principles of immunocytochemistry used in experimental neuroanatomy are essentially the same as when the technique was first introduced by Coons and Kaplan in the 1950s (2). An antibody is raised against a specific neurochemical; the antibody preparation (whether produced in a whole animal or as a monoclonal antibody), is incubated with the experimental tissue where it binds to the molecules against which it is directed. It is the bound antibody that is then localized in the tissue thus revealing the sites of the specific neurochemical. The bound antibodies can be revealed either by direct or by indirect methods (2). In the former, the antibody itself is conjugated to a label that enables it to be visualized in the microscope; for instance it may be labelled with a fluorescent molecule. In the indirect methods the primary antibody is not labelled but the tissue is incubated with a *secondary* antibody preparation (raised in a different species) that is directed against the primary antibody. The secondary antibody binds to the primary antibody thus marking the position of the antigen of interest. The secondary antibody can be localized by conjugation of markers to the antibody itself, for instance, a fluorescent molecule or gold particles (see Chapter 6), or it can be labelled with a substance that can give rise to coloured or electron dense marker for instance horseradish peroxidase (HRP) or biotin (that can be reacted with an avidin–biotin–peroxidase complex, see *Protocol 9*). An alternative to the use of *labelled* antibodies, are unlabelled antibody procedures, e.g. the peroxidase anti-peroxidase (PAP) method (3) (see below), in which the antigen is localized by markers immunologically bound to the antibodies.

Successful immunocytochemistry at the level of the electron microscope requires a careful balance between conditions that favour the detection of the antigen and conditions that favour the maintenance of ultrastructural integrity. This chapter will deal with the choice of appropriate fixatives, the methods available to enhance the penetration of the immunoreagents, and the reduction of non-specific staining. It will also describe some of the standard methods for detecting the antibodies and possible ways to enhance their detection. The object of this chapter is not to deal exhaustively with the subject of immunocytochemistry but rather to describe basic and simple procedures for immunocytochemistry at the electron microscope level. For more detailed discussions of the principles and practice of immunocytochemistry the reader is referred to recent monographs (3–6). The reader is also referred to Chapter 3, *Protocol 2* and Chapter 10, *Protocols 7* and *9* which deal with the immunocytochemical localization of PHA-L and Lucifer Yellow.

2. Sequence of procedures in pre-embedding immunocytochemistry

The sequence of events or procedures for the preparation of neuronal tissue for pre-embedding immunocytochemistry at the electron microscopic level follow.

(a) Perfuse–fix the animal with appropriate fixative (*Protocols 1* and *2*, see also Chapter 1, *Protocols 2* and *3*).
(b) Remove brain, cut areas of interest into blocks.

(c) Cut sections, preferably on a vibrating microtome at 50–100 μm (Chapter 1, *Protocol 4*).
(d) *Optional*. Carry out procedures to reduce background staining (*Protocols 6* and *7*).
(e) *Optional*. Carry out procedures to enhance penetration of immuno-reagents (*Protocols 3–5*).
(f) *Optional*. Further background reduction by incubation in normal serum derived from species of origin of the secondary antibody.
(g) Subject sections to immunocytochemistry (*Protocols 8* and *9*).
(h) *Optional*. Enhance the signal by the double bridge technique.
(i) Reveal the immunoreactive sites by peroxidase reaction (*Protocols 8, 10*, and *11*).
(j) Post-fix sections for electron microscopy in osmium tetroxide (Chapter 1, *Protocol 7*).
(k) Dehydrate sections and flat-embed in an electron microscopic resin on microscope slides (Chapter 1, *Protocol 8*).
(l) Examine the sections in the light microscope, re-embed areas of interest, cut ultrathin sections, and examine in the electron microscope (see Chapter 1).

3. Fixation

Fixation of the tissue for immunocytochemistry is not only required for preservation purposes but also to fix the antigen in position in the tissue so that it can be localized by the antibody, however the degree of fixation should be such that the antibody still recognizes the antigen. Taking these points into consideration generally involves a compromise, as optimal conditions for good ultrastructural preservation are generally not the optimal conditions for retaining antigenicity. This is particularly true for immunocytochemistry at the electron microscopic level.

The fixation procedure required for pre-embedding immunocytochemistry is dependent on the nature of the antigen under study. Small molecules, (e.g. amino acids) do not induce antibody formation unless they are conjugated to a large carrier protein. In this case antibodies are produced which recognize the neurochemical of interest, conjugated with formaldehyde or glutaraldehyde to a carrier molecule such as bovine serum albumin or keyhole limpet haemocyanin. The antibody is not specific to the neurochemical itself but rather to a modified derivative formed in the tissue during fixation. It is therefore vital that fixation conditions should aim to produce the same modified derivative in the tissue. Commercially obtained antibodies usually specify the optimum fixation conditions. When non-conjugated antigens are being located, paraformaldehyde based fixatives are generally recommended as they penetrate the tissue quickly preventing movement of the antigen from its natural site as well as leaving the conformational state of the antigen unchanged. For light microscopic immunocytochemistry paraformaldehyde alone can be used as the fixative. However glutaraldehyde, which is necessary for electron microscopic studies, has two functional aldehyde groups that cross-link amino groups resulting in restricted rotation and conformational changes in proteins, changes that probably reduce the antigenicity. With this fixative it is therefore a question of establishing how much glutaraldehyde can be tolerated before the antibody fails to recognize the antigen. A number of fixatives that have been used extensively in the study of the nervous system are described below (Sections 3.1 and 3.2).

The animals should be fixed by perfusion, the practical details of which are described in detail in Chapter 1, *Protocol 3* (see also Chapter 10, *Protocol 2*). Before beginning the perfusion with the fixative it is necessary to remove the blood from the circulatory system by pre-perfusing the animal with a vascular rinse consisting of 0.9% sodium chloride solution, calcium-free Tyrode's solution (see Chapter 1, Appendix 1), or some other physiological salt solution. The anticoagulant heparin, can be added to these solutions at a concentration of 50 U/ml. The duration and the rate of perfusion of the animal are important for subsequent immunoreactions and for the preservation of the tissue. The conditions vary for different antibodies and different antigens but as a general rule immunostaining for electron microscopy should be attempted first with those fixatives listed in Section 3.1. The perfusion with fixative is preceded by the vascular rinse for 30 to 90 seconds followed by a mixture of paraformaldehyde and glutaraldehyde, usually dissolved in 0.1 M phosphate buffer pH 7.4 (PB) (Chapter 1, *Protocol 1*) at a rate of approximately 10–20 ml/min. For a 250 g rat a total of about 300 ml are administered over a period of about 15 to 30 minutes. The brain is then removed from the skull and placed in the same fixative for a further one to two hours if necessary, before placing in PB or PBS until it is convenient to cut sections. The amounts of fixative and rates of perfusion will vary for different species.

The more commonly used aldehyde-based fixatives suitable for pre-embedding immunohistochemistry can be divided into two groups according to the nature of the antibody and antigen, those containing low concentrations of glutaraldehyde and those containing high concentrations of glutaraldehyde. For other fixatives that are suitable for immunocytochemistry refer to more specialized publications (3–6).

3.1 Paraformaldehyde-based fixatives with low concentrations of glutaraldehyde

Paraformaldehyde-based fixatives with low concentrations of glutaraldehyde are the most commonly used for pre-embedding immunohistochemistry at the electron microscopic level. Refer to Chapter 1, *Protocol 2* for a detailed description of the preparation of paraformaldehyde/glutaraldehyde fixatives. Rates of fixative flow and amounts of fixative are applicable to 200–300 g rats.

(a) 4% paraformaldehyde, 0.1% glutaraldehyde in PB for 10 min followed by 3% paraformaldehyde in PB for 5 min. Rate: 20 ml/min, 15 min total. The 10 min exposure to glutaraldehyde-containing fixative is sufficient to give reasonable ultrastructure. This is often the fixative of choice in the first instance and has proved optimal in our hands for choline acetyltransferase immunocytochemistry (7, 8).

(b) 4% paraformaldehyde, 0.01–0.5% glutaraldehyde in PB. Rate: 10–20 ml/min for approximately 15–30 min (300 ml).

(c) 4% paraformaldehyde, 0.05% glutaraldehyde, 0.2% picric acid in PB (*Protocol 1*) (9). Rate: 10–20 ml/min for 15–30 min (300 ml). The presence of the picric acid which acts as a fixative of proteins, compensates for the small amount of glutaraldehyde. Aldehyde mixtures including picric acid have proven successful for the ultrastructural localization of several antigens (10, 11).

(d) 4% paraformaldehyde, 0.1% glutaraldehyde in PB for 8 min (160 ml, 20 ml/min), followed by 4% paraformaldehyde in 0.1 M sodium hydrogen carbonate buffer, pH 10.4 for 15 min (300 ml, 20 ml/min, (12, 13)). Paraformaldehyde is a more efficient fixative in alkaline conditions, however efficient fixation hinders the penetration of the fixative into the tissue. The logic of this method is therefore to allow rapid entry of the fixative into the tissue followed by increasing the reactivity of the paraformaldehyde to speed the fixation.

Protocol 1. Preparation of mixed aldehyde fixative with picric acid (9)

For the preparation of 600 ml of 0.05% glutaraldehyde, 4% paraformaldehyde, and approximately 0.2% picric acid, in 0.1 M sodium phosphate buffer, pH 7.4. (See *Safety note 1* in Chapter 1, p. 5.)

Method

1. Prepare a saturated solution of picric acid in distilled water by stirring excess picric acid for several hours in water. Allow to settle and filter appropriate amount before use.[a]
2. Dissolve 24 g paraformaldehyde in 200 ml distilled water, add 300 ml 0.2 M phosphate buffer, and 1.2 ml 25% glutaraldehyde solution. (See Chapter 1, *Protocol 2* for details.)
3. Add 90 ml of saturated picric acid.
4. Make up to 600 ml with distilled water.

[a] **Safety note 1**. Caution should be exercised with picric acid as it is explosive in its dry state. Wash all contaminated surfaces and materials with excess water.

3.2 Aldehyde-based fixatives with high concentrations of glutaraldehyde

Aldehyde-based fixatives with high concentrations of glutaraldehyde are suitable for antibodies that recognize antigens conjugated to glutaraldehyde. They have the advantage that tissue preservation is good but the disadvantage that there is poor penetration of immunoreagents into the tissue. An example of such an antiserum is that against dopamine, developed by Geffard and colleagues (14). Dopamine may be released very rapidly under conditions of stress, such as hypoxia, resulting in a loss of specific cell and fibre staining; it is therefore an example of an antigen for which it is necessary to ensure that the fixative reaches the brain very rapidly. *Protocol 2* thus describes a fixation regime for an antiserum that requires a high concentration of glutaraldehyde and very rapid fixation.

Protocol 2. Perfuse–fixation using high concentrations of glutaraldehyde, e.g. for the dopamine antiserum (15), (see *Safety note 1* in Chapter 1, p. 5)

5% glutaraldehyde, 1% sodium metabisulphite in 0.05 M sodium cacodylate buffer (pH 7.5).

Materials

- 0.1 M sodium cacodylate, pH 7.5 (pH adjusted with HCl) (BDH)[a]
- sodium metabisulphite ($Na_2S_2O_5$) (Sigma)
- glutaraldehyde

Method

1. Prepare 1 litre of fixative by mixing:
   - sodium metabisulphite — 10 g
   - 0.1 M sodium cacodylate buffer, pH 7.5 — 500 ml
   - 25% glutaraldehyde — 200 ml
   - distilled water — up to 1 litre
2. Perfuse through the aorta with 1% sodium metabisulphite or calcium-free Tyrode's solution at 37 °C for 30–90 sec at a rate of 50–100 ml/min (about 100 ml), (see Chapter 1, *Protocol 3*, for details of perfusion).
3. Perfuse with 1 litre of 5% glutaraldehyde and 1% sodium metabisulphite in 0.05 M sodium cacodylate buffer, pH 7.5 (about 50–100 ml per min for 10–20 min).
4. After removal of the brain post-fix for 45 min in same fixative at 4 °C.

[a] **Safety note 2**. Sodium cacodylate contains arsenic and is highly toxic. Wear gloves at all times when handling.

3.3 Post-fixation

After perfusion, the brain is removed from the skull (Chapter 1, *Protocol 3*) and the whole brain or blocks of tissue including the regions of interest may be post-fixed. Post-fixation is particularly important if the initial perfusion was poor; this will be apparent when the brain is removed as it will appear pink and will be soft to the touch. Post-fixation of blocks of tissue including the region of interest will allow the tissue to be cut without difficulty and may aid the subsequent immunoreaction. The time required for this process is variable depending on the fixative used, the quality of the perfusion, and the nature of the tissue. There is some variation in the appropriate time for post-fixation, for example, a complete rat brain which has been perfused well using fixative (b) above will be adequately post-fixed after one to two hours, whereas cat spinal cord usually needs at least six hours' post-fixation. The optimal time in a particular experimental situation should be established empirically.

3.4 Preparation of blocks and sectioning of tissue

The usual method of sectioning fixed brain for immunocytochemistry at the electron microscopic level is to use the vibrating microtome (see Chapter 1, *Protocol 4* for details). The sections are cut at 50–100 μm and placed in vials in which they should be able to move freely with shaking in 1–2 ml of solution. The sections can be cut and collected in phosphate buffer or phosphate-buffered saline (see Chapter 1, *Protocol 1*).

The sections are now processed for immunocytochemistry. Optimal staining occurs when there is binding of the immunoreagents throughout the thickness of the tissue section, but to achieve this is it may be necessary at this point to carry out procedures that enable the immunoreagents to penetrate more easily into the tissue. Depending upon the antibody preparation and the fixative, it may be necessary to carry out procedures that reduce background staining.

4. Enhancement of the penetration of immunoreagents

Having selected a fixation regime that will result in good ultrastructural preservation it may be necessary to disrupt membrane integrity to some extent, to allow the entry of the large molecules (150–500 kd) of the immunoreagents into the tissue. Without such treatment immunostaining will be limited to the most superficial layers of the sections and in the most extreme cases, to only the outer one or two microns of the sections.

4.1 Detergents

The most commonly used system to aid penetration of the immunoreagents into tissue sections is the incubation with the detergent Triton X-100

(*Protocol 3*), although other detergents have been used, e.g. ethylene glycol (Photoflo, Kodak) (16). Triton X-100 acts by dissolving the lipid layers of membranes and thus allows larger molecules to pass. For light microscopy it is usual to include the Triton at a concentration of up to 0.5% in the buffer used for preparing the immunoreagents and washing the sections. The concentrations used to enhance the penetration of immunoreagents into sections prepared for electron microscopy are far lower (0.05–0.1%) as Triton and detergents in general have marked detrimental effects on ultrastructure. The time of exposure to the detergent should also be kept to a minimum; it should not exceed 30 minutes. This inevitably means that the degree of penetration is less than that seen in light microscopic preparations. However, even such short exposures to low concentrations of detergent can have a detrimental effect on ultrastructure. Triton X-100 dissolves fairly readily if added drop-wise from a pipette whilst stirring vigorously. It is convenient to keep a stock solution of 1–10% at 4°C.

Protocol 3. Enhancement of penetration of immunoreagents with detergents

1. Prepare a 0.05% solution of Triton X-100 from the stock solution in PBS, or in 10% normal serum in PBS.
2. Add about 2 ml to each vial of sections, i.e. sufficient to cover the sections, and shake gently at room temperature for 30 minutes.
3. Wash 3 × 10 min in PBS.

4.2 Freeze-thaw

It is possible to enhance the penetration of immunochemicals by mechanically disrupting the tissue. This can be achieved by freezing the section and then allowing it to thaw. As with treatment with detergents, the procedure has detrimental effects on ultrastructure of the tissue, the freezing procedure therefore, is designed to produce small ice crystals that cause only limited damage to the tissue. In order to produce small ice crystals the tissue is first equilibrated with a strong sucrose solution. Freezing of the tissue is then carried out in two stages, with an exposure first to cold isopentane and then liquid nitrogen.

Protocol 4. Freeze-thaw of tissue sections

Materials

- sucrose
- glycerol

- 0.2 M phosphate buffer pH 7.4 (Chapter 1, *Protocol 1*)
- isopentane (2-methylbutane)
- liquid nitrogen (stored in a Dewar flask)
- plastic beakers which stack into each other and have lips
- mesh baskets[a]
- Petri dishes
- paint brushes
- plastic tweezers with securing ring

Method

1. Prepare cryoprotectant: 25 g sucrose, 10 ml glycerol, 25 ml 0.2 M phosphate buffer pH 7.4, make up to 100 ml with distilled water.[b]
2. Place the sections in the cryoprotectant and shake gently until they sink (about 1 hour).
3. In a fume cupboard, pour some liquid nitrogen into a plastic beaker and place this in the top of the Dewar flask. Pour some isopentane into a second beaker and place this in the first.
4. Take a vial of sections and pour into a mesh basket in a Petri dish.
5. Place the Petri dish on a dark background and gently flatten the sections with a paint brush.
6. Use the plastic tweezers to grasp the mesh basket and slide the ring down to hold it firmly.
7. Wearing protective gloves, gently lift the basket from the Petri dish, taking care that the sections are not disturbed. Drain off the excess cryoprotectant by dabbing on absorbent paper.
8. Lower the mesh basket into the cold isopentane and wait for the sections to freeze. The sections turn white when they are frozen.
9. Remove them from the isopentane and place in the liquid nitrogen for about 10–15 sec.
10. Allow the sections to thaw in cryoprotectant or PBS and then use the paint brush to transfer them into a vial of buffer. Wash the sections several times in PBS or PB.

[a] To make mesh baskets cut a ring of plastic about 1 cm high and with a diameter of 4–5 cm from a convenient source, such as a plastic beaker, stretch a piece of fine nylon mesh, hold in place with an elastic band and glue with in position with cyanoacrylate glue.

[b] This solution may be stored for several months at −23°C.

4.3 Enzyme digestion

Increasing the penetration of immunoreagents by enzyme digestion relies on the partial digestion of protein molecules that make up the membrane wall (17). The procedure involves the incubation of the tissue sections with the enzyme pronase. As with all procedures that are designed to increase the penetration of immunoreagents a balance has to be achieved between the degree of increased penetration and the maintenance of structural integrity. An additional factor that has to be taken into consideration with proteolytic enzyme digestion is that the enzyme may destroy the antigen that is the subject of the study. Thus the procedure may not be appropriate for every antigen. It has been successfully applied to the ultrastructural localization of choline acetyltransferase immunoreactive terminals in the substantia nigra (8) and cortex (18).

Protocol 5. Enzyme digestion

Materials

- pronase (Protease, P6911 Sigma)
- 0.05 M Tris-HCl buffer (pH 7.4)

Method

1. Prepare the enzyme solution just prior to use. Dissolve 0.01 g pronase in 100 ml of the Tris-buffer. Dilute this solution 1:10 with Tris-buffer to give a final concentration of 0.001%.
2. Replace the buffer in the vial containing the sections with sufficient enzyme solution to cover the sections.
3. Shake gently at room temperature for 5–10 min.
4. Stop the reaction by filling the vial with ice-cold Tris-buffer and wash the sections several times in ice-cold Tris-buffer.
5. Wash the sections several times in PB or PBS.

---

5. Reduction of background staining

Background staining occurs either when the antibody recognizes antigenic sites other than the one to which it was raised, for example when a particular amino acid sequence occurs in a molecule other than the desired antigen, or where other immunoreagents become bound in a non-specific way to the tissue. The degree of background staining depends on a number of factors including the specificity of the antibody, the purity of the immunoreagents, and the structure of the tissue.

5.1 Borohydride treatment

The use of fixatives with high concentrations of glutaraldehyde is often desirable in immunocytochemical studies as it results in better preservation of ultrastructure of the tissue, and indeed for some antigens or antibody preparations it is necessary. However with a number of antibodies the benefit is often offset not only by the decreased penetration of the immunoreagents, but also by the increase in background staining. Glutaraldehyde has two aldehyde groups each of which can form Schiff base linkages with free amino groups. These restrict the rotation and thus the tertiary structure of proteins. It is possible to reverse this reaction by using sodium borohydride and reduce the double bonds to single bonds which are able to rotate again, thus permitting greater penetration of large molecules through the membrane. It is not known why, with some antibodies, high levels of glutaraldehyde result in increased background staining, but it has been suggested that the main role of borohydride treatment in reducing background staining, is the reduction of excess aldehyde groups (19).

Protocol 6. Reduction of background staining with sodium borohydride

1. Make a fresh 1% solution of sodium borohydride in water, PB, or PBS.
2. Remove the buffer from the vials of sections and add about 5 ml sodium borohydride solution. Bubbles of gas will be evolved from the tissue. Incubate for 5–10 min.[a]
3. Pour the sections into a mesh basket (see footnote to *Protocol 4*), and rinse many times in buffer until evolution of gas bubbles has ceased.
4. Transfer all sections to a vial containing PB or PBS.

[a] At this stage poorly fixed tissue may become badly disrupted and if in doubt about tissue integrity process only one or two trial sections first.

5.2 Endogenous peroxidase activity

A further source of background staining is that resulting from endogenous peroxidases in the tissue. An example is seen when erythrocytes have not been adequately flushed from the tissue prior to perfusion with the fixative, although this may not be an important source since it is restricted to erythrocytes and can usually be eliminated by pre-perfusing for longer with saline or Tyrode's solution. Such staining is unlikely to result in confusion as the erythrocytes are immediately recognizable, as are another source of endogenous peroxidase, the pericytes. In general endogenous enzymes, including for instance cytochrome oxidase, are destroyed by the perfusion–fixation and they are usually only a problem, therefore, in poorly fixed tissue. In this case it is possible that enzymes which are not specifically peroxidases, such as catalase, may be able to use the hydrogen peroxidase as a substrate or react with the chromogen to produce a reaction product. When the tissue is reacted to demonstrate the peroxidase complex associated with the immunoreaction, these non-specific enzymes also produce reaction product. However, it is possible to reduce the amount of staining produced by endogenous peroxidases by reacting them before the start of the immunocytochemical procedure. This is usually done with a mixture of methanol and hydrogen peroxide although other inhibitors of peroxidases may be used.

Protocol 7. Inhibition of endogenous peroxidase activity

1. Prepare a solution containing 10% methanol and 3% hydrogen peroxide in PBS.
2. Remove the PBS from the vials containing the sections and add the methanol/hydrogen peroxide mixture. Bubbles of gas will be evolved.
3. Incubate for 5 min.
4. Wash with PBS several times until the bubbles cease to arise.

5.3 Non-specific staining

Non-specific staining can result from the binding of the primary antibody to tissue sites or by antibodies being absorbed by the tissue in non-immunological bonds. Both of these can be minimized by pre-treatment with normal serum from the species which donates the secondary antibody. The tissue is incubated in 10% normal serum in PBS for 30 minutes. The incubation is carried out immediately prior to the immunocytochemical protocols and if the tissue is to be treated with Triton X-100 it may be carried out at the same time. Furthermore, 1% normal serum from the species of origin of the secondary antibody can be included in the buffer used to wash the sections and dilute the antisera.

6. Immunocytochemistry

Two standard immunocytochemical methods that have proved successful for electron microscopy as well as light microscopy will be described, the peroxidase anti-peroxidase technique (3), and the avidin–biotin–peroxidase technique (20). They are both indirect methods, i.e. the primary antibody is not directly labelled, instead a secondary antibody binds to the primary antibody and it is this secondary reagent that is labelled or binds to a label. The advantages of using indirect methods as opposed to directly labelling the primary antibody are:

(a) that it acts as an amplification step—more than one molecule of the secondary antibody will bind to the primary antibody;

(b) it obviates the necessity to subject valuable, and usually scarce, primary antiserum to a chemical reaction.

In both of the methods that are described the enzyme, horseradish peroxidase, is incorporated in the final layer of the reaction and is used to localize the antigenic sites by standard histochemical techniques.

Figure 1 diagrammatically illustrates the two techniques. Immunocytochemistry is based on immunological principles involving antibody/antigen reactions. The antibodies involved usually belong to the immunoglobulin G class (IgG) which themselves can act as antigens in different species. Both the methods utilize unlabelled primary antibodies which, during incubation with the sections, bind to the specific antigen. The amount of antibody that binds is directly related to the time of incubation which varies between 12 hours and several days. The species of origin of the primary antibody is designated x in the figure. The next stage involves a secondary antibody which binds to the primary antibody. The secondary antibody is raised in a different species, designated y in the diagram, against the IgG of species x.

6.1 The peroxidase anti-peroxidase method (unlabelled antibody) *Protocol 8* (3)

In the case of the peroxidase anti-peroxidase method, the secondary antibody is applied in excess so that only one limb of the divalent antigen binding (Fab) fragment becomes bound to the primary antibody. This results in 'spare' Fab fragments that are available for the third layer or step of the technique. The third step involves incubation with the PAP complex, which consists of an antibody raised against HRP and then reacted with HRP to form an antibody/antigen complex. The antibody in this complex is raised in the same species as the primary antibody, i.e. species x, it will thus be recognized by the free Fab fragments of the second antibody. The antigen will therefore be localized by the presence of the enzyme, HRP. The PAP method is referred to as an unlabelled antibody method, as none of the antibodies are chemically conjugated to the marker molecules, rather the marker molecule is immunologically bound.

6.2 The avidin–biotin–peroxidase method (labelled antibody) *Protocol 9* (20)

In the case of the ABC method a different principle is applied. The secondary antibody is similarly raised in a different species, against immunoglobulin G of the species of origin of the primary antibody, but in this case the secondary antibody is itself labelled. The label is biotin, but for other labelled antibody techniques the secondary antibody may be labelled with HRP or colloidal gold (see Chapter 6). The biotinylated secondary antibody recognizes and binds to the primary antibody. The secondary antibody, and therefore the

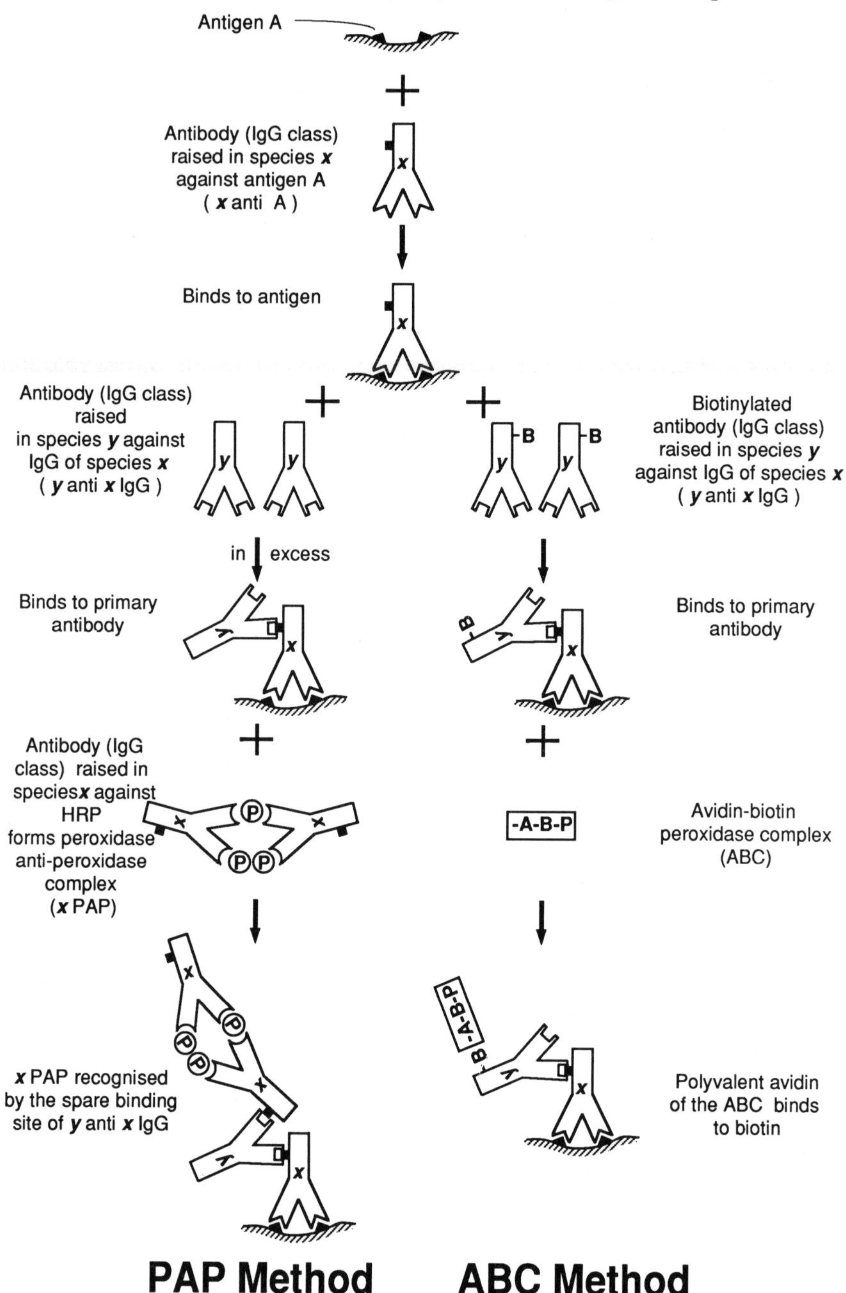

Figure 1. Diagram to illustrate two indirect pre-embedding immunocytochemical methods, the PAP (peroxidase anti-peroxidase) method and the ABC (avidin–biotin–peroxidase complex) method. See text for detailed explanation. (This figure was kindly prepared by W. M. Christie and S. H. Hood.)

primary antibody bound to the antigen, is then localized by taking advantage of the fact that the biotin binds with a high affinity to the glycoprotein, avidin. The avidin is applied in the form of a complex with biotin and HRP, i.e. the avidin–biotin–peroxidase complex which, by virtue of the polyvalent nature of avidin, binds to the biotin conjugated to the secondary antibody.

6.3 Histochemical localization of the antigenic sites

In both the PAP method and the ABC method the antigenic sites are then localized by the enzymatic properties of HRP. The HRP catalyses the breakdown of H_2O_2 and in doing so will oxidize a large number of compounds. A substance is therefore included in the reaction mixture that becomes coloured and insoluble upon oxidation. The most commonly used substances in peroxidase histochemistry are derivatives of benzidine. With these derivatives the free bonds of the oxidation product react with each other to form insoluble phenazine polymers. The reaction products have characteristic colours, subcellular location, and texture.

6.4 Incubations for immunocytochemistry

Incubations for immunocytochemistry can be conveniently carried out in glass scintillation vials that should be placed on a shaker for the entire procedure. When changing solutions it helps to remove two vials from the shaker at a time and allow sections to settle before pipetting out the solution with a disposable plastic pipette. To ensure adequate rinsing between immunocytochemical incubations, the following procedure can be adopted. Remove immunochemical solution and fill vial to the top with the rinsing solution. When all vials have been filled start immediately on the next rinse, during this and subsequent rinses, remove solution, replace with 2–3 ml rinsing solution, replace vial on shaker with clean cap. To ensure all traces of the last immunochemical are removed from the walls of the vial, pipette solutions against the vial walls. To ensure against cross contamination make sure that if *different* immunochemicals have been used at one stage that *different* pipettes are used to remove the solutions.

Protocol 8. Immunocytochemistry using the peroxidase anti-peroxidase method (*Figure 1*)

Materials

- PBS (Chapter 1, *Protocol 1*)
- Tris-HCl buffer (0.05 M, pH 7.4) (TB)
- phosphate buffer (0.1 M, pH 7.4) (PB)
- primary antibody (raised in species *x* against the antigen of interest)

Protocol 8. *Continued*

- secondary antibody (raised in species *y* against IgG of species *x*)
- peroxidase anti-peroxidase complex (raised in species *x*)
- normal serum (from species *y*)
- sodium azide
- 3,3′-diaminobenzidine tetrahydrochloride (DAB, Sigma) (see *Safety note 3*)
- hydrogen peroxide (30% solution, Sigma)

Method

All incubations should be carried out on a rotary shaker. For short incubation times carry out at room temperature, for long incubation times carry out at 4°C.

1. Wash sections in PBS, up to 6 × 10 min to remove all traces of fixative. (Any pre-incubation procedure will substitute for some of the washing time.)
2. Incubate in primary antibody at 4°C for 12–72 h diluted in PBS. This diluent may contain 0.01% sodium azide as a preservative and 1% normal serum derived from the species of the secondary antibody. The optimal dilution varies for different antibodies; if there is no recommended dilution then test a series of different dilutions, e.g. 1:500–1:5000.
3. Rinse 2–4 × 15 min in PBS at room temperature. The primary antibody solution may be saved, stored at 4°C, and reused until signal begins to weaken.
4. Incubate in secondary antibody (raised in species *y* against IgG of the species of origin of the primary antibody, i.e. species *x*, *Figure 1*) diluted 1:50 in PBS ±1% normal serum, for 1–18 h.
5. Rinse 2–4 × 15 min in PBS at room temperature.
6. Incubate with peroxidase anti-peroxidase complex (species of origin of the primary antibody) at a dilution of about 1:100 in PBS for 1–18 h.
7. Rinse 3 × 10 min in PBS at room temperature.
8. Rinse 2 × 10 min in TB at room temperature.
9. Transfer vials of sections on the shaker to a fume cupboard. Take necessary safety precautions for handling suspect carcinogenic substances (see *Safety note 3*). Incubate for 10–20 min at room temperature in a solution of 0.05% DAB in TB.[a] Usually 2.5 ml per vial.
10. Add 1% hydrogen peroxide, (i.e. 1:30 dilution of stock H_2O_2) to give a final concentration in incubation medium of 0.01%, (i.e. 25 μl per 2.5 ml DAB solution). Incubate for a further 5–15 min, monitoring reaction under a dissection microscope.[b]

11. Rinse 3 × 10 min in TB.

12. Rinse 3 × 10 min in phosphate buffer (0.1 M, pH 7.4).

Safety note 3. Derivatives of benzidine, e.g. DAB, are suspect carcinogens and should be handled accordingly and appropriate protective clothing worn. These compounds may be inactivated by reacting with sodium hypochlorite solution (chlorine bleach) (minimum 8% chlorine, diluted 1:1 with water). All waste solutions and contaminated materials (use disposable items preferably) should therefore be placed in a waste container of excess bleach. After at least 30 min, the inactivated solution should be washed down the sink with excess water. All contaminated materials should be washed extensively.

[a] DAB solution can be stored frozen as a 5% solution in water in appropriately sized aliquots, (e.g. 0.5 or 1.0 ml). Add 0.5 ml 5% DAB to 50 ml TB and filter before use.
[b] Different chromogens can be used (see Section 7.1), or staining may be intensified or modified to produce different coloured reaction products.

Protocol 9. Immunocytochemistry using the avidin–biotin–peroxidase complex (ABC) method (*Figure 1*)

Materials

- PBS (Chapter 1, *Protocol 1*)
- Tris-HCl buffer (0.05 M, pH 7.4)
- phosphate buffer (0.1 M, pH 7.4)
- primary antibody (raised in species *x* against the antigen of interest)
- biotinylated secondary antibody (raised in species *y* against IgG of species *x*) (Vector Laboratories)
- avidin–biotin–peroxidase complex (Vector Laboratories)
- normal serum (from species *y*)
- sodium azide
- 3,3′-diaminobenzidine tetrahydrochloride (DAB, Sigma) (see *Safety note 3*)
- hydrogen peroxide (30% solution, Sigma)

Method

All incubations should be carried out on a rotary shaker. For short incubation times carry out at room temperature, for long incubation times carry out at 4°C.

1. Follow steps **1–3** of *Protocol 8*.

Protocol 9. *Continued*

2. Incubate in biotinylated secondary antibody at a dilution of about 1:200 in PBS for 1–18 h.
3. Rinse 2–6 × 10 min in PBS.
4. Prepare avidin–biotin–peroxidase complex according to manufacturers' instruction. In the case of kits from Vector Laboratories mix solution A (avidin DH), with solution B (biotinylated peroxidase), and PBS in the ratios 1:1:100. Allow to react for 30 min.
5. Incubate sections in the avidin–biotin–peroxidase complex for 1–18 h.
6. Follow steps **7–12** of *Protocol 8*.

The above protocols are basic procedures for immunocytochemistry, the exact conditions and times of incubation will vary according to many factors including the antigen under study, the antibody preparation, and the degree of fixation of the tissue. The optimal conditions in a particular situation should be arrived at empirically. The reader is referred to Chapter 3, *Protocol 2*, Chapter 10, *Protocols 7* and *9*, and Chapter 11 where immunocytochemical protocols for specific applications are dealt with.

6.5 Characteristics of the DAB reaction product

The DAB acts as an electron donor during the peroxidase reaction and on oxidation, polymerizes to produce a precipitate which is insoluble both in aqueous and alcoholic media. It is clearly visible as an amorphous brown material in the light microscope (*Figure 2A*). Reaction of tissue with osmium tetroxide, i.e. after preparation for electron microscopy (see Chapter 1) results in the formation of a dark brown reaction product in the light micro-

Figure 2. Sections of the rat brain stained immunocytochemically by the ABC or PAP method using DAB as the chromogen for the peroxidase reaction. (A) is a light micrograph showing cell bodies (arrows) containing the amorphous DAB reaction product. The neuropil also contains axonal fibres and boutons (some of which are indicated by arrowheads). Some of the stained boutons surround unstained cell bodies (asterisks). (Rat cortex stained for parvalbumin immunoreactivity using the ABC method; Bennett and Bolam unpublished observations.) (B) is an electron micrograph of a dendrite (den) that contains the DAB immunoreaction product. Note that the reaction product is electron dense and associated with the membranes of intracellular organelles including mitochondria and microtubules. (Rat medial globus pallidus stained for choline acetyltransferase immunoreactivity using the PAP method.) (C) is an electron micrograph of vesicle-filled axonal boutons (b) containing DAB reaction product. Note that the immunostained boutons are electron dense compared to the non-immunoreactive bouton (asterisk), and have the floccular reaction product attached to the outer membrane of vesicles and mitochondria and the inner surface of the plasma membrane. (Rat entopeduncular nucleus stained by the PAP method to reveal substance P immunoreactivity.) Scale markers: (A) 10 μm, (B) 1 μm, (C) 0.5 μm.

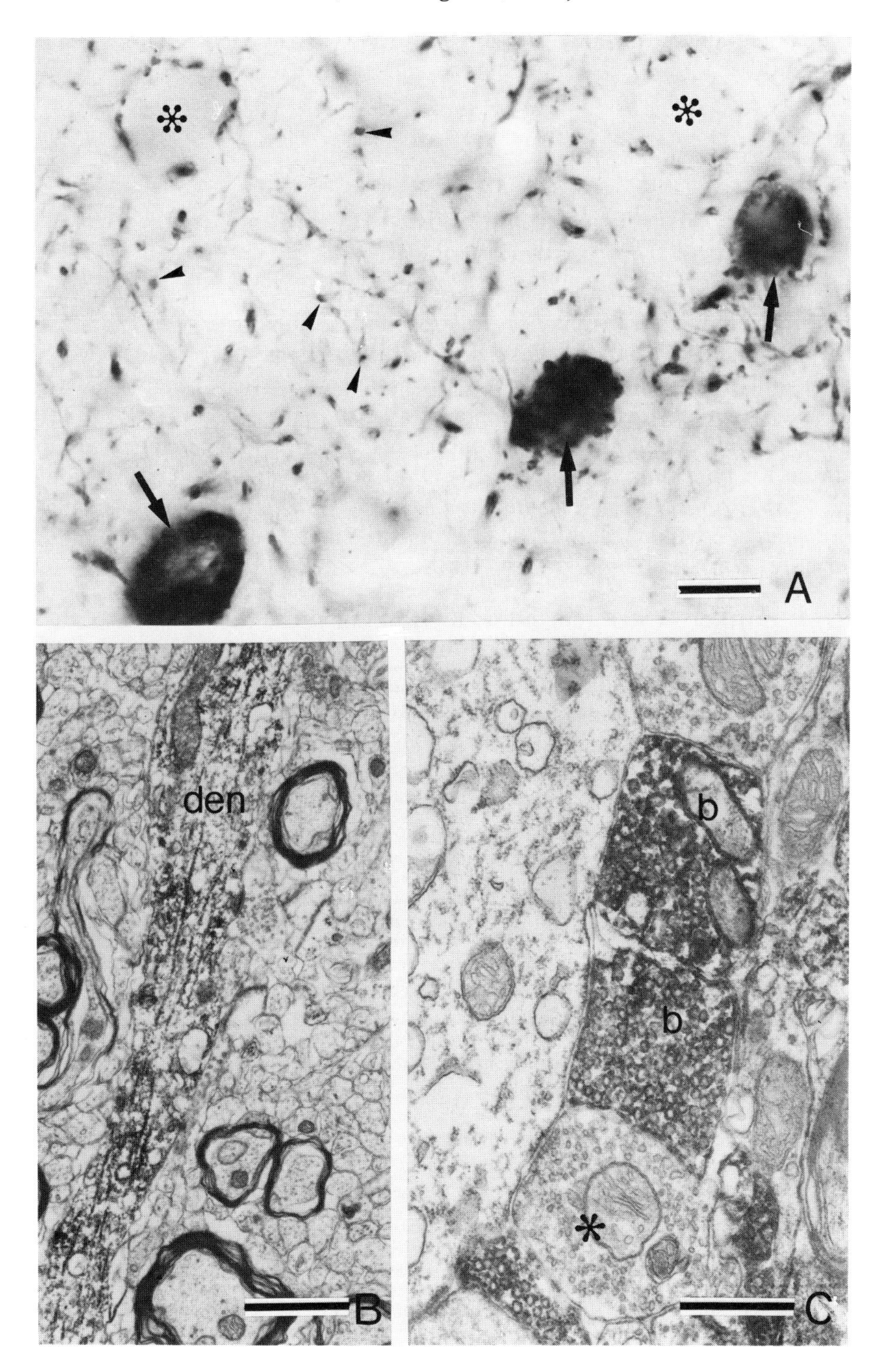
A
den
B
b
b
C

scope that is electron dense and thus clearly visible in the electron microscope (*Figures 2B, C* and *3B*). It appears as an homogeneous electron dense substance associated with the internal surface of the plasma membrane of stained structures and the external surface of subcellular organelle membranes (*Figures 2B, C* and *3B*).

6.6 Alternative chromogens and intensification methods for immunocytochemistry

In addition to DAB, other substances that produce reaction products with different characteristics may be used as chromogens in the peroxidase reactions. The use of chromogens that have different characteristics at both the light and the electron microscopic levels are of particular importance in double immunocytochemical protocols in which the marker is HRP for both antigens (see Chapter 10). Two examples are given, a non-carcinogenic substitute for benzidine derivatives (21) (*Protocol 10*), and a salt of benzidine (22, 23) (*Protocol 11*) (see *Safety note 4*, p. 123). The immunocytochemical procedures are identical to those in *Protocols 8* and *9* but *Protocols 10* and *11* substitute for steps **9–10**.

6.6.1 Hanker–Yates reagent as a chromogen for the immunoperoxidase reaction

This method was developed for localizing retrogradely-transported HRP (21) and was subsequently used for localizing intracellularly injected HRP (see Chapter 10). In this method aromatic amines and phenols are oxidized to form osmiophilic melanin-like polymers. The precipitate is dark brown/black in the light microscope and electron dense in the electron microscope. The reaction product is present throughout immunoreactive structures. It is similar to, but somewhat denser than that formed when DAB is used as a chromogen (24). The advantage of this method is the non-carcinogenic nature of the reagent. The disadvantage, however, is a relatively high background tissue staining. The reaction product can also be too dense in the electron microscope even without intensification.

Protocol 10. Hanker–Yates reagent with cobalt intensification as a chromogen for the immunoperoxidase reaction

Materials

- 0.1 M sodium cacodylate buffer, pH 7.4 (see *Protocol 2*)
- 0.1 M sodium cacodylate buffer, pH 5.1 (as above, but adjust pH with concentrated HCl)
- Hanker–Yates reagent (pyrocatechol/*p*-phenylenediamine, Sigma)
- cobalt chloride

- nickel sulphate
- hydrogen peroxide

Method

1. Wash sections for 2 × 10 min in 0.1 M sodium cacodylate buffer (pH 7.4).
2. Incubate at room temperature in several changes (10–15 min total) of a mixture consisting of:
   - 0.15% pyrocatechol/*p*-phenylenediamine (Hanker–Yates reagent, Sigma)
   - 0.6% cobalt chloride
   - 0.4% nickel sulphate
   - in 0.1 M sodium cacodylate buffer (pH 5.1)
3. Rinse 2 × 10 min in sodium cacodylate buffer (0.1 M, pH 7.4).
4. Incubate the sections for a further 15–20 min in 0.15% pyrocatechol/*p*-phenylenediamine containing 0.01% H_2O_2 (1 ml 1% H_2O_2 per 100 ml).
5. Rinse 2 × 10 min in sodium cacodylate buffer (0.1 M, pH 7.4).

6.6.2 Benzidine dihydrochloride (BDHC) as a chromogen for immunoperoxidase reaction (23)

Benzidine dihydrochloride forms a blue reaction product which turns dark blue/black or grey after osmium treatment. It is in the form of large granules or crystals within the labelled structures (*Figure 3A*). In the electron microscope the BDHC reaction product is electron dense and crystalline in appearance. The granules or crystals are not associated with any particular subcellular structure but are found scattered throughout the cytoplasm (*Figure 3B*). Occasionally reaction product is lost during the processing, leaving 'holes' within the labelled structures.

Safety note 4. Benzidine and its salts (including BDHC) are recognized carcinogens and should be treated with extreme caution. The substance should only be handled wearing protective clothing and in a fume cupboard. As with the benzidine derivatives, benzidine itself and salts of benzidine can be inactivated by reacting with chlorine bleach (sodium hypochlorite solution). All waste solutions, washings, and all contaminated materials should be placed in a large beaker or bucket containing excess bleach. After at least 30 minutes the inactivated solution can be washed down the sink with large volumes of water and materials washed extensively with water. Local Safety Officers should be consulted for local codes of practice for carcinogenic substances.

In the United Kingdom, it is forbidden by law (Control of Substances

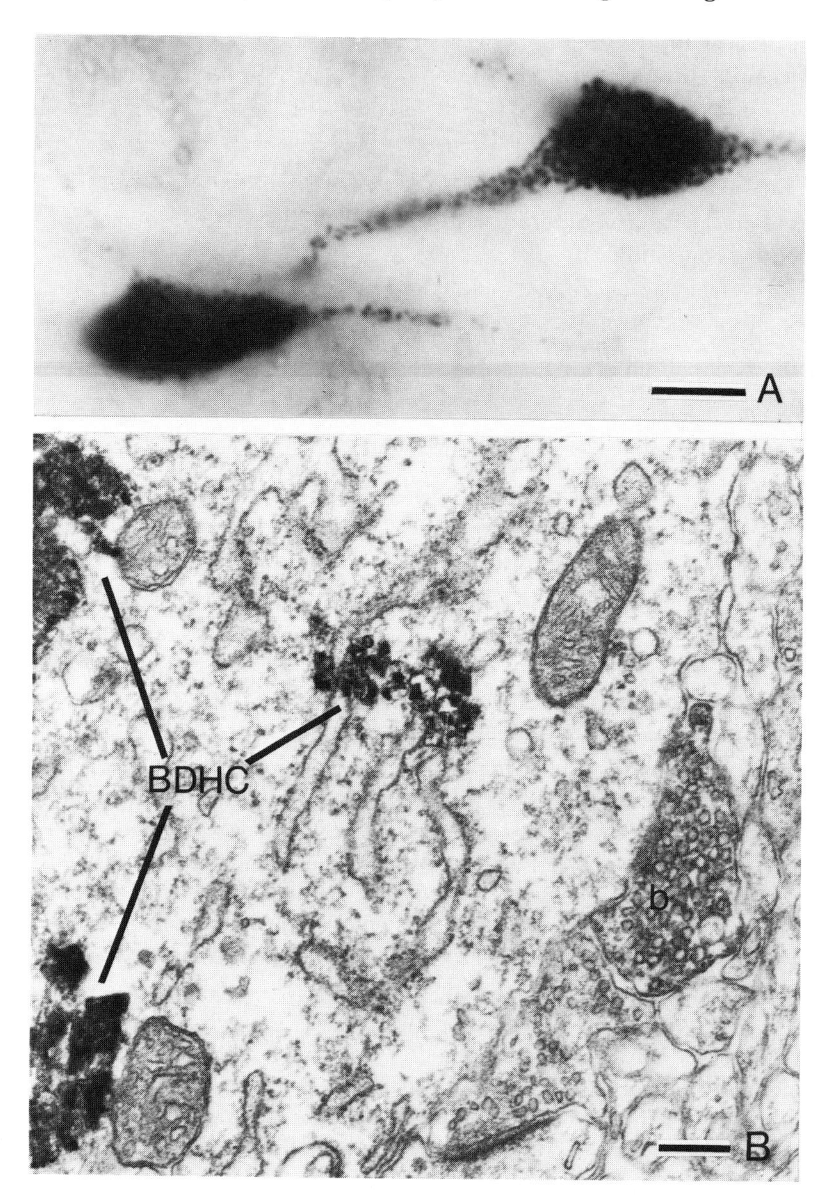

Figure 3. Sections of the rat striatum stained by the PAP method using BDHC as the chromogen for the peroxidase reaction. (A) is a light micrograph of two immunostained neurones that contain the BDHC reaction product. Note the granular nature of the reaction product and compare to the amorphous nature of the reaction product formed when DAB is used as the chromogen (*Figure 2A*). (B) is an electron micrograph of part of the cell body of a neurone that contains the BDHC immunoreaction product. Note the granular nature and electron density of the crystals of reaction product (BDHC) which shows no selective association with subcellular structures. This section was immunostained by a double

Hazardous to Health Regulations, 1988, COSHH) to use or import benzidine and its salts. Exemption certificates can be granted, applications should be lodged to the Health and Safety Executive through local safety officers.

Protocol 11. Benzidine dihydrochloride (BDHC) as a chromogen for immunoperoxidase reaction (see *Safety note 4*)

Materials

- 0.2 M phosphate buffer, pH 6.0–6.8
- 0.01 M phosphate buffer, pH 6.0–6.8
- 0.1 M phosphate buffer, pH 7.4
- sodium nitroprusside
- benzidine dihydrochloride (BDHC)[a]
- hydrogen peroxide

Method

1. Wash sections 2 × 10 min in phosphate buffer, pH 7.4.
2. Wash sections 2 × 10 min in 0.01 M phosphate buffer, pH 6.0–6.8.
3. Incubate for 10 min in reaction mixture prepared in the following manner:
   - dissolve 25 mg sodium nitroprusside in 95 ml distilled water
   - add 10 mg of BDHC[a] and stir until dissolved
   - add 5 ml of 0.2 M phosphate buffer (pH 6.0–6.8) to give a final concentration of 0.01 M
4. Add 20–40 μl of a 1:100 dilution of H_2O_2 (i.e. 0.3%) per 2.5 ml of reaction mixture, to each vial. Incubate for 1–10 min.[b] Monitor under a dissection microscope and stop reaction before background staining occurs, and before the solution turns blue.
5. Rinse 3 × 10 min in phosphate buffer (0.01 M, pH 6.0–6.8).
6. Osmium tetroxide treatment (Chapter 1, *Protocol 8*) should be carried out in phosphate buffer 0.1 M at the lower pH (6.8)

[a] BDHC is available from Sigma in sealed vials. Phosphate buffer containing sodium nitroprusside is added to the vial by means of a syringe and hypodermic needle thus avoiding any contact with the BDHC in powder form.

[b] If the reaction occurs too quickly, the amount of hydrogen peroxide can be reduced.

---

peroxidase method to reveal a second antigen using DAB as the chromogen (see Chapter 11, *Protocol 7*). A bouton apposed to the cell body contains the DAB reaction product (b). This micrograph illustrates the difference between the BDHC and DAB reaction products. Both micrographs are from sections of the rat striatum immunostained to reveal choline acetyltransferase immunoreactivity. The electron micrograph was also stained to reveal substance P immunoreactive boutons. Scale markers: (A) 12.5 μm, (B) 0.25 μm.

7. Enhancement of immunostaining

The signal produced by the immunocytochemical reaction can be enhanced either by increasing the number of marker molecules at the antigenic site, or by carrying out procedures that increase the amount of, or the intensity of, the reaction product.

Increasing the number of marker molecules at the antigenic site, i.e. amplification of the signal, is brought about by many of the procedures that have already been described. Thus the use of indirect methods increases the number of marker molecules as one molecule of bound primary antibody has several antigenic sites on it, and will therefore be bound by several molecules of the secondary antibody. Similarly, the use of the PAP method gives a marked amplification, since each molecule of secondary antibody binds a PAP complex which includes several (probably three) molecules of horseradish peroxidase.

7.1 Double bridge method

A further amplification step, referred to as the double bridge method, can be included in the PAP method by applying a second layer of the secondary antibody and a second layer of the PAP complex. Since the PAP complex is presumably bound to only one molecule of the secondary antibody (see *Figure 1*), then incubation with the secondary antibody again will result in the binding to the free antigenic sites on the immunoglobulins of the PAP complex. Provided the secondary antibody is again in excess, then free Fab fragments will be available to bind further PAP complexes. In the double bridge method it is convenient to use the *same* secondary antibody and PAP solutions used in the original incubations, and to expose the sections to these solutions for about one hour each, with appropriate washes between (steps **4–7** in *Protocol 8*).

7.2 Intensification of the immunoreaction product

Several methods are available for the intensification of the reaction product formed in peroxidase reactions most of which depend on the fact that metal ions can intensify the reaction product. The most commonly used system is to include either cobalt chloride ($CoCl_2$, at a concentration in the range of 0.01–0.02%) (see also Chapter 2), or ammonium nickel sulphate ($(NH_4)_2SO_4 . NiSO_4 . 6H_2O$; at a concentration in the range of 0.15–0.4%) (see Chapter 2, Chapter 9, *Protocol 9*, Chapter 11, *Protocol 4*) in the peroxidase reaction mixtures. The consequence of the presence of cobalt or nickel ions is a more intense reaction product that is blue/black in colour as opposed to the brown reaction product formed when DAB is used alone. Following treatment with osmium tetroxide, although the blue/black colour is sometimes retained in intensely stained neurones, it is usually the case that the reaction product takes on a brown colour similar to that produced by DAB alone.

8. Preparation of immunostained sections for electron microscopy

On completion of the immunostaining the sections that are for light microscopic analysis alone, are mounted on to gelatin-coated microscope slides, dehydrated, and coverslips applied (Chapter 1, *Protocols 5* and *6*). Those sections for electron microscopy are post-fixed in osmium tetroxide (Chapter 1, *Protocol 7*), dehydrated, and flat-embedded in electron microscopic resin on microscope slides (Chapter 1, *Protocol 8*), After the resin has set the sections are in a permanent form. They are examined in the light microscope for structures that contain the immunoreaction product and recorded and examined in the electron microscope as described in Chapter 1.

9. Controls

It is particularly important to carry out controls in immunocytochemical experiments because of the non-specific staining that may occur (see above) and because of the possibility of cross-reactivity of the immunoreagents. The most important control is to adsorb the primary antibody to the antigen against which it is directed. The adsorbed antiserum is then used in place of the non-adsorbed primary antiserum. This procedure should abolish all staining; any staining that remains is due to non-specific binding of the primary antibody, specific binding of contaminating immunoglobulins, or true cross-reactivity of the antiserum, i.e. it recognizes a site that occurs on more than one molecule. These possibilities should be taken into consideration when examining the sections. It is not always possible to adsorb the antiserum against the antigen because of limited availability of purified antigen, the 'second line' control is therefore to either omit altogether the primary antibody and substitute it with an equivalent dilution of normal serum, or to react a series of sections with increasing dilutions until all staining is lost. This control indicates that the staining is a result of the primary antibody preparation, it does not tell us about the specificity of the antiserum. Similarly omission of the secondary antibody or the PAP or ABC will tell whether either of the reagents or which step in the procedure is giving rise to non-specific staining. If non-specific staining occurs take precautions described above and obtain 'cleaner' immunoreagents.

References

1. Gerfen, C. R. and Sawchenko, P. E. (1984). *Brain Res.*, **343,** 144.
2. Coons, A. H. and Kaplan, M. H. (1950). *J. Exp. Med.*, **91,** 1.

3. Sternberger, L. A. (1979). *Immunocytochemistry*. J. Wiley and Sons, New York.
4. Bullock, G. R. and Petrusz, P. (ed.) (1982). *Techniques in Immunocytochemistry*. Academic Press, London.
5. Cuello, A. C. (ed.) (1983). *Immunohistochemistry*. J. Wiley and Sons, New York.
6. Polak, J. M. and Varndell, I. M. (ed.) (1984). *Immunolabelling for Electron Microscopy*. Elsevier Science Publishers, Amsterdam.
7. Izzo, P. N. and Bolam, J. P. (1988). *J. Comp. Neurol.*, **269**, 219.
8. Bolam, J. P., Francis, C. M., and Henderson, Z. (1991). *Neurosci.*, **41**, 483.
9. Somogyi, P. and Takagi, H. (1982). *Neurosci.*, **7**, 1779.
10. Somogyi, P., Priestley, J. V., Cuello, A. C., Smith, A. D., and Takagi, H. (1982). *J. Neurocytol.*, **11**, 779.
11. Freund, T. F. (1989). *Brain Res.*, **478**, 375.
12. Berod, A., Hartman, B. K., and Pujo, J. F. (1981). *J. Histochem. Cytochem.*, **29**, 844.
13. Eldred, W. D., Zucker, C., Karten, H. J., and Yazulla, S. (1983). *J. Histochem. Cytochem.*, **31**, 285.
14. Geffard, M., Buijs, R. M., Seguela, P., Pool, C. W., and LeMoal, M. (1984). *Brain. Res.*, **294**, 161.
15. Buijs, R. M., Geffard, M., Pool, C. W., and Hooneman, E. M. D. (1984). *Brain Res.*, **323**, 65.
16. Wouterlood, F. G., Sauren, Y. M. F. H., and Pattiselanno, A. (1988). *J. Chem. Neuroanat.*, **1**, 65.
17. Finley, J. C. W. and Petrusz, P. (1982). In *Techniques in Immunocytochemistry* (ed. G. R. Bullock, and P. Petrusz), pp. 239–49. Academic Press, London.
18. Beaulieu, C. and Somogyi, P. (1991). *J. Comp. Neurol.*, **304**, 666.
19. Kosaka, T., Nagatsu, I., Wu, J-Y., and Hama, K. (1986). *Neurosci.*, **18**, 975.
20. Hsu, S. M., Raine, L., and Fanger, H. (1981). *J. Histochem. Cytochem.*, **29**, 577.
21. Hanker, J. S. and Yates, P. E. (1977). *Histochem. J.*, **9**, 789.
22. Lakos, S. and Basbaum, A. I. (1986). *J. Histochem. Cytochem.*, **34**, 1047.
23. Levey, A. I., Bolam, J. P., Rye, D. B., Hallanger, A. E., Demuth, M., Mesulam, M. M., and Wainer, B. H. (1986). *J. Histochem. Cytochem.*, **34**, 1449.
24. Maxwell, D. J., Christie, W. M., and Somogyi, P. (1989). *Neurosci.*, **33**, 169.

6

Immunocytochemistry II: post-embedding staining

C. A. INGHAM

1. Introduction

Post-embedding immunocytochemistry involves carrying out immunocytochemical techniques on tissue which has been fixed, dehydrated, and embedded in a material suitable for cutting sections for subsequent light or electron microscopy, (e.g. wax, celloidin, resin). It is beyond the scope of this chapter to discuss all the available techniques and so it will concentrate on post-embedding methods applied to material which has been prepared in the conventional manner for electron microscopy, including post-fixation with osmium tetroxide and embedding in epoxy resin. Many antigens do not survive this treatment; their antigenicity may be affected by osmium tetroxide treatment, by resin infiltration (possibly due to interactions of the antigen with epoxy groups), and by heat (1–3). However, amino acids such as γ-aminobutyric acid (GABA), glutamate, aspartate, taurine, glycine, and glutamine have been successfully localized using these methods (4).

It is possible to employ specialized post-embedding methods to examine more sensitive antigens. Peptide distribution can be analysed at the light and electron microscopical level using tissue embedded in conventional epoxy resins but not treated with osmium tetroxide (5). For antigens which are sensitive to epoxy resin infiltration, hydrophilic acrylic embedding media such as Lowicryl K4M and LR White are alternatives (6–8). Readers should refer to the referenced papers for details about the above techniques.

The post-embedding method on epoxy resin embedded material can be applied at the light microscope level using 0.5–1 μm semi-thin sections, and at the electron microscope level using 80–150 nm thin sections.

As with all immunocytochemical methods a number of different markers can be used to visualize the location of the antigens. The method of choice for post-embedding semi-thin immunocytochemistry is the immunoperoxidase technique, using a biotinylated secondary antibody and an avidin–biotin–peroxidase complex, followed by peroxidase histochemistry using diaminobenzidine as the chromogen. The method of choice for post-embedding thin section immunocytochemistry is the immunogold technique. Colloidal gold adsorbed to a secondary antibody is the method described in this chapter (9), however, gold adsorbed to protein A is an alternative method (6).

1.1 Why use post-embedding immunocytochemistry?

There are several advantages to using post-embedding rather than pre-embedding immunocytochemistry (Chapter 5).

(a) Penetration problems (see Chapter 5) are minimized because sections are only 80–1000 nm thick.

(b) Minimizing penetration problems means that tissue can be fixed optimally for electron microscopy so that ultrastructural preservation is good. This greatly aids analysis and interpretation.

(c) Material that has been embedded and stored can be immunostained retrospectively. This can be particularly useful for double labelling techniques, such as intracellular filling (see Chapters 9 and 10). It also means techniques can be optimized and repeated in the same material without having to prepare more animals.

(d) Serial sections of the same tissue can be processed in different ways to examine the same structures using other antisera and control solutions.

(e) Quantification is possible because penetration problems are minimized. The immunogold technique results in a particulate end product which can be quantified easily.

(f) The immunostaining procedure takes only a few hours to complete compared to several days for pre-embedding immunocytochemistry.

There are, however, some disadvantages to the method.

(a) It is not applicable to all antigens. Although specialized techniques can be employed to localize more sensitive antigens (see above), the quality of ultrastructural preservation is often diminished which means that one of the main attributes of the technique ((b) above) is then lost.

(b) To enable successful immunostaining to be performed, the epoxy resin embedding media has to be oxidized and osmium tetroxide has to be removed from the tissue. This introduces variability into the reaction; different material reacts differently to the treatment, and there appears to be some variability between different post-embedding experiments. Consequently, it is only possible to make comparisons between different animals and between different post-embedding experiments after rigid controls. This is particularly important if quantification is carried out.

(c) The removal of osmium tetroxide (b) results in lowered contrast in the electron microscope which can cause difficulty with analysis and interpretation.

1.2 Applications

In experimental neuronatomy, post-embedding immunocytochemistry is used for exactly the same reasons as pre-embedding immunocytochemistry (Chapter 5), i.e. to visualize the distribution of neurochemicals. These are often neurotransmitter related compounds; the transmitter itself, the synthetic or breakdown enzymes for that transmitter, or the post-synaptic receptor sites.

2. Fixation

This is critical to the success of the method. The methods described in this chapter apply to antisera which recognize antigen conjugated to bovine serum albumin with glutaraldehyde (10, 11). The GABA antiserum recognizes, in part, the linkage of GABA to glutaraldehyde (11, 12). It is important to create identical cross-linking in the tissue to be examined which means introducing a glutaraldehyde based fixative into the tissue rapidly. In practice, the optimal method involves a rapid clearing of the blood vessels via the aorta with calcium free Tyrode's solution (30–60 sec) (see Chapter 1, Appendix 1), followed by a mixed aldehydes perfusion. The optimum fixative is 2.5% glutaraldehyde, 1% paraformaldehyde in sodium phosphate buffer, pH 7.4. The aldehyde mix is reasonably flexible, although it is inadvisable to reduce glutaraldehyde concentrations to below 1%. Details of preparation of these solutions and of the actual perfusion method are given in Chapter 1, *Protocols 2* and *3* as are details of safety precautions (*Safety note 1*, p. 5). The rate of perfusion should be between 10 and 50 ml/min for a 200–300 g rat, and each animal should receive at least 500 ml of fixative. Use a fast rate for the first 5–10 min (40–50 ml/min) followed by a slower rate for an additional 20 min (10–15 ml/min). Post-fix the brain for at least one to two hours in the same fixative (this time may vary for different material, e.g. cat spinal cord requires eight hours' post-fixation). After post-fixation the tissue should be placed in 0.1 M sodium phosphate buffer, pH 7.4 (PB) at 4°C until sectioning or preparation of blocks. This can be overnight if necessary.

3. Preparation of tissue (see Chapter 1, *Protocol 4*)

Prepare the fixed tissue by cutting 50–100 μm sections on a vibrating microtome, (e.g. Vibratome—Lancer) or by preparing standard EM size blocks of tissue from the region of interest. Vibratome sections allow other techniques to be performed before dehydration (see Chapter 11) and allow more accurate selection of areas of interest. Post-fix with osmium tetroxide (Chapter 1, *Protocol 7*), dehydrate, and embed sections or blocks in a conventional resin (we use Durcupan, Fluka) (Chapter 1, *Protocol 8*). Carry out light microscopic analysis and photomicroscopy before re-embedding areas of interest (see Chapter 1).

4. Post-embedding immunocytochemistry on semi-thin sections using the immunoperoxidase technique

This procedure involves mounting semi-thin sections on glass slides and then taking them through solutions which etch the resin and remove osmium tetroxide, followed by immunocytochemicals and peroxidase histochemicals. This is carried out by processing either the whole slide or just the sections on the slide (by dropping small amounts of the solutions on to the top of the sections). Finally the sections are dehydrated and coverslips applied. The following protocol uses diaminobenzidine tetrahydrochloride as the chromogen in the peroxidase histochemistry, but other chromogens can be employed. The immunoperoxidase procedure has been discussed in detail in Chapter 5. Preparing glass microscope slides coated in gelatin, and cutting semi-thin sections are described in *Protocol 1*.

Protocol 1. Coating slides with gelatin, and cutting semi-thin sections (see also Chapter 1, *Protocol 5*)

1. [a]Mix equal volumes of:
   - 1% gelatin (heat gently to dissolve)
   - 2% paraformaldehyde (see Chapter 1, *Protocol 2*)

   Warm whilst stirring until the solution is clear. This solution can be kept for several months at 4°C.
2. Mark 3–4 small circles close together with a diamond pencil on the reverse side of microscope slides for later positioning of sections.
3. Reheat gelatin mixture until it forms a clear solution. Quickly, take a cotton bud soaked in the gelatin mixture and draw over the region of the slide which is to be used for mounting the sections (approximately 1 × 4 cm rectangle). This restricted coating helps to prevent the flow of solutions away from the mounted sections.
4. Dry on hot plate (hand-hot).
5. Cut 0.5–1 μm semi-thin sections on to distilled H_2O using an ultramicrotome and a glass knife. Several sections can be taken from a good part of the knife but look out for the first signs of score marks and should these occur move to a new part of the knife, or a new knife. Transfer sections to droplets of H_2O overlying the scored circles on the gelatin-coated slides. Place on a hot plate (hand-hot) to dry. Place about three sections on each droplet unless it is important to know the order of a series when sections can be placed singly in sequence along the slide.

It is not practical to take more than three slides through the staining procedure at one time unless large quantities of immunochemicals are available. In the latter situation staining dishes can be used.

[a] Note that an alternative subbing solution is to mix equal volumes of egg albumin powder and glycerol (filtered and stored at 4°C with a crystal of thymol added) which is smeared on to the slides as described above and dried in an oven at 56°C.

4.1 Immunocytochemistry for semi-thin sections

The following are required for immunocytochemistry on semi-thin sections (*Figure 2A*).

- oven (56°C)
- Coplin jars (approximately three)
- at least three glass Petri dishes (112 × 20 mm)
- saturated ethanolic NaOH (see below)
- sodium metaperiodate ($NaIO_4$)
- Tris and phosphate-buffered saline (TPBS—0.01 M Tris-HCl buffer, pH 7.5, 0.01 M PB, pH 7.4, 0.9% NaCl)
- primary antiserum raised in species *x* (we have used GABA antiserum kindly provided by Dr P. Somogyi)
- biotinylated secondary antibody raised in species *y* against IgG's from species *x* (Vector Laboratories)
- normal serum from species *y*, i.e. the species in which secondary antibody was raised (N*y*S) (Scottish Antibody Production Unit, SAPU)
- avidin–biotin–peroxidase complex (Vector Laboratories)
- 0.05 M Tris-HCl buffer pH 7.5 (TB)
- diaminobenzidine tetrahydrochloride (DAB, Sigma) (see *Safety note 3* in Chapter 5, p. 119)
- 0.1 M sodium phosphate buffer, pH 7.4 (PB)

Protocol 2. Immunocytochemistry on semi-thin sections (see *Figure 2A*)

1. Prepare a saturated solution of ethanolic NaOH at least two to three days prior to the experiment by adding excess NaOH pellets (stirring) to 100 ml of absolute ethanol. Stir until NaOH forms a solid lump, when stirring becomes impossible. The solution is ready to use when it turns brown.

Steps **2–8**: *carry out in staining dishes or Coplin jars.*

2. Immerse slides in saturated ethanolic NaOH (removes resin) for 1 h.

Protocol 2. *Continued*

3. Drain well and wash in fresh 100% ethanol for 5 × 3 min.
4. Wash in distilled H_2O for 5 × 2 min.
5. Place in 1% sodium metaperiodate (removes osmium tetroxide) for 7 min.
6. Wash in distilled H_2O for 5 × 2 min.
7. Wash in TPBS for 2 × 10 min.
8. Dry slides around the sections with a tissue and place flat in a humid chamber.[a]

Steps **9–18**: *apply drops of the following solution to the sections.*

9. Normal serum of appropriate species (N*y*S), 20% in TPBS for 20 min.
10. TPBS for 3 × 10 min.
11. Antiserum raised in species *x* against antigen of interest (dilution varies for different antisera) in 1% N*y*S in TPBS, overnight at 4°C.
12. TPBS for 3 × 10 min.
13. Biotinylated *y* anti *x* immunoglobulin G, diluted 1:200 in 1% N*y*S in TPBS for 1 h.
14. TPBS for 3 × 10 min. Make up avidin–biotin–peroxidase complex (see step **15**) during this wash, as it needs to stand for 30 min before use.
15. Avidin–biotin–peroxidase complex in 1% N*y*S in TPBS (1:50) for 1 h.
16. TPBS for 3 × 10 min.
17. 0.1 M PB for 4 × 5 min.
18. 0.05 M TB for 2 × 5 min.

Steps **19–22**: *carry out in Coplin jars or staining dishes*

19. Incubate in 0.05% DAB in TB for 20 min. Take the necessary safety precautions as described in Chapter 5, *Safety note 3*, p. 119.
20. Add 1% H_2O_2 to the DAB incubation solution to make a final concentration of 0.01%, (e.g. 500 μl 1% H_2O_2 to 50 ml 0.05% DAB). Incubate 6–10 min.
21. Wash in TB for 4 × 5 min.
22. Wash in PB for 4 × 5 min.
23. Lay slide flat in a Petri dish and apply 1% osmium tetroxide in PB for 10 min. Take necessary safety precautions as described in Chapter 1, *Safety note 3*, p. 13.
24. Wash in PB for 4 × 5 min.
25. Wash in H_2O for 5 min.

26. Dehydrate and mount with standard LM mountant, (e.g. DPX)—see Chapter 1, *Protocol 6*.

[a] High humidity is maintained by placing tissue paper soaked in water around the edge of the dish and by keeping it closed whenever possible. The slides are placed flat so that droplets of the solutions can be pipetted on to the top of the sections. Use approximately 500 μl of each solution per slide. The solution should stay as one single droplet covering the area with sections on it but should not cover the whole slide (to avoid using large volumes of the immunochemicals). The solutions can be removed by picking up the slide (it helps to have the slide sitting on Parafilm or Plasticene) and pouring the solution away. A little of the washing solution can be pipetted gently over the sections at this point before replacing the slide in the humid Petri dish (having dried off excess liquid from around the sections).

5. Post-embedding immunocytochemistry of thin sections using the immunogold technique

This procedure involves cutting thin sections, mounting them on coated single-slot grids (gold or nickel), and then incubating the sections by floating the grids on droplets of the various solutions which results in the deposition of gold particles at immunoreactive sites (see *Figure 1*). The immunogold technique is the method of choice to localize immunoreactive sites as it allows good resolution of immunopositive structures which are not obscured by the gold particles. Immunoperoxidase techniques can be used but the electron dense reaction product obscures the ultrastructural details of immunoreactive processes and it cannot be quantified easily. As in the semi-thin method, before applying the immunochemicals, the resin is oxidized and osmium is removed. Epoxy resins are hydrophobic but if the alkane side chains are oxidized to alcohols, aldehydes, and acids, a hydrophilic gel may form on the

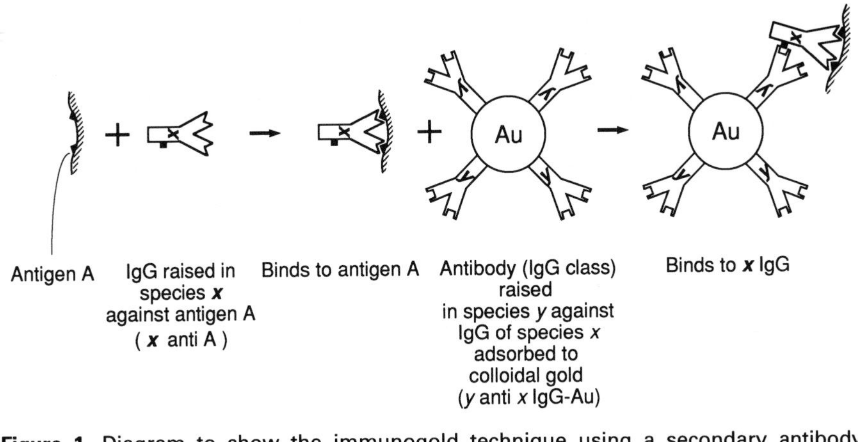

Figure 1. Diagram to show the immunogold technique using a secondary antibody adsorbed to colloidal gold.

surface of the section allowing the immunoreaction to take place (2). The grids have to be made from an inert metal so that they are not oxidized during these procedures. Gold grids, although more expensive and very delicate, are generally preferable to nickel grids as the latter magnetize very easily which makes them difficult to handle. The immunogold method is then carried out by floating the grids on the antiserum followed by colloidal gold adsorbed to a secondary antibody (*Figure 1*). Thus, the antigenic site is localized in the electron microscope by the presence of gold particles. The size of the gold particles can vary. They should be large enough to be seen reasonably easily in the electron microscope, but small enough not to obscure intracellular components that may be of interest. For labelling synaptic boutons, 15 nm diameter colloidal gold appears to be the optimal choice. Different sized gold particles can be used to localize more than one antigen in the same tissue (6).

5.1 Cutting thin sections for post-embedding immunocytochemistry

A diamond knife is ideal for cutting sections suitable for post-embedding immunocytochemistry because long unbroken series of sections are generally required. Glass knives can be used but serial sections can not be collected reliably.

When starting this technique it is advisable to collect series of sections as pairs mounted alternately on coated (see Chapter 1, *Protocol 10*) copper single-slot grids and gold single-slot grids. The sections mounted on the copper grids are not immunostained but are examined in the electron microscope after lead staining (see Chapter 1, *Protocol 11*). This aids orientation when immunostained sections are examined. This can be vital if the contrast of the immunostained sections is very low (due to removal of the osmium tetroxide, step **3** below). Similarly, if the material has been already stained using another method, (e.g. by a peroxidase reaction using DAB as the chromogen), the electron dense reaction product is bleached to some extent during the post-embedding procedure, and peroxidase stained structures often have to be identified from neighbouring non-immunostained sections. Short series of two or three sections are also required when using more than one antiserum or control solution, that is in cases where it is important to study the *same* structure under different staining conditions. In other situations it is preferable to have long series of sections on the same grid so that structures can be followed through many serial sections.

Sections should be cut slightly thicker than is normally acceptable for electron microscopy. Silver/gold sections (100–150 nm) should be cut in preference to grey/silver sections (80–100 nm). When added to the thickness of the grid coating the sections should look gold/purple. The extra thickness increases the contrast in the electron microscope but should be varied to achieve optimum results for all material.

5.2 Post-embedding immunogold technique for thin sections

The following are required for post-embedding immunogold staining (*Figure 2B*).

- diamond knife—optional (Diatome)
- copper and gold grids
- large diameter glass Petri dishes (112 × 20 mm), at least three
- small glass vials, (15 ml), approximately 10
- disposable, plastic syringes (2 × 10 ml, 5 × 5 ml)
- Millipore swinnex disc filter holders (size 13 mm), box of 10
- Millipore swinnex disc filter holders (size 25 mm), box of 12
- MF-Millipore membrane filters for above (pore size 0.22 μm)
- periodic acid (H_5IO_6)
- sodium metaperiodate ($NaIO_4$)
- Tris and phosphate-buffered saline (TPBS—0.01 M Tris-HCl buffer, pH 7.5, 0.01 M PB, pH 7.4, 0.9% NaCl)
- primary antiserum raised in species *x* against antigen of interest (we have used GABA antiserum kindly provided by Dr P. Somogyi, and glutamate antiserum kindly provided by Drs O. P. Ottersen and J. Storm-Mathisen)
- secondary antiserum raised in species *y* against IgG's found in species *x* adsorbed to colloidal gold, e.g. 15 nm diameter (Janssen Life Sciences)
- normal serum (from species in which secondary antibody was raised (N*y*S))
- polyethylene glycol

All water used should be double distilled or membrane filtered. This and all solutions except antisera, must be filtered using Millipore (or equivalent) filters (0.22 μm pore size). Use a 10 ml syringe with a 25 mm filter unit for filtering water, and a 5 ml syringe with the 13 mm filter unit for all other solutions. Antisera should always be diluted with filtered solutions, but the antisera themselves should not be filtered. Most of the steps are carried out by floating the grids (sections down) on small droplets (40–50 μl each) of the various solutions. The droplets are placed on pieces of Parafilm in large Petri dishes. When buffers are used as diluents or for washes, the Petri dish must be kept humid to avoid evaporation and subsequent crystal formation on the grids. The humidity is maintained by keeping moist tissue paper in the dish. For the same reason care should be taken to avoid contact of the solutions with the side of the grid which has no sections on it. The minimum number of Petri dishes is three; this allows two steps to be prepared in advance. As soon as grids have been removed from one Petri dish the used droplets are absorbed with tissue paper and fresh Parafilm placed in the dish which is then

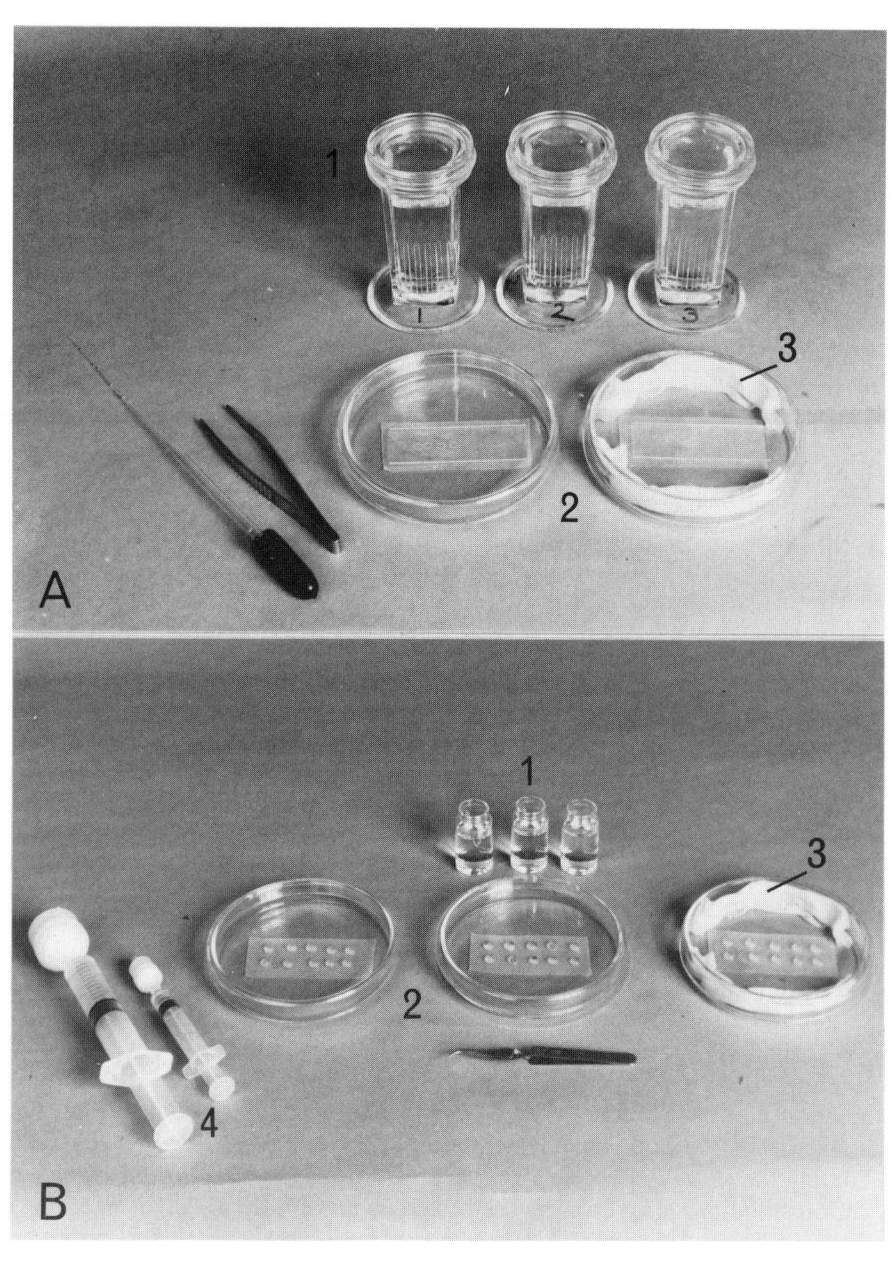

Figure 2. Apparatus for post-embedding immunocytochemistry. (A) Post-embedding immunocytochemistry on semi-thin sections. (1)—three Coplin jars, (2)—two Petri dishes, in which glass slides are placed on Parafilm. Moist tissue paper (3) keeps one Petri dish humid. (B) Post-embedding immunocytochemistry on thin sections. (1)—glass vials containing filtered water for washing, (2)—glass Petri dishes in which droplets of solutions are sitting on Parafilm. Moist tissue paper (3) keeps one Petri dish humid. (4)—disposable syringes attached to Millipore filters. Gold single-slot grids are floating on the droplets in the middle Petri dish.

ready for addition of the next set of droplets. Some of the rinsing steps are carried out by immersing the grids in small vials of water, after which excess water is dried off the forceps and the grid with tissue and filter paper. Grids should be placed on the droplets at regularly spaced time intervals, (e.g. 20 sec) to allow for washing at the end of the step. Once experienced in the procedure it is possible to process 10–12 grids in one experiment (try six for the first run). The procedure is slightly modified from that developed by Somogyi and Hodgson (13). At the start of the experiment each grid to be immunostained should be identified and its position noted. It is important that all glassware and containers are clean.

Protocol 3. Post-embedding immunogold staining for thin sections (see *Figure 2B*)

Place grids, sections down, at 20 sec intervals on to droplets of the following solutions.

1. Filtered 1% periodic acid. Periodic acid oxidizes the resin to allow access of the immunochemicals. Vary time to achieve optimal results; try 10 min at first.
2. Wash; pick up each grid in turn and dip it in three vials of filtered H_2O (approximately five quick dips in each). Dry forceps with tissue and/or filter paper (especially the drop between the ends as H_2O collects here) and place on droplet of H_2O.[a]
3. 1% filtered sodium metaperiodate for 10 min.[b]
4. Repeat step **2**.
5. Filtered TPBS for 2 × 10 min. From this stage onwards keep the Petri dish humid.
6. Filtered 5% normal serum (N*y*S) in TPBS for 30 min.
7. Filtered 1% normal serum (N*y*S) in TPBS for 10 min.
8. Primary antiserum diluted[c] in filtered 1% N*y*S in TPBS for 1–3 h.
9. Filtered 0.05% polyethylene glycol in 0.05 M Tris-HCl buffer pH 7.5 (PEG/TB) for 4 × 10 min.
10. Gold-labelled secondary antibody diluted 1:10 in filtered PEG/TB, for 1.5–2 h.[d]
11. Wash grids in five vials of filtered H_2O, as in step **2**, and then float on a drop of H_2O.
12. Stain with 1% aqueous uranyl acetate (optional if *en bloc* stained already) for 15 min–1 h.
13. Rinse under a stream of distilled H_2O from a wash bottle.

Protocol 3. *Continued*

14. Stain sections with lead citrate ((14), see Chapter 1, *Protocol 11*).

[a] If the water is not removed, the grid tends to stick to the forceps and can flip over as well as being difficult to place on the next droplet.
[b] This solution removes osmium tetroxide which hinders the immunoreaction but as a consequence contrast in the electron microscope is reduced. The time and concentration (up to about 9%) can be varied to achieve maximum staining with an acceptable loss of contrast.
[c] Optimal dilution should be determined empirically. Primary antisera usually in region of 1:1000.
[d] Polyethylene glycol helps to prevent aggregates of gold particles forming. Alternative diluents can be used such as 1% bovine serum albumin, 0.5% Tween 20 in 0.05 M Tris-HCl buffer.

6. Control procedures for semi-thin and thin section immunocytochemistry

As with all immunocytochemistry it is important to verify the specificity of the technique. Some of these procedures have been discussed already in Chapter 5. The advantage of post-embedding immunocytochemistry for control procedures is that serial sections of a single structure can be processed on different slides or grids under different experimental conditions. For the semi-thin technique it is usual to process one slide for the control sections to avoid the possibility of mixing solutions. For thin sections, two or three sections should be mounted in series and then alternate grids processed with the control or experimental incubation media. This allows the same structure, (e.g. synaptic bouton) to be examined under the different conditions.

6.1 Omission of the primary antiserum

Incubate sections in the diluent only at step **11**, *Protocol 2* for semi-thin sections, and step **8**, *Protocol 3* for thin sections, otherwise treat the control sections in exactly the same way as the test sections. There should be no staining of the control sections.

6.2 Substitution of the primary antiserum

The primary antiserum is substituted by one or each of the following at the same dilution as the original primary antiserum.

(a) Normal serum from the species in which the primary antiserum was raised.
(b) Antiserum adsorbed to antigen of interest. This ensures that the primary antiserum is specifically recognizing the antigen of interest. In the case of antisera which recognize a glutaraldehyde conjugated substance the

appropriate antigen is likewise glutaraldehyde conjugated. Structures that are immunoreactive in adjacent serial sections processed with normal antiserum should not be labelled; in fact as in Section 6.1 there should be no labelling whatsoever.

(c) Antiserum adsorbed to inappropritae but similar antigens which may cross-react with the antiserum. In this case immunostaining should be similar in the control and experimental sections. If the immunostaining is weaker in these controls then cross-reaction should be suspected, and primary antiserum adsorbed to the suspect antigen/antigens should be used routinely.

6.3 Test sample

Once a particular tissue/block has been found to give good results with the post-embedding technique it can be used as a positive control to compare with other tissue, acting as a control against any errors made in individual experimental runs.

6.4 Sandwich test sections

The use of sandwich test sections is a method developed by Ottersen ((15), also see review by Ottersen (4)) for testing amino acid antisera. In brief, the technique involves the production of brain macromolecules conjugated with a known concentration of various amino acids (GABA, glutamate, taurine, glycine, aspartate, and glutamine) in the presence of glutaraldehyde and then freeze dried. These amino acid–glutaraldehyde–brain macromolecule complexes are embedded in resin, sections are cut (5 μm for subsequent semi-thin immunostaining, 2 μm for subsequent thin section immunostaining). These sections are piled on top of a resin support alternated with sections of the same thickness from brain tissue prepared for electron microscopy in the normal way. This resulting pile of sections (macromolecule conjugated to different amino acids alternating with normal brain tissue) is re-embedded, and sections (semi-thin or thin) are cut at right angles to the original sections so that all layers of the sandwich appear on each section. Sections prepared in this way can be routinely included in semi-thin or thin post-embedding immunocytochemistry. The only macromolecule conjugate to be labelled should be that conjugated to the relevant amino acid. This control is particularly important for evaluating antisera to antigens which are widely distributed in nervous tissue.

A second type of multilayered sandwich block can be constructed by preparing a series of antigen–glutaraldehyde brain protein conjugates with different antigen concentrations ranging from low, (e.g. 0.1 mmol/litre) to high, (e.g. 154 mmol/litre). This can be used to examine the relationship between concentration of antigen and numbers of gold particles (16).

6.5 Test runs

All new material and new antisera should be processed initially in test runs to establish the optimum conditions. The optimum conditions can vary with different fixation procedures and so it is advisable to test all new tissue. The following parameters should be examined:

- times of incubation and dilution of antisera
- time in ethanolic NaOH or periodic acid
- time of incubation and concentration of sodium metaperiodate.

7. Analysis and interpretation

Immunopositive structures in the semi-thin technique are recognized by the brown reaction product formed when DAB is used as the chromogen. Both immunoreactive boutons and cell bodies can be identified. Serial sections should be examined to establish consistent labelling (*Figure 3*). In *Figure 3* GABA-immunoreactive punctate structures are scattered throughout the neuropil and are generally darker than the immunoreactive cell bodies. Both types of immunoreactive structures are easily distinguishable from pale non-immunoreactive structures.

Structures that are immunopositive in the immunogold procedure are recognized by the relatively high concentrations of gold particles overlying them compared to other structures (*Figure 4*). The presence of a uniform scattering of immunogold particles over the tissue implies non-specific staining. In order to assess labelling the following checklist can be followed.

(a) Is the distribution of gold particles overlying the tissue heterogeneous? (see *Figures 4, 5*).

(b) Are specific structures associated with gold particles?

(c) Find a structure which you believe to be labelled in one section and examine it in several serial sections. Is the labelling consistent? Repeat this for a number of structures (see *Figure 4*).

(d) Find a structure which you believe to be unlabelled and follow it through serial sections to check that the lack of gold particles is consistent (see *Figure 4*).

(e) Quantify the density of gold particle labelling over different structures (see below) and compare them using statistical analysis (Section 7.1.3). Do this in random and serial sections. This is particularly important with substances that have a metabolic role as well as a neurotransmitter role, (e.g. glutamate).

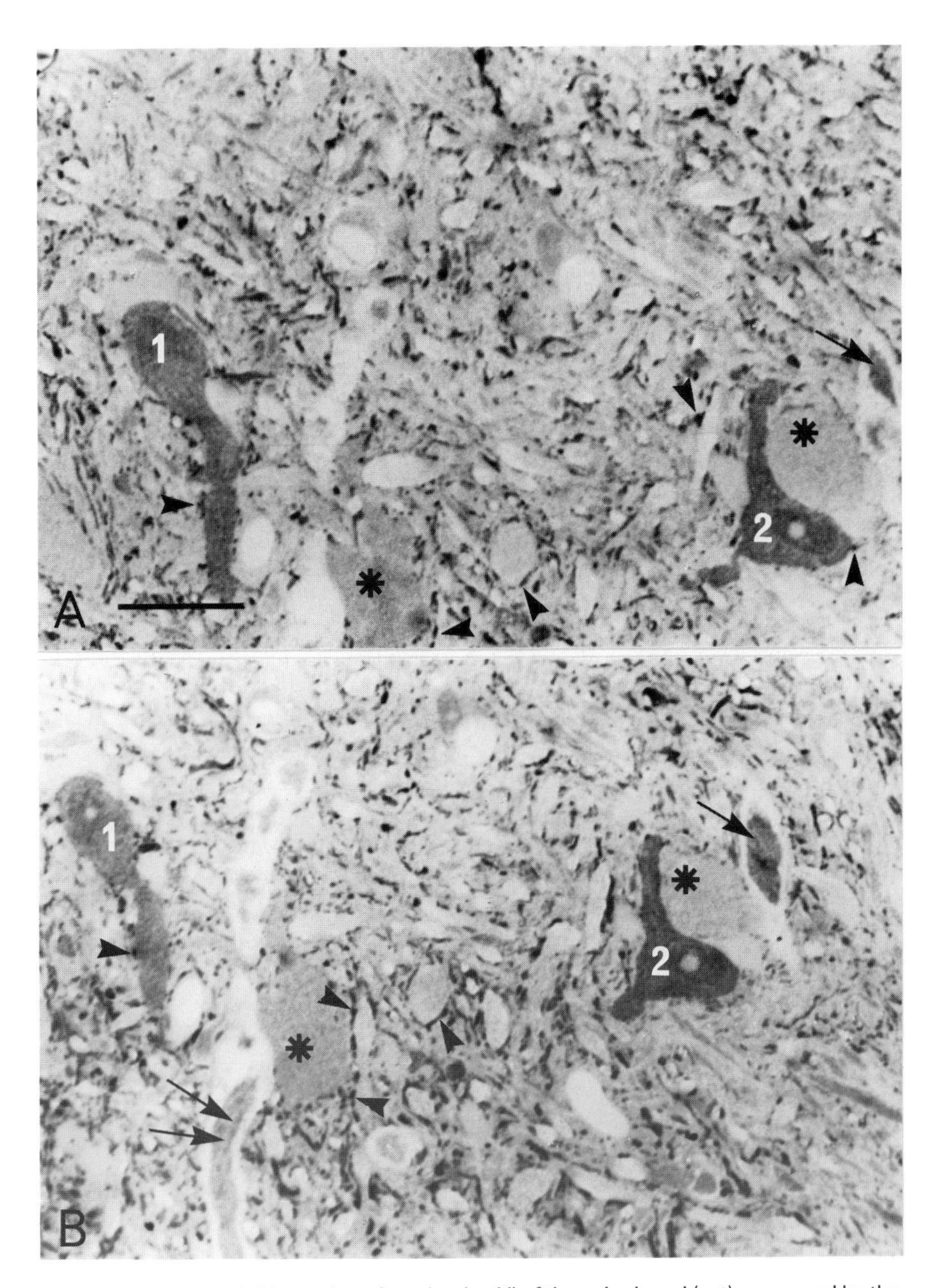

Figure 3. Serial semi-thin sections from lamina VI of the spinal cord (cat) processed by the post-embedding immunocytochemical method to reveal GABA. Many immunoreactive punctate structures, some of which are indicated by arrowheads, are scattered throughout the tissue and surround immunoreactive and non-immunoreactive structures. Two immunoreactive cell bodies (1, 2) with primary dendrites are visible in both (A) and (B). Non-immunoreactive cells are also present (asterisks). Large immunoreactive (single arrow) and non-immunoreactive (two arrows) myelinated axons are also visible. Scale bar = 25 μm. (The material used for these photographs was kindly provided by Dr. D. J. Maxwell.)

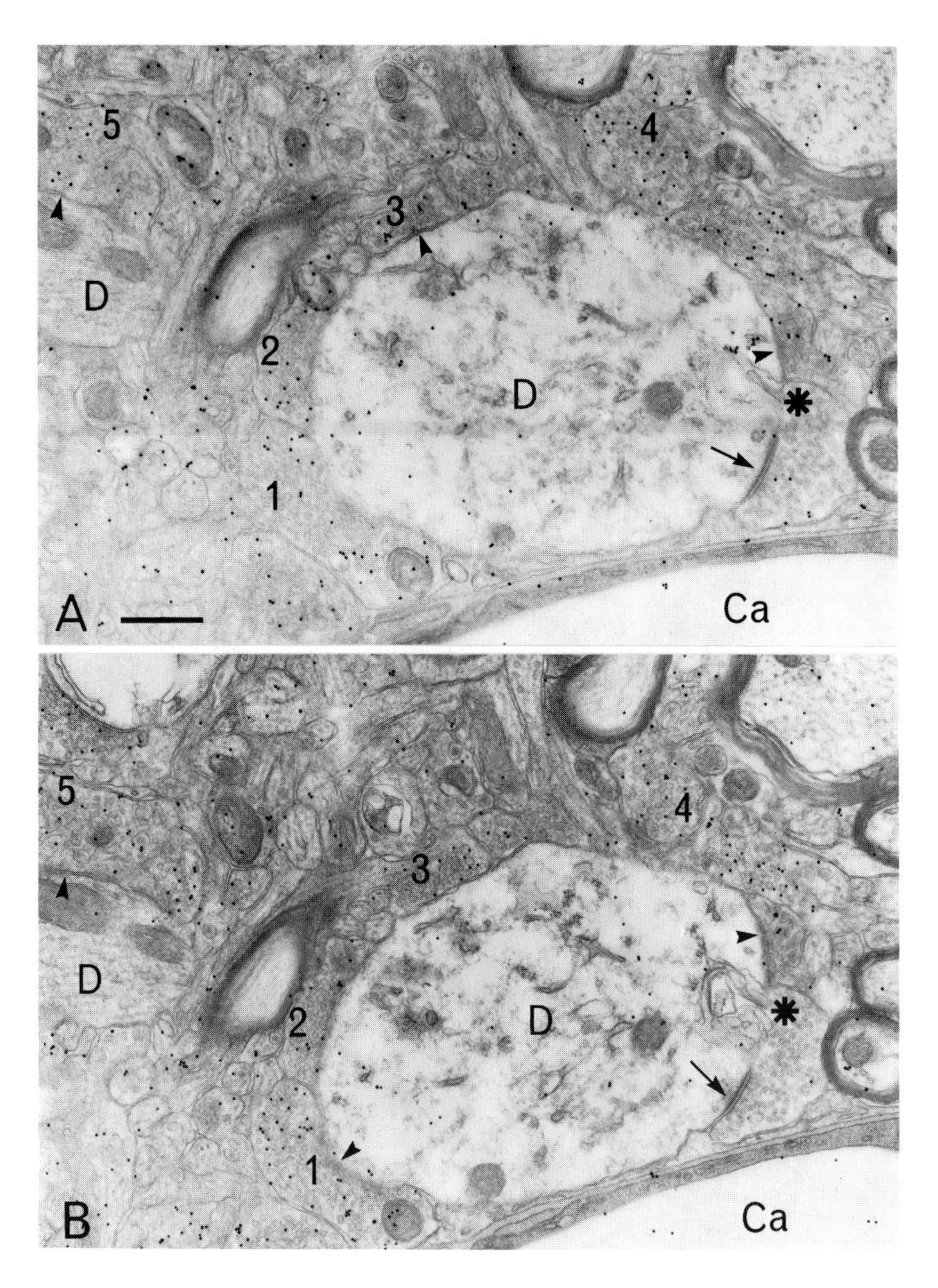

Figure 4. Post-embedding GABA immunocytochemistry on two serial sections from the rat globus pallidus. GABA-positive structures are those that have a high concentration of immunogold particles overlying them in both sections. The labelling is concentrated over vesicle-containing structures, some of which are in symmetrical synaptic contact (arrowheads) with dendritic shafts (D). Some of the labelled boutons are numbered (1–5) for correlation in both (A) and (B). A non-immunoreactive bouton (asterisk) makes asymmetrical synaptic contact (arrow) with the dendrite. A blood capillary (Ca) has very few gold particles overlying it. Scale bar = 0.5 μm.

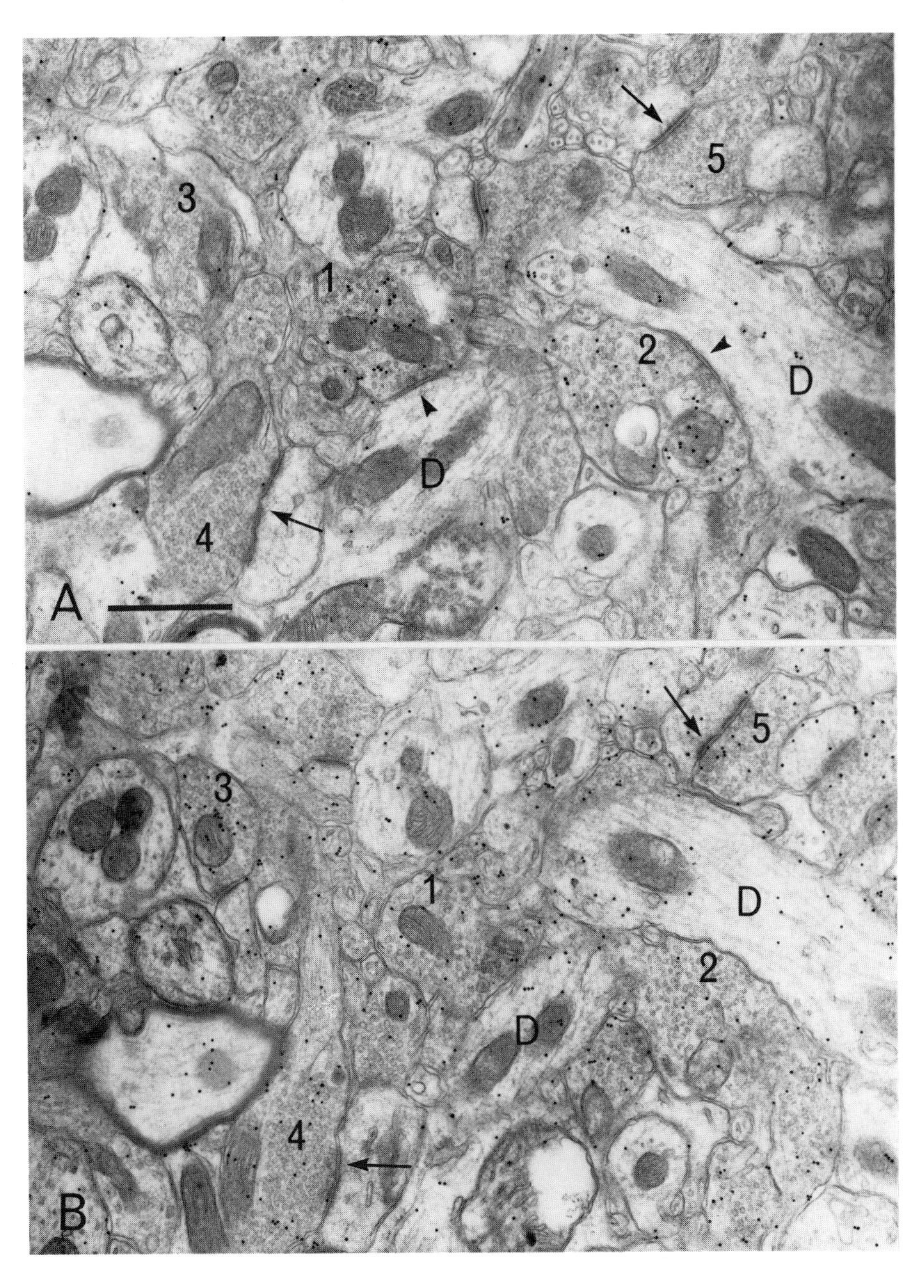

Figure 5. Post-embedding immunocytochemistry on two serial sections from the rat neostriatum stained with GABA antiserum (A) and glutamate antiserum (B). Boutons 1 and 2 make symmetrical synaptic contacts (arrowheads) with dendritic shafts (D) and are GABA-immunoreactive (A) but are not glutamate-enriched (B). Gold particles are scattered over many structures in (B) due to the presence of metabolic glutamate, however some structures have more gold particles over them than others. Many boutons in asymmetrical contact with spines (arrows) including boutons 3–5 are not labelled after the GABA immunogold process (A), but have a high density of gold particles overlying them after glutamate immunogold labelling (B). Scale bar = 0.5 μm. (Ingham, Storm-Mathisen, and Ottersen, unpublished.)

7.1 Quantitative analysis of immunogold labelling

7.1.1 Methods for calculating density of gold particles

The density of immunogold labelling is calculated by counting gold particles within a measured area, and is expressed as number of gold particles/μm^2. The tools required for this calculation range from very basic to extremely sophisticated. All that is required is a way of measuring areas and counting particles. Some examples of possible equipment follow.

(a) A planimeter, manual counter and calculator can be employed, and for small numbers of calculations are quite adequate.

(b) A digitizing tablet hooked up to a computer with software able to calculate areas. The particles can be counted manually, on or off the computer depending on the software, followed by density calculation. The range of equipment available within this group is high, starting from relatively cheap options using IBM type computers to more custom-made systems such as the IBAS–Kontron–videoplan system, or site developed software such as that described by Blackstad *et al.* (17) which has been designed specifically for analysing immunogold material. The latter software is available on request on a non-commercial basis.

(c) A digitized image relayed to a computer using a high resolution scanner (from electron micrographs), or a video camera (from electron micrographs, negatives, or directly from the electron microscope). Regions are traced with a mouse or light pen, and the area of these regions are calculated by the computer. Particle counts are also entered into the computer and densities calculated.

(d) As above, but additional automatic counting of particles is carried out using for example, density thresholding (e.g. Apple Macintosh computer with Image 1.32VDM software—Perceptics Corp.) or alternative more complex image analysis custom developed software using large workstations, e.g. SUN (Sun Microsystems).

7.1.2 Analysis

Confirmation of positive immunostaining of a particular structure using the immunogold method requires that gold particle density is significantly more than the background gold particle density, i.e. quantification. In the case of metabolic substances a potential neurotransmitter role of that substance in structures has to be demonstrated by showing a significantly higher density in that structure compared with other structures. Several approaches to this analysis should be taken to ensure an unbiased analysis. All approaches are based on making statistical comparisons (Section 7.1.3) of immunogold labelling density over groups of morphologically defined structures. This will be described for an experiment examining the question of immunolabelling in synaptic boutons, but it could apply to any structure.

(a) Take approximately 20 random electron micrographs from one or more immunogold labelled sections at a high enough magnification to assess some morphological features of the boutons, such as membrane specializations, vesicle shape, post-synaptic target etc. but low enough to sample a reasonable number of boutons (a magnification of × 16 500 is routinely used in this laboratory). This sample of tissue can be used to make the following calculations.

i. Compare the average gold particle density over all the tissue with that over blood capillary lumens. The latter can be considered to be the true background or non-specific label. If specific labelling is present the average gold particle density over all the tissue should be higher than that over blood capillaries. It is possible to take this background away from labelling over all other structures (4) to get a more accurate measure of specific label. The background label should be low, a density of 1 particle/μm^2 or less is optimal, however higher backgrounds than this are acceptable. Instead of calculating the overall tissue density by counting all the gold particles on all the photographs, randomly generated 1 μm^2 areas can be acquired by dropping a correctly sized frame from a consistent height above the photograph (18). It must be borne in mind that overall tissue labelling includes specific labelling and therefore the more specific labelling there is the higher the overall tissue labelling will be.

ii. Compare the average gold particle density over vesicle containing structures with that over all the tissue and with that over dendrites, neuronal cell bodies, glial cells, and blood capillary lumens. This will determine whether or not vesicle containing structures have a higher gold particle labelling density than other structures. It may also be possible to determine whether or not boutons fall into different populations according to their labelling pattern and morphology (19).

iii. Compare average gold particle density over different populations of synaptic boutons defined for example by the symmetry of the synaptic specialization. Compare these densities with those found over the post-synaptic structures. This can be used to establish that certain morphologically defined structures, e.g. asymmetrical or symmetrical synaptic boutons have more gold particles over them than other structures and hence establish specific labelling.

iv. There may be some other form of labelling in the tissue, such as pre-embedding immunolabelling, intracellular labelling, retrograde, or anterograde labelling—see Chapter 11. In this case the average density of gold particles over labelled structures can be compared with that over non-labelled structures.

(b) Take as many serial sections as possible through specific structures.

i. Pick out synaptic boutons which appear to be labelled in the first section, photograph them in each section of the series together with the post-synaptic targets (*Figure 4*), and calculate the average gold particle density over both structures. Compare this with the average gold particle density over boutons considered to be unlabelled in the first section and with their post-synaptic targets. This will establish the consistency of the labelling and hence its specific nature.

ii. Examine serial sections on a number of grids (two to three sections per grid) which have been processed alternately for immunogold labelling of two different antigens such as GABA and glutamate (*Figure 5*). Carry out the above analysis (*i*) with both antisera. A morphological label can be attached to these boutons, e.g. asymmetric or symmetric, similarly post-synaptic structures can be subdivided according to morphological criteria. As above this will establish the consistency of the two labels and hence specificity.

7.1.3 Statistical analysis

The above methods require descriptive and comparative statistics with at least the capacity for carrying out Student's *t*-tests to compare two sets of data. To compare more than two sets of data a one-way analysis of variance can be carried out followed by multiple comparison procedures such as the Scheffé test. It is most convenient to be able to use a statistical package on the raw data using the same computer (or network) on which densities were calculated.

8. Trouble-shooting

When a method does not work it is often difficult to find the cause especially when its a new technique to a laboratory. To bypass some of the inevitable teething problems *Tables 1* and *2* show some of the problems that may be encountered and how to combat them.

Acknowledgements

Many thanks for the useful discussions with and contributions from Dr Paul Bolam, Dr David Maxwell, Sue Hood, and Frieda Christie. The research presented in this chapter was supported by the Wellcome Trust, UK.

Table 1. Problems encountered using the semi-thin post-embedding immunoperoxidase technique

Effect	Problem	Action
Score marks on sections.	Glass knife imperfect.	Use new section of knife.
		Use new knife.
Sections folded on slide.	Picking up technique at fault.	Adjust technique.
Sections disappear from slide.	Sections not securely fixed to the slide.	Adjust drying conditions (longer or hotter?)
		Improve coating technique.
	Too much etching.	Reduce time in ethanolic NaOH.
No immunostaining or pale immunostaining.	Insufficient etching.	Increase etching time.
	Insufficient osmium removal.	Increase time in sodium metaperiodate.
	Faulty immunochemicals.	Test different antibodies.
	Faulty visualization.	Check DAB, H_2O_2 etc.
	Fixation inappropriate.	Perfuse another animal.
Background staining high.	Faulty immunochemicals.	Check immunochemicals.
	Non-specific antibody.	Test different antibodies.
	Incubation times in immunochemicals too long.	Vary incubation times.
	Incubation times in DAB too long.	Shorten incubation time.
	Fixation inappropriate.	Perfuse another animal.

Table 2. Problems encountered in the thin section immunogold technique

Effect	Problem	Action
Sections disappear from grids.	Sections inadequately fixed to grids.	Dry grids for longer with hair dryer. Leave overnight before immunostaining.
Sections folded	Picking up technique at fault.	Practise picking up sections, if picking up from above, try from underneath.
Contrast so poor in the EM that structures are not identifiable.	Sections too thin. Too much osmium removed. Too little contrast staining.	Cut thicker sections (gold). Cut down time in sodium metaperiodate. Increase staining time with lead citrate. Stain with uranyl acetate on grids (1% aqueous for 15 min–1 h) after immunogold labelling. Decrease objective aperture size in EM.
Gold particles scattered over tissue but not associated with any particular structures.	Immunochemicals faulty. Grid processed on the wrong side. Too little resin removed. Too little osmium removed.	Try new immunochemicals. Repeat with another grid. Increase time in periodic acid. Increase time in sodium metaperiodate. Increase concentration of sodium metaperiodate.
High density of gold particles scattered all over tissue.	Primary antiserum too concentrated. Gold labelled IgG too concentrated.	Reduce concentration of antiserum. Reduce concentration of IgG.
Patches of high density of gold deposits not related to structure.	Insufficient washing at some stage.	Increase washing at all stages.
Gold particles clustered into aggregates.	Gold-labelled IgG too old.	Try new gold-labelled IgG.
Uneven labelling.	Too little resin removed. Too little osmium removed. Bubbles on droplets of immunochemicals.	Increase time in periodic acid. Increase time in sodium metaperiodate. Move grids around on droplets.
Crystalline deposits on grids.	Buffer dried out on top side of grid. Grids not washed enough.	Keep Petri dishes humid. Don't allow top side of grid to come in contact with solutions. Wash grids more.

References

1. Larsson, L-I. (1983). In *Handbook of Chemical Neuroanatomy Vol 1. Methods in Chemical Neuroanatomy* (ed. A. Bjorklund and T. Hokfelt), pp. 147–209. Elsevier, Amsterdam.
2. Causton, B. E. (1984). In *Immunolabelling for Electron Microscopy* (ed. J. M. Polak and I. M. Varndell), pp. 29–36. Elsevier, Amsterdam.
3. Newman, G. R. and Jasani, B. (1984). In *Immunolabelling for Electron Microscopy* (ed. J. M. Polak and I. M. Varndell), pp. 53–70. Elsevier, Amsterdam.
4. Ottersen, O. P. (1989). *Anat. and Embryol.,* **180,** 1.
5. Varndell, I. M., Tapia, F. J., Probert, L., Buchan, A. M. J., Gu, J., De Mey, J., Bloom, S. R., and Polak, J. M. (1982). *Peptides,* **3,** 259.
6. Bendayan, M. (1984). *J. Electron Microsc. Technol.,* **1,** 243.
7. Valentino, K. L., Crumrine, D. A., and Reichardt, L. F. (1985). *J. Histochem. Cytochem.,* **33,** 969.
8. Timms, B. G. (1986). *Am. J. Anat.,* **175,** 267.
9. van den Pol, A. N. (1984). *Quart. J. Exp. Physiol.,* **69,** 1.
10. Storm-Mathisen, J., Leknes, A. K., Bore, A. T., Vaaland, J. L., Edminson, P., Haug, F-M. S., and Ottersen, O. P. (1983). *Nature (Lond.),* **301,** 517.
11. Hodgson, A. J., Penke, B., Erdei, A., Chubb, I. W., and Somogyi, P. (1985). *J. Histochem. Cytochem.,* **33,** 229.
12. Somogyi, P., Hodgson, A. J., Chubb, I. W., Penke, B., and Erdei, A. (1985). *J. Histochem. Cytochem.,* **33,** 240.
13. Somogyi, P. and Hodgson, A. J. (1985). *J. Histochem. Cytochem.,* **33,** 249.
14. Reynolds, E. S. (1963). *J. Cell Biol.,* **17,** 208.
15. Ottersen, O. P. (1987). *Exp. Brain Res.,* **69,** 167.
16. Ottersen, O. P. (1989). *J. Chem. Neuroanat.,* **2,** 57.
17. Blackstad, T. W., Karagulle, T., and Ottersen, O. P. (1990). *Comput. Biol. Med.,* **20,** 15.
18. Maxwell, D. J., Christie, W. M., and Somogyi, P. (1989). *Neurosci.,* **33,** 169.
19. Bogan, N., Mennone, A., and Cabot, J. B. (1989). *Brain Res.,* **505,** 257.

7

Histochemistry of endogenous enzymes

S. R. VINCENT

1. Introduction

Enzyme histochemistry is the art of performing biochemical reactions on tissue sections, thereby providing the precise localization of particular enzymes. Given the cellular complexity of the nervous system, histochemical methods have played a key role in the biochemical dissection and mapping of various neurochemically distinct cell types. Enzyme histochemistry, like other histochemical techniques, is always a compromise between preserving enzyme activity and maintaining adequate histological structure. Thus aldehyde fixation is often used for two purposes, to preserve cellular morphology, and to prevent diffusion of otherwise soluble enzymes. However, it must always be borne in mind that such fixation can inhibit or destroy enzyme activity.

The enzyme histochemical methods outlined below are all designed to be performed on brain sections obtained from animals that have been vascularly perfused with an aldehyde fixative (see Chapter 1, *Protocol 3*). Although these techniques will all work with a standard 4% paraformaldehyde fixation, some require the addition of glutaraldehyde for optimum staining (see Chapter, *Protocol 2* for preparation of fixatives). These techniques are also compatible with sections obtained with a cryostat or freezing microtome, although some are greatly improved by using unfrozen, vibrating microtome sections. In addition, the use of glutaraldehyde fixation together with vibrating microtome sectioning usually provides the optimum preservation of structure for the ultrastructural localization of these various enzymes.

2. Cholinesterases

Although acetylcholine was the first neurotransmitter to be identified, it is only recently that the anatomical localization of central cholinergic neurones has been defined. This has been made possible by the purification of the synthetic enzyme choline acetyltransferase, and the generation of specific antibodies to this marker. Prior to these achievements, attempts were made to determine the distribution of potential cholinergic pathways by the histochemical localization of the enzyme responsible for the breakdown of acetylcholine, acetylcholinesterase. In light of the new immunohistochemical data, it is now possible to appreciate how accurate these earlier enzyme histochemical attempts often were (1).

2.1 Acetylcholinesterase

The original histochemical methods for acetylcholinesterase of Koelle (2) and Karnovsky and Roots (3) resulted in a diffuse staining pattern when applied to the central nervous system. Well defined axons and cell bodies were not readily apparent. These techniques have been refined over the years, and in particular two sensitive modifications of the Karnovsky and Roots procedure have been introduced. Both are based on the enhancement of the visibility of the Hatchett's brown [$Cu_2Fe(CN)_6$] formed in this method, and they thereby provide sensitive and detailed staining of acetylcholinesterase (AChE) positive fibres and cells. One of these techniques relies on silver-enhancement (4), while the second (5) makes use of the ability of Hatchett's brown to catalyse the oxidative polymerization of 3,3′-diaminobenzidine by H_2O_2, which can be detected using the peroxidase method introduced by Karnovsky and Roots (6). The latter technique appears to be the simplest, cleanest, and most robust, and is thus detailed below (see *Figure 1A, B*). This method is readily adaptable to ultrastructural studies by the use of glutaraldehyde in the fixation step, and treatment with osmium following the histochemical reaction.

Protocol 1. Acetylcholinesterase histochemistry

Fixation

Animals are perfused with an aldehyde fixative in phosphate buffer. Optimum results are obtained with a mixture of 4% paraformaldehyde and 1% glutaraldehyde in phosphate buffer, followed by post-fixation in 4% paraformaldehyde for one day at 4°C. (See Chapter 1, *Protocol 2* for preparation of fixatives and *Protocol 3* for perfusion–fixation. See also *Safety note 1*, p. 5.)

Materials

- maleic buffer (0.1 M maleic acid, pH to 6.0 with NaOH)
- 5 mM potassium ferricyanide, $K_3Fe(CN)_6$
- 40 mM copper sulphate
- 100 mM sodium citrate
- Tris-buffer (50 mM Tris base, pH to 7.4 with HCl)
- 3,3′-diaminobenzidine (10 mg/ml aqueous stock solution stored frozen in 0.5 ml aliquots)

- nickel ammonium sulphate
- solution A: mix together in this order; 6.5 ml maleic buffer, 0.5 ml sodium citrate, 1.0 ml copper sulphate, 1.0 ml water, 1.0 ml potassium ferricyanide
- solution B: 5–30 mg acetylthiocholine iodide/10 ml maleic acid buffer[a]

Method

1. Wash sections for 5 min in maleic buffer.
2. Pre-incubate sections for 30 min at room temperature in solution A diluted 1:100 in maleic buffer.
3. React sections for 30 min at room temperature in 98 ml maleic buffer, containing 1 ml solution A, and 1 ml solution B.
4. Wash sections in Tris-buffer, two times, 1 min.
5. Incubate in 19.5 ml Tris-buffer with one aliquot (5 mg in 0.5 ml H_2O) 3,3'-diaminobenzidine, and 200 mg nickel ammonium sulphate, 5 min at room temperature.
6. Add 20 μl of 1% H_2O_2 and react for 10–15 min at room temperature.
7. Rinse sections in Tris-buffer, mount on to subbed slides (Chapter 1, *Protocol* 5), dehydrate, and apply a coverslip with Permount (Chapter 1, *Protocol 6*).

[a] The concentration of substrate, i.e. acetylthiocholine iodide can be varied (5–30 mg) depending on the sensitivity required in a particular experiment or for a particular cell type.

2.1.1 Appearance of staining

The acetylcholinesterase method should result in an intense blue/black staining of both fibre networks and cell bodies containing the enzyme. There should be no non-specific or background staining present. The reaction product is stable, and stained sections can be dehydrated through organic solvents, or treated with osmium and processed for electron microscopy.

2.1.2 Controls

Reactions performed in parallel without substrate (acetylthiocholine), or in the presence of acetylcholinesterase inhibitors, (i.e. 0.1 mM 1,5-bis-(4-allyldimethyl-ammonium-phenyl)pental-3-one dibromide, BW284c51; Sigma, or 10 mM physostigmine (eserine sulphate; Sigma)) should produce no positive staining. Also, in tissues containing high levels of other esterases, it may be necessary to pre-incubate the sections for 30 min in the presence of the non-specific esterase inhibitor *N,N'*-bis-(1-methylethyl)-pyrophosphorodiamidic anhydride (50 μM iso-OMPA), and also include it in the reaction.

2.2 The pharmacohistochemical method

An important variation of the acetylcholinesterase method was introduced by Koelle and his colleagues (7), and refined and applied to the brain by Lynch

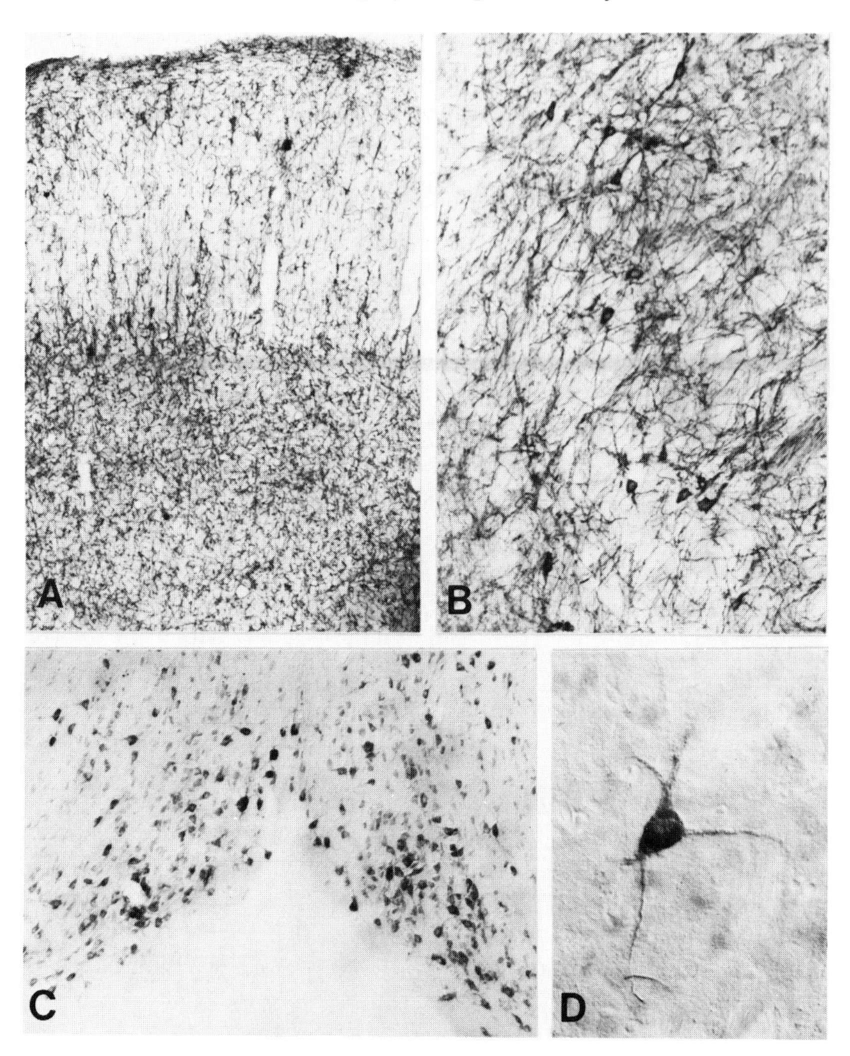

Figure 1. Acetylcholinesterase histochemistry. The coupled peroxidase method reveals dense fibre networks in the cerebral cortex (A), and cell bodies in the basal forebrain (B). The pharmacohistochemical method illustrates the intensely stained cells of the nucleus of the diagonal band (C) and the striatum (D).

et al. (8), and Butcher *et al.* (9). The method is based on the *in vivo* poisoning of acetylcholinesterase with an irreversible inhibitor such as diisopropylphosphofluoridate (DFP). This abolishes all staining, however, after a few hours (usually four to eight) sufficient amounts of new enzyme will be synthesized on the ribosomes in the cell soma and major dendrites of the cells expressing the acetylcholinesterase gene to allow histochemical detection. Histochemical staining at this time will therefore result in the staining of cell bodies, without the intense neuropil staining that normally obscures the cell bodies (see *Figure 1C, D*). This method has been of great value in mapping cholinergic neurones, which are often intensely stained relative to the neuropil by this pharmacohistochemical method. In addition, it is readily extended to the electron microscopic level (10). However, the results must be interpreted with caution since some non-cholinergic cells including the catecholamine neurones in the locus coeruleus and substantia nigra, are also intensely stained. Also some cell groups now known to be immunoreactive for choline acetyltransferase, and thus thought to be cholinergic, do not stain intensely by this method. The pharmacohistochemical method is usually applied to the original Karnovsky and Roots staining procedure (3), as outlined below. The coupled peroxidase method described above can allow the visualization of both cell bodies and fibres in untreated animals.

Protocol 2. Acetylcholinesterase pharmacohistochemistry

Materials

- DFP stock solution at 2.0 mg/ml in peanut oil. DFP is highly toxic, see *Safety note 1*
- atropine sulphate
- acetylthiocholine iodide
- 0.1 M maleic buffer, (pH to 6.0 with NaOH)
- 0.1 M sodium citrate
- 30 mM copper sulphate
- 5 mM potassium ferricyanide

Method

1. Rats are given an intra-muscular injection of DFP (2.0 mg/kg), followed by an intra-peritoneal injection of atropine sulphate (5.0 mg/kg).
2. After an appropriate survival time (2–12 h, often 4 h is optimal) deeply anaesthetize animals and perfuse with an aldehyde fixative, often 4% paraformaldehyde plus 1% calcium chloride (see Chapter 1, *Protocols 2* and *3*). The brains can be post-fixed in the same solution at 4°C for up to 2 days and then cut on a vibrating microtome (Chapter 1, *Protocol 4*), or soaked in 15% sucrose and cut on a cryostat. Sections can either be stained free-floating, or mounted on to subbed slides (Chapter 1, *Protocol 5*) and dried prior to staining.
3. Incubate sections for 4–12 h at room temperature in a freshly prepared reaction medium containing:

   5.0 mg acetylthiocholine iodide
   6.5 ml sodium maleate buffer

Protocol 2. *Continued*

0.5 ml sodium citrate
1.0 ml copper sulphate
1.0 ml H_2O
1.0 ml potassium ferricyanide

4. Stop the reaction by rinsing in buffer or distilled water, after which the sections can be mounted, dehydrated, and a coverslip applied (Chapter 1, *Protocol 6*).

Safety note 1. DFP is highly toxic by ingestion, inhalation, and absorption through the skin. Handle *only* in a fume cupboard and wear appropriate protective clothing. Consult local safety officer before use.

2.2.1 Appearance of staining

Following the pharmacohistochemical method neurones expressing acetylcholinesterase are stained orange/brown in colour by the deposition of Hatchett's brown at the site of reaction. Neurones can be intensely, moderately, or weakly stained. The longer the time between DFP treatment and fixation, the more newly synthesized acetylcholinesterase will be available, and the further from the cell body it will have travelled. Thus at longer time intervals cells will stain more intensely, however greater neuropil staining will also result. The Hatchett's brown reaction product is osmiophillic and stable, sections can thus be processed for electron microscopy.

2.3 Pseudocholinesterases

In addition to acetylcholinesterase, the nervous system contains an additional activity termed non-specific, or pseudocholinesterase which preferentially hydrolyses butyrylcholine and other higher choline esters. This activity can be examined using the histochemical methods developed for acetylcholinesterase, substituting 0.1 mM propionylthiocholine or butyrylthiocholine as substrate, and including a specific acetylcholinesterase inhibitor such as 0.1 mM BW284c51.

3. Monoamine oxidase (MAO)

Many biogenic amines are metabolized to their corresponding aldehydes by the action of monoamine oxidase. This includes the catecholamines dopamine, noradrenaline, and adrenaline, as well as serotonin. In addition, certain methylated metabolites of neurotransmitters are also substrates. These include the dopamine metabolite 3-methyltyramine, and the primary histamine metabolite *t*-methylhistamine. Thus monoamine oxidase plays a major role in the catabolism of amine neurotransmitters.

Two forms of monoamine oxidase have been described based on their substrate and inhibitor specificities (11). Monoamine oxidase A uses 5-hydroxytryptamine preferentially as substrate, and can be irreversibly inhibited by low concentrations of clorgyline. The B form of monoamine oxidase is inhibited by low concentrations of deprenyl, and can preferentially utilize phenylethylamine and benzylamine as substrates. Recent molecular biological studies have identified distinct genes encoding these two isoforms (12).

Both types of monoamine oxidase catalyse the oxidative deamination of amines. This process requires molecular oxygen and produces hydrogen peroxide along with the corresponding aldehyde as products. Thus two main techniques have been used for MAO histochemistry, based on the assay of these two products. The first was the tetrazolium technique using tryptamine as substrate, developed by Glenner *et al.* (13). This method allowed the first description of MAO-positive cells in the brain (14). Although this method has been improved over the years, results on the nervous system have not been particularly useful, since it results in rather diffuse images. This procedure is also only applicable to substrates which generate an active aldehyde upon oxidation.

The second method, originally developed by Graham and Karnovsky (15), is based on coupling the generation of H_2O_2 by MAO to a peroxidase detection system. This method was greatly improved by the use of 3,3′-diaminobenzidine instead of semicarbazol dyes (16). In combination with aldehyde fixation and vibrating microtome sectioning, this technique provides robust and distinct staining of various aminergic cell groups and can be used at both the light and electron microscopic levels (17). Further refinements to the technique involve the use of selective substrates and inhibitors allowing the discrimination of MAO A and B at the histochemical level (18).

This histochemical method has proven to be very useful for the light and electron microscopic examination of particular aminergic cell groups (see *Figure 2*). In particular the adrenaline and noradrenaline containing neurones of the pons and medulla, the serotonin neurones of the raphe, and the histaminergic neurones of the tuberomammillary nucleus are beautifully stained by this technique (19). This method has also allowed the cellular localization of the MAO activity responsible for the oxidation of various exogenous substrates, including the neurotoxin 1-methyl-4-phenyl-1,2,3,6-tetrahydropyridine (MPTP) (20).

Protocol 3. Monoamine oxidase histochemistry

Fixation

Optimum results are obtained using sections cut on a vibrating microtome (Chapter 1, *Protocol 4*) after perfusion (Chapter 1, *Protocol 3*) with a fixative containing both paraformaldehyde and glutaraldehyde (Chapter 1, *Protocol 2*).

Protocol 3. *Continued*

Mixtures containing 1% paraformaldehyde plus 1% glutaraldehyde, or 4% paraformaldehyde plus 2% glutaraldehyde have been used successfully.

Materials

- horseradish peroxidase (Sigma, Type III)
- tyramine hydrochloride
- sodium azide
- nickel ammonium sulphate
- 3,3′-diaminobenzidine (10 mg/ml aqueous solution stored frozen in 0.5 ml aliquots)
- Tris-HCl buffer (50 mM Tris, pH 7.4)

Method

1. Prepare reaction solution containing:
    - 10 mg horseradish peroxidase
    - 0.5 mg 3,3′-diaminobenzidine
    - 60 mg nickel ammonium sulphate
    - 10 ml Tris-buffer
    - an appropriate substrate (the most common substrate for demonstrating both MAO A and B is 7.5 mg tyramine hydrochloride)
2. Incubate sections with shaking at 4°C for 3–12 h.
3. Stop the reaction by rinsing the sections in Tris-buffer, after which they can be mounted, dehydrated, cleared, and a coverslip applied (Chapter 1, *Protocols 5 and 6*).

3.1 Appearance of staining

This monoamine oxidase histochemical method results in intense blue/black staining of positive neuronal cell bodies and major dendrites. In fact a Golgi-like image of these cells can be obtained using vibrating microtome sections. However, axons and terminal fields are not readily stained.

3.2 Controls

Omission of the substrate, or inhibition of MAO activity by pre-incubating the sections with an inhibitor such as 0.1 mM pargyline hydrochloride for 15 minutes prior to the histochemical reaction should block all staining. To selectively inhibit MAO-A or MAO-B, pre-incubate the sections for 15 minutes and include in the reaction mixture 0.1 μM clorgyline or deprenyl, respectively.

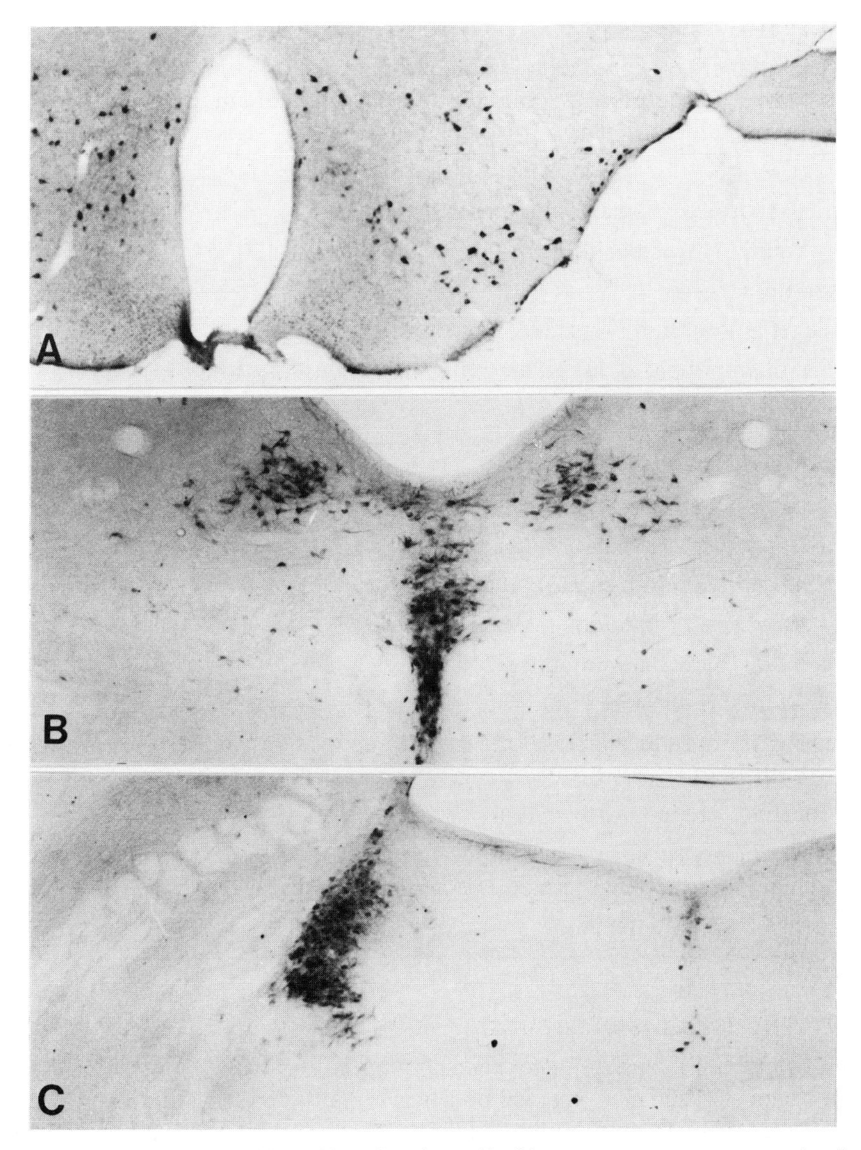

Figure 2. Monoamine oxidase histochemistry. Positive neurones are present in the tuberomammillary nucleus (A), the dorsal raphe (B), and the locus ceruleus (C).

4. Nitric oxide synthase (NADPH-diaphorase)

The NADPH-diaphorase histochemical technique was first shown to stain specific neurones by Thomas and Pearse in the early sixties (21, 22). Twenty years later, this technique experienced a renaissance when it was shown that in aldehyde fixed material it could selectively stain particular populations of neurones in a Golgi-like manner (23, 24). This led to the widespread use of this technique for experimental and neuropathological studies (see *Figure 3*). The enzyme responsible for the neuronal NADPH-diaphorase reaction has recently been identified as nitric oxide synthase (25). This will no doubt lead

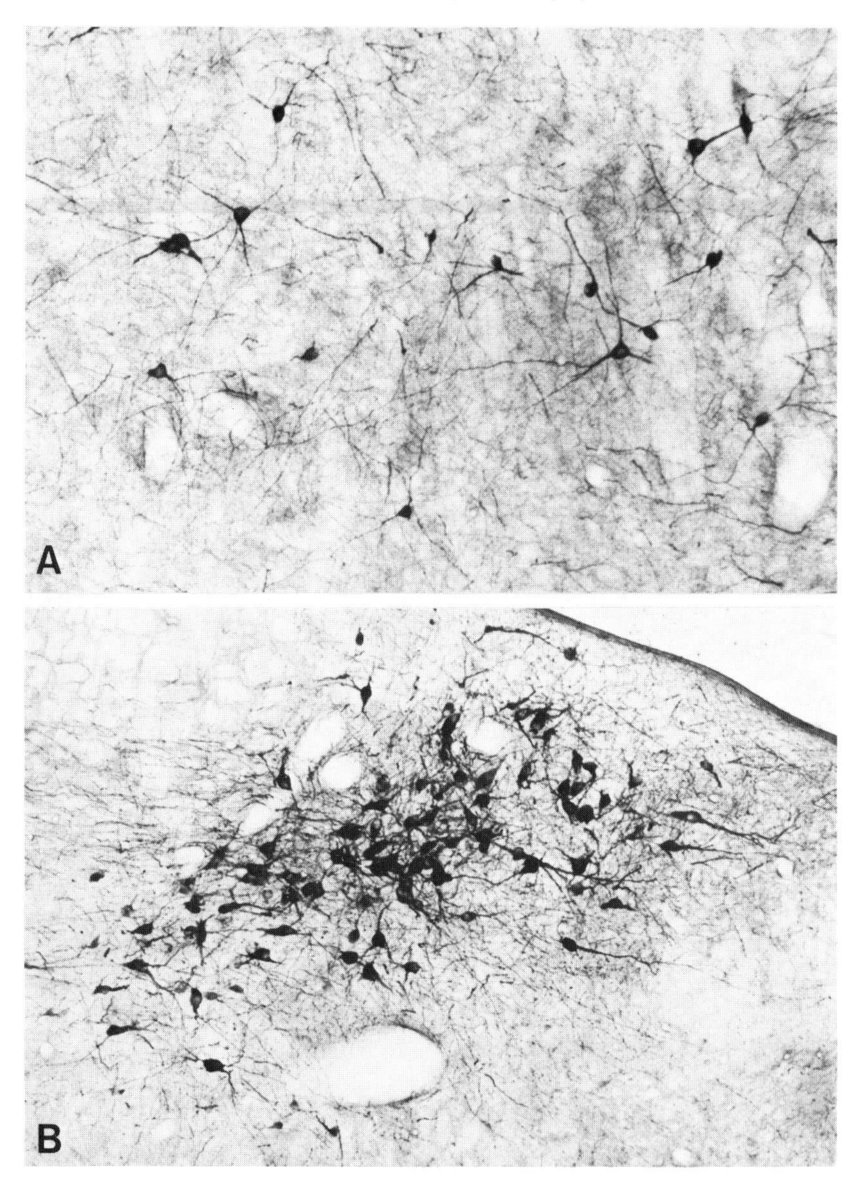

Figure 3. Nitric oxide synthase activity demonstrated with the NADPH diaphorase histochemical method in medium aspiny neurones in the striatum (A), and in the cholinergic neurones of the mesopontine tegmentum (B).

to even greater interest in this extremely simple histochemical method, since it now makes it possible to visualize those neurones synthesizing the newly discovered cellular messenger nitric oxide.

Protocol 4. NADPH-diaphorase histochemistry

Fixation

Sections can be obtained from material fixed by immersion in 4% paraformaldehyde, or following vascular perfusion with an aldehyde mixture (Chapter 1, *Protocol 3*). Glutaraldehyde can be tolerated up to 2% in the perfusion solution (Chapter 1, *Protocol 2*). Following fixation, sections are soaked in 15% sucrose, sectioned on a cryostat or vibrating microtome, and stained either free-floating or mounted on gelatin-coated slides (Chapter 1, *Protocol 5*).

Materials

- β-NADPH (nicotinamide adenine dinucleotide phosphate, reduced form, tetrasodium salt, Sigma)
- nitroblue tetrazolium (Sigma)
- 20 mM sodium phosphate buffer, pH 7.4, containing 0.3% Triton X-100[a]

Method

1. Prepare a reaction mixture containing:
   - 10 mg β-NADPH
   - 1 mg nitroblue tetrazolium
   - in 10 ml phosphate buffer, pH 7.4
2. Incubate the sections at 37°C until desired level of staining is reached (30–60 min).
3. Stop reaction by rinsing sections in PBS, after which they can be mounted (if free-floating), and dried at room temperature.
4. Rinse sections in distilled water, and air-dry overnight.
5. Soak in xylene and apply a coverslip with Permount.

[a] For electron microscopy the Triton X-100 should be omitted or markedly reduced.

The use of glutaraldehyde fixative in the perfusion, and osmium treatment (Chapter 1, *Protocol 7*) after the reaction allows the NADPH-diaphorase technique to be used for electron microscopic studies (26) (see Chapter 1 for details of preparation for electron microscope). In addition, this robust method can be performed on sections previously processed by immunohistochemical techniques (27) (see Chapter 5), and is compatible with other enzyme histochemical methods including acetylcholinesterase (28).

4.1 Appearance of staining

The NADPH-diaphorase reaction results in a dark blue staining of positive cell bodies, dendrites, axons, and terminal fields. The formazan reaction product is not water soluble, however it is soluble in various organic solvents. In particular, alcohol-containing solutions will result in the formation of formazan crystals which can obscure the fine localization of the enzyme. For this reason, air-drying followed by immersion directly in xylene is recommended for clearing prior to the application of coverslips. If treated this way the staining is permanent and stable.

5. GABA-transaminase

The amino acid GABA was first identified in brain in 1950, and has since been shown to be the major inhibitory neurotransmitter in the mammalian brain. It is formed by the decarboxylation of glutamate, a reaction catalysed by the enzyme glutamate decarboxylase. This enzyme is selectively expressed in cells which synthesize GABA, and antibodies to it have provided an immunohistochemical method with which to localize GABAergic neurones.

The catabolism of GABA proceeds via a specialized metabolic pathway associated with the Krebs cycle, termed the GABA shunt. In the first step, GABA is deaminated by the enzyme GABA-transaminase to yield succinate semialdehyde, with α-ketoglutarate acting as the acceptor of the amino group, thereby forming glutamate as a co-product. The glutamate formed may act to replenish the precursor pool for GABA synthesis. The second step in GABA metabolism involves the oxidation of succinate semialdehyde to the Krebs cycle intermediate, succinic acid, catalysed by the enzyme succinate semialdehyde dehydrogenase.

A tetrazolium method for the histochemical detection of GABA-transaminase activity was developed by Van Gelder (29). This method actually indicates the activity of succinate semialdehyde dehydrogenase by detecting the NAD^+-dependent oxidation of the succinate semialdehyde formed by the GABA-T reaction. The reduced NADH formed in this reaction can then reduce a tetrazolium dye to a visible formazan. The NADH cannot reduce nitroblue tetrazolium (NBT) directly, and so an intermediary electron carrier, phenazine methosulphate (PMS) is also included in the reaction. Thus the overall histochemical procedure is actually based on 4 steps:

- GABA + α-ketoglutarate → glutamate + succinate semialdehyde
- succinate semialdehyde + NAD^+ → succinate + NADH
- NADH + PMS^+ → NAD^+ + PMSH
- PMSH + NBT → PMS^+ + formazan

Thus the histochemical reaction requires the inclusion of GABA, α-ketoglutarate, NAD, PMS, and NBT, and the overall reaction is:

GABA + α-ketoglutarate + NBT → glutamate + succinate + formazan

Since the succinate formed in this reaction can be further oxidized by endogenous succinate dehydrogenase catalysing the reduction of NBT, it is also necessary to include malonate, an inhibitor of this enzyme in the reaction mixture.

The method of Van Gelder was originally applied to unfixed cryostat sections, but the diffuse nature of the resulting reaction product limited its utility. The method was subsequently improved by the use of aldehyde fixation (Chapter 1, *Protocols 2* and *3*) (30) and vibrating microtome sections (Chapter 1, *Protocol 4*) (31). This together with the development of a pharmacohistochemical method, analogous to that employed for acetylcholinesterase, allows the visualization of GABA-T synthesizing cell bodies (31, 32) (see *Figure 4D*).

Protocol 5. GABA-transaminase histochemistry

Fixation

Perfusion (Chapter 1, *Protocol 3*) is performed with 80 ml of ice-cold phosphate-buffered saline (Chapter 1, *Protocol 1*), followed by 150 ml of 2% paraformaldehyde and 2% glutaraldehyde (Chapter 1, *Protocol 2*). The brain is immediately removed, sectioned on a vibrating microtome (Chapter 1, *Protocol 4*), and collected in 0.1 M phosphate buffer, pH 7.4.

Materials

1. Prepare a pre-incubation solution in 50 mM Tris-HCl, pH 8.6, containing:
- 5 mg/ml α/ketoglutarate
- 1 mg/ml β-NAD^+
- 0.5 mg/ml malonate
- 0.05 mg/ml potassium cyanide

2. Prepare a reaction solution in pre-incubation solution containing:
- 1 mg/ml GABA
- 1 mg/ml nitroblue tetrazolium
- 0.005 mg/ml phenazine methosulphate

Method

1. Soak sections at 37°C in pre-incubation solution for 15 min in order to use up any endogenous substrates.

Protocol 5. *Continued*

2. Add fresh reaction solution containing the substrate, NBT and PMS and react at 37 °C for 45 min in the dark.
3. Stop the reaction by transferring the sections to PBS, after which they can be mounted, dehydrated, and a coverslip applied (Chapter 1, *Protocol 6*).

5.1 Appearance of staining

The formazan seen with the GABA-transaminase reaction is identical to that produced by the NADPH-diaphorase reaction. Sections should be handled in a similar manner after processing. The GABA-T positive cell bodies are, however, often somewhat obscured by the intense neuropil staining seen with this technique, and if they are the main focus of interest, the pharmacohistochemical method should be employed.

5.2 Controls

Sections should be incubated without substrate (GABA) or in the presence of a GABA-T inhibitor, (i.e. 1 mM amino-oxyacetic acid, AOAA Sigma).

For the pharmacohistochemical method, rats are injected intra-venously with an irreversible GABA-T inhibitor (60 mg/kg gabaculine), and examined 12 hours later using the standard method.

6. Fluoride-resistant acid phosphatase (FRAP)

Histochemical studies of the rat and mouse sensory system have been greatly aided by the discovery of an extralysosomal fluoride-resistant form of acid phosphatase in some dorsal root ganglia neurones (33). The FRAP reaction can use thiamine monophosphate as a substrate, and this has led to the suggestion that the FRAP reaction is due to the enzyme thiamine monophosphatase (34, 35). However, since it can also use a number of other monophosphate esters (36), its endogenous substrate remains a mystery. Double staining studies have demonstrated that FRAP is a specific marker for a population of small diameter primary sensory neurones that is largely distinct from those containing the neuropeptides substance P and somatostatin (37, 38). FRAP has also been shown to stain the adrenaline containing (PNMT-positive) chromaffin cells of the rat adrenal gland (39) and a subpopulation of sympathetic neurones (36). A similar enzyme is likely to be present in other species but it has only been detected histochemically in the rat and mouse (see *Figure 4*). The method is readily extended to the electron microscope by using glutaraldehyde in the fixation step, and treatment with osmium (Chapter 1, *Protocols 7–11*) following the histochemical reaction.

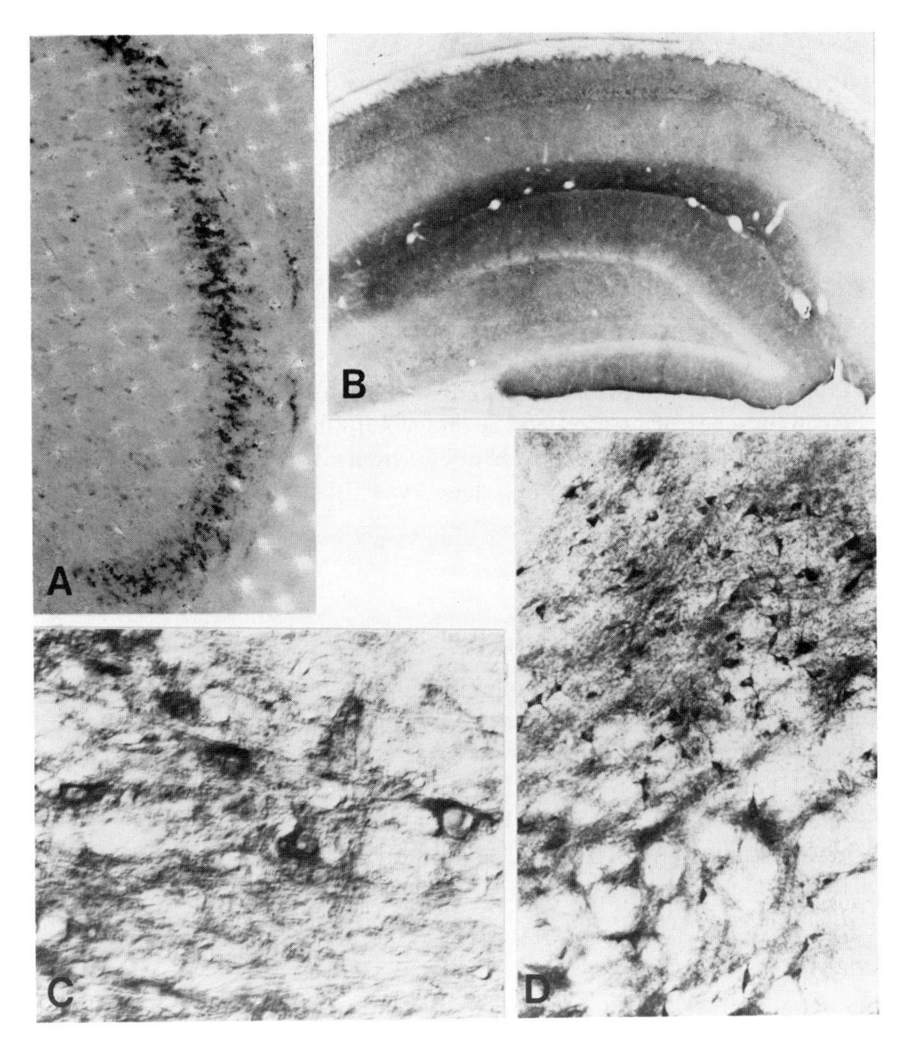

Figure 4. Fluoride-resistant acid phosphatase in the substantia gelatinosa of the rat spinal cord (A). Cytochrome oxidase in the neuropil of the rat hippocampus (B) and in cell bodies in the red nucleus (C). GABA-transaminase containing neurones in the globus pallidus detected using the pharmacohistochemical technique (D).

Protocol 6. FRAP histochemistry

Fixation

Animals can be perfused (Chapter 1, *Protocol 3*) with an aldehyde fixative (Chapter 1, *Protocol 2*) in phosphate buffer. Glutaraldehyde fixatives up to 5% are tolerated, but a simple 4% paraformaldehyde fixation is often used, except for when electron microscopy is the goal.

Protocol 6. *Continued*

Materials

- 1.25% sodium β-glycerophosphate
- 20 mM Tris-maleate buffer, pH 5.0
- 0.2% lead nitrate
- sodium fluoride
- 1% ammonium sulphide

Method

1. Prepare reaction solution consisting of 10 ml sodium β-glycerophosphate, 10 ml buffer, 10 ml water, and 20 ml lead nitrate. 0.3 mM NaF is included to inhibit lysosomal acid phosphatase activity.
2. Incubate sections for 30 min at 37°C.
3. Rinse the sections in distilled water and treat with 1% ammonium sulphide for 15 sec at room temperature.
4. Dehydrate and apply coverslip (Chapter 1, *Protocol 6*).

It is possible to substitute thiamine monophosphate as substrate, and since this is not a substrate for the lysosomal acid phosphatase, it is not necessary to include sodium fluoride in the reaction.

6.1 Appearance of staining

Following immersion in the ammonium sulphide solution, the FRAP-positive cells will appear black against a light brown background. The reaction product is stable and sections can be dehydrated or processed for electron microscopy.

7. Cytochrome oxidase

Cytochrome oxidase is the terminal enzyme in the mitochondrial electron transport chain, transferring electrons from reduced ferrocytochrome c to molecular oxygen, thereby forming water. This is associated with ATP formation by coupled oxidative phosphorylation. The activity of cytochrome oxidase appears to be a useful marker for metabolic activity in the nervous system, complementing the 2-deoxyglucose technique (40). It appears that cytochrome oxidase activity in the mitochondrial oxidative phosphorylation pathway varies with the metabolic activity of the cell, in response to the neurone's need for ATP.

Seligman *et al.* (41) devised a histochemical technique based on the oxidative polymerization of 3,3′-diaminobenzidine which accepts electrons from cytochrome c. In order for the reaction to proceed, cytochrome c must be continually re-oxidized by cytochrome oxidase, and thus the technique provides a detection method for this enzyme. The modified method developed by Wong-Riley (42) has become very popular and is outlined here (see *Figure 4*). It is interesting to note that the localization seen using this method corresponds clearly to that seen immunohistochemically using antibodies to cytochrome oxidase (43, 44).

Protocol 7. Cytochrome oxidase histochemistry

Fixative

Animals are perfused (Chapter 1, *Protocol 3*) with an aldehyde mixture (Chapter 1, *Protocol 2*) (usually 4% paraformaldehyde and 1% glutaraldehyde) in phosphate buffer. The brain is removed and post-fixed at 4°C for 1 h. Sections to be cut frozen are incubated in 15% sucrose overnight. If a vibrating microtome (Chapter 1, *Protocol 4*) is used, sections can be cut immediately.

Materials

Reaction solution consisting of:

- 0.06% 3,3′-diaminobenzidine
- 0.02% cytochrome c (Sigma Type III)
- 4.5% sucrose
- in 0.1 M phosphate buffer pH 7.4.

Method

Incubate sections at 37°C in the dark until desired staining is achieved (often 2 h). The sections are then rinsed, mounted if free-floating, dehydrated, and coverslip applied (Chapter 1, *Protocol 6*).

7.1 Appearance of staining

The cytochrome oxidase reaction product is a diffuse orange/brown precipitate. Individual nerve fibres are difficult to discern and cell bodies are not sharply stained. The reaction product is stable, and the sections can be dehydrated or treated with osmium tetroxide for electron microscopy.

7.2 Controls

The substrate, cytochrome c can be left out, or cytochrome oxidase can be poisoned with 100 mM potassium cyanide.

References

1. Shute, C. C. D. and Lewis, P. R. (1963). *Nature,* **199,** 1160.
2. Koelle, G. B. (1954). *J. Comp. Neurol.,* **100,** 211.
3. Karnovsky, M. J. and Roots, L. (1964). *J. Histochem. Cytochem.,* **12,** 219.
4. Hedreen, J. C., Bacon, S. J., and Price, D. L. (1985). *J. Histochem. Cytochem.,* **33,** 134.
5. Tago, H., Kimura, H., and Maeda, T. (1986). *J. Histochem. Cytochem.,* **34,** 1431.
6. Graham, R. C. and Karnovsky, M. J. (1966). *J. Histochem. Cytochem.,* **14,** 291.
7. Nichols, C. W. and Koelle, G. B. (1967). *Science,* **155,** 477.
8. Lynch, G. S., Lucas, P. A., and Deadwyler, S. A. (1972). *Brain Res.,* **45,** 617.
9. Butcher, L. L., Talbot, K., and Bilezikjain, L. (1975). *J. Neural. Trans.,* **37,** 127.
10. Satoh, K., Staines, W. A., Atmadja, S., and Fibiger, H. C. (1983). *Neurosci.,* **10,** 1121.
11. Johnston, J. P. (1968). *Biochem. Pharmacol.,* **17,** 1285.
12. Bach, A. W. J., Lam, N. C., Johnson, D. C., Abell, C. W., Bembenek, M. E., Kwan, S. W., Seeburg, P. H., and Shih, J. C. (1988). *Proc. Natl Acad. Sci. USA,* **85,** 4934.
13. Glenner, G. G., Burtner, H. J., and Brown, G. W. Jr. (1957). *J. Histochem. Cytochem.,* **5,** 591.
14. Shimizu, N., Morikawa, N., and Okada, M. (1959). *Z. Zellforsch.,* **49,** 389.
15. Graham, R. C. and Karnovsky, M. J. (1965). *J. Histochem. Cytochem.,* **13,** 604.
16. Kishimoto, S., Himura, H., and Maeda, T. (1983). *Cell. Molec. Biol.,* **29,** 61.
17. Maeda, T., Imai, H., Arai, R., Tago, H., Nagai, T., Sakumoto, T., Kiahama, K., Onteniente, B., and Kimura, H. (1987). *Cell. Molec. Biol.,* **33,** 1.
18. Kitahama, K., Arai, R., Maeda, T., and Jouvet, M. (1986). *Neurosci. Lett.,* **71,** 19.
19. Arai, R., Kimura, H., and Maeda, T. (1986). *Neurosci.,* **19,** 905.
20. Nakamura, S. and Vincent, S. R. (1986). *Neurosci. Lett.,* **65,** 321.
21. Thomas, E. and Pearse, A. G. E. (1961). *Histochemie,* **2,** 266.
22. Thomas, E. and Pearse, A. G. E. (1964). *Acta Neuropath.,* **3,** 238.
23. Scherer-Singler, U., Vincent, S. R., Kimura, H., and McGeer, E. G. (1983). *J. Neurosci. Meth.,* **9,** 229.
24. Hope, B. T. and Vincent, S. R. (1989). *J. Histochem. Cytochem.,* **37,** 653.
25. Hope, B. T., Michael, G. J., Knigge, K. M., and Vincent, S. R. (1991). *Proc. Natl Acad. Sci. USA,* **88,** 2811.
26. Vincent, S. R., Johansson, O., Hökfelt, T., Skirboll, L., Elde, R. P., Terenius, L., Kimmel, J., and Goldstein, M. (1983). *J. Comp. Neurol.,* **217,** 252.
27. Vincent, S. R., Staines, W. A., and Fibiger, H. C. (1983). *Neurosci. Lett.,* **35,** 111.
28. Vincent, S. R. and Johansson, O. (1983). *J. Comp. Neurol.,* **217,** 264.
29. Van Gelder, N. M. (1965). *J. Neurochem.,* **12,** 231.
30. Hyde, J. C. and Robinson, N. (1976). *Histochem.,* **46,** 261.
31. Vincent, S. R., Kimura, H., and McGeer, E. G. (1980). *Neurosci. Lett.,* **16,** 345.
32. Nagai, T., McGeer, P. L., and McGeer, E. G. (1983). *J. Comp. Neurol.,* **218,** 220.
33. Gerebtzoff, M. A. and Maeda, T. (1968). *C.R. Soc. Biol. (Paris),* **162,** 2032.

34. Inomata, K. and Ogawa, K. A. (1979). *Acta Histochem. Cytochem.,* **12,** 337.
35. Knyihar-Csillik, E., Bezzegh, A., Boti, S., and Csillik, B. (1986). *J. Histochem. Cytochem.,* **34,** 363.
36. Dodd, J., Jahr, C. E., Hamilton, P. N., Heath, M. J. S., Matthew, W. D., and Jessell, T. M. (1983). *Cold Spring Harbor Symp. Quant. Biol.,* **48,** 685.
37. Dalsgaard, C.-J., Ygge, J., Vincent, S. R., Ohrling, M., Dockray, G. J., and Eldge, R. (1984). *Neurosci. Lett.,* **51,** 139.
38. Nagy, J. I. and Hunt, S. P. (1982). *Neurosci.,* **7,** 89.
39. Vincent, S. R., Schultzberg, M., and Dalsgaard, C.-J. (1982). *Brain Res.,* **253,** 325.
40. Wong-Riley, M. (1989). *Trends Neurosci.,* **12,** 94.
41. Seligman, A. M., Karnovsky, M. N., Wasserkrug, H. L., and Hanker, J. S. (1968). *J. Cell Biol.,* **38,** 1.
42. Wong-Riley, M. (1979). *Brain Res.,* **171,** 11.
43. Hevner, R. F. and Wong-Riley, M. (1989). *J. Neurosci.,* **9,** 3884.
44. Karmy, G., Carr, P. A., Yamamoto, T., Chan, S. H. P., and Nagy, J. I. (1991). *Neurosci.,* **40,** 825.

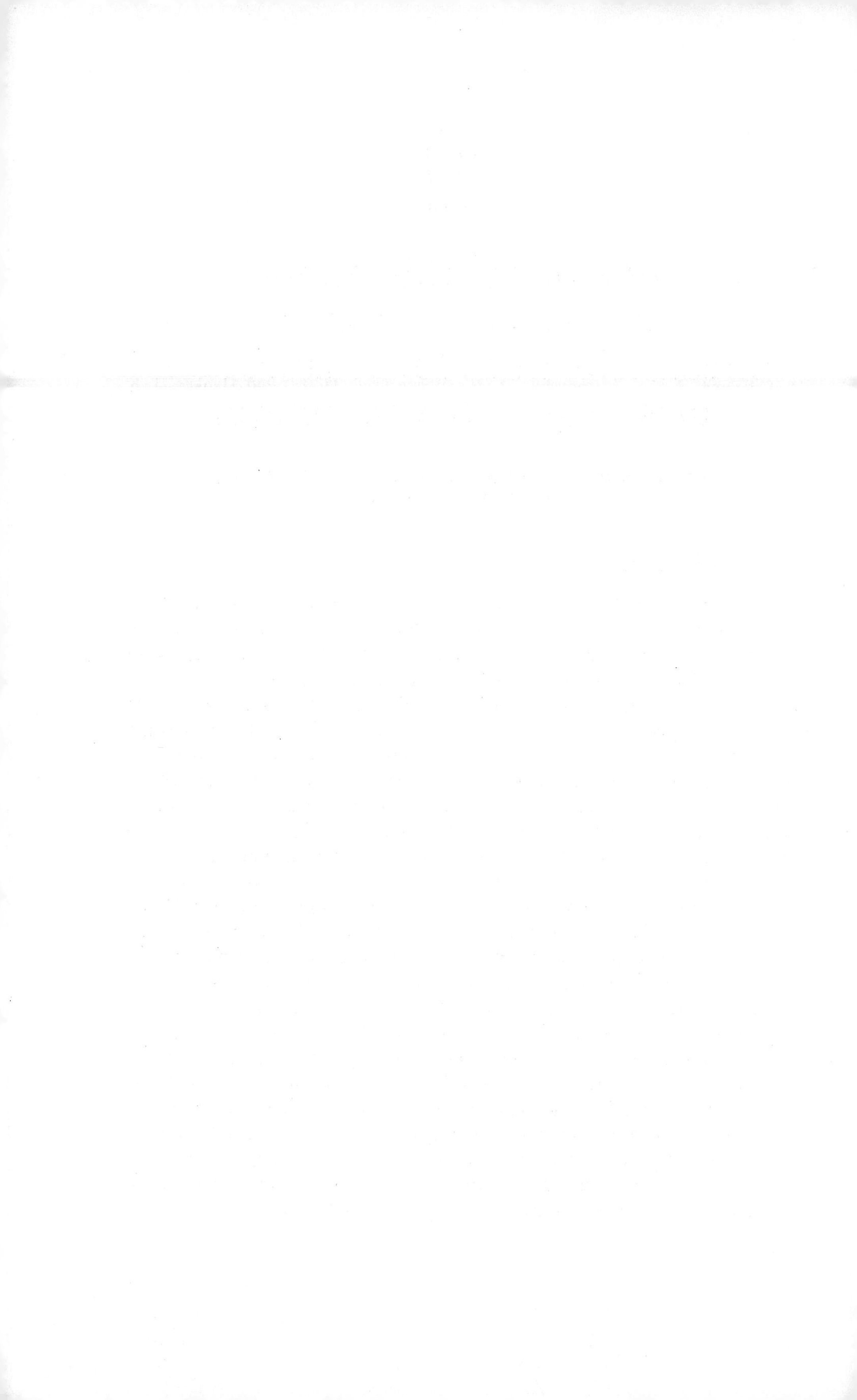

8

In situ hybridization histochemistry with oligonucleotides for localization of messenger RNA in neurones

CHARLES R. GERFEN, W. SCOTT YOUNG, III,
and PIERS EMSON

1. Introduction

In situ hybridization histochemical (ISHH) localization of messenger RNA transcripts (mRNA) provides a powerful technique for characterizing the biochemical phenotype of neurones in the brain (1). With the growing list of characterized mRNAs encoding proteins and neuropeptide precursors the utility of ISHH for the study of neural system organization and function has increased at a phenomenal rate. Included in the list of available probes are those directed against a variety of neurotransmitter and neuropeptide receptors, including G-protein coupled receptors and ion channel receptors, proteins of various signal transduction systems, neurotransmitter synthetic enzymes, and neuropeptides. It is thus possible with ISHH techniques to characterize neurones on the basis of their expression of neurotransmitter receptors, signal transduction systems linked to these receptors, and the neurotransmitter/neuropeptides they may use for synaptic signalling. When ISHH is combined with retrograde axonal tracing techniques the additional information of the neuroanatomical connections of neurones may be added to their neurochemical characteristics. Additionally, levels of mRNA transcripts in neurones are sometimes regulated either during development or in the adult by alterations in the functional state of the neurones. Quantitative ISHH techniques provide the ability to measure changes in levels of mRNA levels in neurones to determine the functional organization of neural systems. In this chapter methods of utilizing oligonucleotides for ISHH localization of mRNA transcripts in neurones will be detailed. Both radiolabelled and non-radiolabelled oligonucleotide methods, combinations of these methods to detect two mRNAs in single histologic brain sections, and a method for quantifying relative levels of mRNAs in neurones will be described.

There are two primary methods for localization of mRNAs in neurones with ISHH techniques, those using synthetic oligonucleotide probes and those using ribonucleotide probes (1). Rather than suggest that one method is better than the other, it should be emphasized that the method to be used should be determined by the experimental question that is to be addressed. Ribonucleotide probes have the benefit of allowing a considerably greater incorporation of radioactive or non-radioactive label per molecule, owing to the longer length of the probes compared with oligonucleotides. This feature alone results in increased sensitivity. An additional advantage of ribonucleotide probes for non-radioactive labelling methods, is that substituted bases used for such labelling are interspersed with normal bases. Thus problems of steric hindrance, which may severely reduce incorporation of substituted bases when added to 'tail' oligonucleotides, are diminished with ribonucleotide probes. Given the clear advantages in sensitivity of ribonucleotide probes it might be questioned why this is not always the method of choice. The simple answer is that techniques for labelling ribonucleotides are somewhat more complicated than those for oligonucleotides, and for many studies oligonucleotides provide nearly identical information.

Oligonucleotide probes offer many advantages. First, with an oligonucleotide synthesizer probes may be made from published sequence data. Second, it is possible to construct an oligonucleotide probe directed against a sequence of a mRNA that is specific for the encoded protein. This is of great utility in being able to construct probes specific to different members of the same protein family. Strategies for determining specificity of probe labelling are relatively simple. One such strategy is to construct probes directed against different regions of the mRNA and to determine if the cells in which such probes are localized are the same. Third, the labelling procedures are relatively straightforward and may be accomplished with a minimum of equipment. Fourth, as will be described, oligonucleotide probes provide a direct means of quantifying relative levels of mRNA expression. One advantage of oligonucleotide probes is that if a standard length of probe is used, for example 48 bases, then the methods of quantification are easily transferable between different probes. The problem of the sensitivity of oligonucleotide probes, compared with the use of ribonucleotide probes, may be overcome in some cases by using multiple oligonucleotide probes directed against a single mRNA transcript to increase the specific labelling for each transcript. None the less, the greater sensitivity of ribonucleotide probes should always remain a determinant in selecting the type of probe to be used for a given experiment.

2. Preparation of brain sections for ISHH

Oligonucleotide probes for ISHH are applied to brain sections that are adhered to glass slides. There are two basic choices for preparation of brain sections, one in which formaldehyde fixation is accomplished by perfusion of the animal (see Chapter 1, *Protocol 3*), and the second in which fresh-frozen brain sections are first adhered to slides and then formaldehyde fixed at a later time. In general the latter method is used, however, for some applications perfusion–fixation is preferable, for example, when ISHH is combined with retrograde axonal tract tracing. In both cases the post-sectioning processing procedures are identical and so the fresh-frozen procedure will be detailed.

Protocol 1. Preparation of brain sections for ISHH

A. *Brain preparation*

1. Kill the animal by carbon dioxide asphyxiation.
2. Remove the brain rapidly and freeze in isopentane (cooled to −70°C on dry ice). For rat brains the time required for freezing is approximately 15–25 sec. This time is relatively critical and requires that the isopentane be sufficiently cold. Keeping the brain in isopentane for this period of time ensures that the entire brain is properly frozen, but keeping the brain in for a longer time may result in 'cracking' of the brain, which should be avoided.
3. Following freezing, remove the brain from the isopentane, dry, wrap in foil, and store at either −20°C, if the brains are to be cut soon, or at −80°C if the brains are to be stored for an extended period prior to cutting.

B. *Sectioning of the brain*

Materials

Glass slides to which brain sections for ISHH are to be adhered should be twice-coated with a solution of chrom alum and gelatin. Heat water plus 1.88 g gelatin (300 bloom swine, Sigma Chemical catalogue number G-2500) in 750 ml total volume while stirring until warm, but do not boil. When gelatin is dissolved, cool, and add 0.188 g chrom alum (chromium potassium sulphate). Dip clean slides, in metal slide rack, into subbing solution, let slides drain and dry, and then repeat (see also Chapter 1, *Protocol 5*).

Method

1. Cut fresh-frozen brains in a cryostat (−16°C) into 4–12 μm thick sections, mount on to twice-coated slides, and dry on a warm plate (35–40°C) for at least 1 min. It is relatively critical to make sure that the sections are well adhered to the slides to ensure that they will not fall off during the ISHH processing.
2. Store brain sections adhered to slides at −20°C until being further processed. It is possible to store sections in this condition for several months.

Protocol 1. *Continued*

C. *Brain section preparation*

Materials

- 4% formaldehyde prepared from paraformaldehyde in 0.9% NaCl solution (saline) (see Chapter 1, *Protocol 2* and *Safety note 1*, p. 5)
- 0.1 M triethanolamine/0.9% NaCl (pH 8.0) (stock solution may be stored at room temperature)
- acetic anhydride (store desiccated at room temperature)

Method

1. Thaw slide mounted sections for 10 min and place in slide racks for histologic processing (all steps at room temperature).
2. Place slides with sections into troughs containing 4% formaldehyde/0.9% saline for 10 min.
3. Rinse slides in 0.9% saline for 5 min.
4. Place slides in 0.25% acetic anhydride in 0.1 M triethanolamine/0.9% NaCl (pH 8.0) for 10 min (add and mix vigorously acetic anhydride immediately before use).
5. Dehydrate slides by passing them for 2 min each through graded dilutions of ethanol in distilled water (v/v) (50%, 70%, 95%, and 2 × 100%).
6. Defat slides for 2 × 5 min periods in chloroform.
7. Rehydrate slides by passing them through 2 × 5 min periods in 100% ethanol, and 1 × 2 min in 95% ethanol.
8. Air-dry slides for 30 min.
9. The sections may be used immediately for ISHH, or stored dry at −20 to −70°C indefinitely.

3. Oligonucleotide labelling

The method described for labelling oligonucleotides with a 'tail' of [^{35}S]dAMPs has been described by Young *et al.* (1, 2). This method involves the addition of [^{35}S]dAMPs to the end of an oligonucleotide with the enzyme terminal deoxtidyl transferase (TdT), called the 'tailing' reaction, followed by the extraction and precipitation of the labelled probe (*Protocol 2*).

There have been many methods developed for the detection of hybridized oligonucleotides using non-radioactive techniques (1–3). The majority of these are variations on the labelling procedures in which radioactive nucleotide 'tails' are added to the probe. In the main, these methods have been used to detect relatively abundant mRNA levels, but have not provided sufficient sensitivity to detect mRNA levels encoding less abundant proteins. One method that has provided some potential utility has been described by Emson and co-workers (4). In this procedure the enzymatic marker alkaline phosphatase is directly conjugated to an oligonucleotide probe. The procedures for synthesis and purification of these probes will not be included in this chapter, however, a protocol for their use and visualization is included.

Protocol 2. Labelling of oligonucleotide probes for autoradiographic localization

Materials

- 5 × tailing buffer: (stored at −20°C) (may be supplied with the TdT), potassium cacodylate (1 M), Tris-HCl (pH 6.6, 125 mM), bovine serum albumin (1.25 mg/ml)
- cobalt chloride ($CoCl_2$, 25 mM): this is supplied with the TdT enzyme and is stored at −20°C
- [^{35}S]dATP: (stored at −20°C). The concentration provided by the supplier is listed as **X** nmol/ml, a final concentration of 1 μM is used in a volume of 50 μl, so the actual volume of [^{35}S]dATP to be used = 50 μl/**X** nmol/ml; i.e. if **X** = 10 nmol/ml then 5 μl of [^{35}S]dATP is used in a 50 μl reaction
- oligonucleotide probes: (stored at 4°C), stock solutions are stored at a concentration of 5 μM
- DNA deoxynucleotidyl transferase (TdT, EC 2.7.7.31): supplied by Boehringer Mannheim at a concentration of 25 U/μl and stored at −20°C
- tRNA: (stored at −20°C), stock solution concentration 27.5 mg/ml
- Tris-EDTA buffer (TE): (10 mM Tris, pH 7.4, 1 mM EDTA, stored at room temperature)
- 4 M NaCl: (stored at room temperature)
- phenol/chloroform/isoamyl alcohol: (50:49:1, stored at 4°C)
- chloroform/1% isoamyl alcohol: (stored at room temperature)
- dithiothreitol (DTT): (5 M, stored at −20°C)

Method

1. Add the following to a 1.5 ml tube on ice:

• water	26 μl
• 5 × tailing buffer	10 μl
• $CoCl_2$	3 μl
• [^{35}S]dATP	~5 μl to make final concentration of 1 μM

Protocol 2. *Continued*

- oligonucleotide — 1 μl (from a stock of 5 μM for a final concentration of 0.1 μM)
- TdT — 4 μl (100 U, Boehringer Mannheim)

2. Place the reaction mixtures in a water bath at 37°C for 5 min.
3. Terminate the enzyme reaction with the addition of 400 μl TE to each reaction mixture.
4. Add 1 μl of tRNA to each tube, which serves as a carrier for the labelled probe.
5. Add 1/20 volume (20 μl) of 4 M NaCl, which will precipitate the probe in step **8**.
6. Phenol extraction: to the reaction mixture add an equal volume of phenol/chloroform/isoamyl alcohol (49:50:1, 450 μl), vortex, centrifuge at 5000 *g* for 3 min, and pipette off the aqueous phase (upper phase) to a new 1.5 ml tube.
7. Chloroform extraction: add 450 μl chloroform (with 1% isoamyl alcohol) to the aqueous reaction mixture, mix the two phases by vortexing, centrifuge at 5000 *g* for 3 min, and pipette the aqueous phase to a new 1.5 ml tube.
8. Precipitation: Add two volumes of ethanol (900 μl) to the aqueous reaction mixture, vortex, place on wet ice for 10 min, and then centrifuge at room temperature for 12 min. Pipette off the ethanol/aqueous mixture, leaving a pellet. Wash the pellet with 1 ml of ice-cold 70% ethanol and pipette off. Resuspend the pellet in 50 μl of TE plus 1 μl DTT (5 M).
9. After 15 min test a sample of 1 μl for radioactivity. A successful labelling reaction gives 500 000–1 000 000 c.p.m./μl. This labelled oligonucleotide solution is stored at 4°C until used for hybridization and is stable for several weeks.

The capability of using ISHH to determine changes in the relative levels of mRNA expression in neurones that occur as a result of functional manipulations may be accomplished with the use of dilution standards. Such standards are prepared as equimolar concentrations of mixtures of radiolabelled and unlabelled oligonucleotide probes, which are applied to separate brain sections. Labelling of such sections, to which have been applied the same molar concentration of oligonucleotide probes, but of known varied specific radioactivity, are compared to determine the relative value of ISHH labelling signals. For a detailed description of this procedure see Gerfen *et al.* (5).

Protocol 3. Preparation of ^{35}S-radioactive oligonucleotide dilution standards

Materials

- same materials used in *Protocol 2*
- non-radioactive dATP

Method

1. Radioactively label oligonucleotide probe according to *Protocol 2*.
2. Simultaneously run an oligonucleotide labelling procedure using non-radioactive dATP substituted for radioactive dATP.
3. Following the precipitation of radioactive and non-radioactive oligonucleotide probes, redissolve each probe in an identical volume (50 μl) of TE.
4. Combine radioactive and non-radioactive oligonucleotide probes in ratios, on a volume basis, to obtain the following dilutions of radioactive probe: non-radioactive probe; 100:0, 80:20, 60:40, 40:60, 20:80.
5. Diluted probes are applied to brain sections on separate slides, which are then processed together according to *Protocol 4*.

4. *In situ* hybridization

The actual process of *in situ* hybridization involves the application of labelled oligonucleotide probes to brain sections which have been prepared to preserve histologic integrity while allowing penetration of the probes into the tissue to hybridize with mRNAs. The specific hybridization of labelled probes to mRNA in the tissue is determined by a combination of the temperature and salt concentration of the wash buffers. The optimal conditions for specific hybridization of a 48 base oligonucleotide are detailed below.

Protocol 4. *In situ* hybridization using radioactively labelled oligonucleotide probes

Materials

- dithiothreitol: (DDT, 5 M, stored at −20°C)
- 20 × SSC: sodium chloride (3 M), sodium citrate (0.3 M) buffer
- hybridization buffer

  50 ml hybridization buffer is prepared by combining the following:

4 M NaCl	7.5 ml
Tris-HCl (1 M, pH 7.5)	4.0 ml

Protocol 4. *Continued*

EDTA (250 mM)	0.8 ml
Na pyrophosphate (10%)	0.5 ml
dextran sulphate (50%)	10 ml
SDS (10%)	1.0 ml
heparin sulphate (0.57 g/10 ml)	0.17 ml
formamide	25 ml
water (sterile distilled)	1.8 ml

Hybridization buffer may be stored at −20°C, but should be thoroughly mixed and warmed prior to use.

Method

1. Add labelled oligonucleotides to hybridization buffer using the following formula. For one to two rat brain sections:
   - hybridization buffer — 50 μl
   - labelled probe (5–10 × 10^5 c.p.m./μl) — 2 μl
   - DTT (5 M) — 1 μl

   This formulation is used in multiples for two sections, a general rule of thumb is 50 μl hybridization buffer mixture for one to two sections per slide, and 100 μl for three to four sections per slide.
2. Vortex hybridization buffer with labelled oligonucleotide probe and DTT, and warm to 37°C in a water bath.
3. Pipette the warmed hybridization buffer mixture on to the brain sections (prepared according to *Protocol 1*), and place a coverslip (either glass or Parafilm) over the mixture making sure that there are no air bubbles over the brain sections.
4. Place the slides in a covered moist container at 37°C for 18–24 h.
5. After incubation remove the coverslips with slides immersed in 1 × SSC.
6. Pass slides through three beakers (or Coplin jars) of 1 × SSC, shaking vigorously to remove excess hybridization buffer.
7. If multiple slides are being processed, collect in a slide rack in 1 × SSC and process through washes together.
8. Wash slides for 4 × 15 min in 2 × SSC/50% formamide at 41°C (or 1 × SSC at 55°C).
9. Place slides in 1 × SSC for 2 × 30 min, rinse briefly in water, and air-dry.

The same basic protocol may be used for *in situ* hybridization using alkaline phosphatase labelled oligonucleotide probes. The differences in the protocol used for radiolabelled probes involve the use of a slightly different hybridization buffer, minus DDT and SDS, which reduce phosphatase activity, and the use of a different wash condition. Both of these modifications are necessary to retain optimal alkaline phosphatase activity.

Protocol 5. *In situ* hybridization using alkaline phosphatase labelled oligonucleotide probes

Materials

Same as *Protocol 4* except that DTT and SDS are not included in the hybridization buffer

Method

1. Add labelled oligonucleotides to hybridization buffer using the following formula. For one to four rat brain sections per slide:
   - hybridization buffer (without SDS) 250 μl
   - labelled probe 2 μl
2. Vortex hybridization buffer with labelled oligonucleotide probe and warm to 37°C in a water bath.
3. Pipette the warmed hybridization buffer mixture on to the brain sections (prepared according to *Protocol 1*). Note: no coverslip is used in this procedure.
4. Place the slides in a covered moist container at 37°C for 18–24 h.
5. After incubation, pass slides through three beakers (or Coplin jars) of 1 × SSC, shaking vigorously to remove excess hybridization buffer.
6. If multiple slides are being processed collect in a slide rack in 1 × SSC and process through washes together.
7. Wash slides for 3 × 30 min in 1 × SSC at 55°C.
8. Place slides in 1 × SSC for 2 × 30 min, rinse briefly in water, and air-dry.

Protocol 6. Visualization of radioactive ISHH labelling

Materials

- Ilford K5 photographic emulsion
- Dektol developer
- Kodak fixer

Protocol 6. *Continued*

Method

1. Under photographic safelight, melt Ilford K5 emulsion at 37°C in slide mailer.
2. Dip sections on slides into emulsion (37°C), drain off excess emulsion.
3. Let emulsion dry completely, box slides into light tight boxes.
4. Expose to photographic emulsion for two to eight weeks (at −20°C).
5. Develop slides in Dektol developer (diluted 1:2 with water) for 2 min at 15°C.
6. Stop photographic reaction in 1% acetic acid (1 min, room temperature).
7. Fix slides in Kodak rapid fix, without hardener (2 min, room temperature).
8. Rinse slides for 30 min in running water.
9. Stain sections in thionin for 1 min, rinse in water for 2 min.
10. Dehydrate slides by passage from water through 1 min rinses each in 50%, 70%, 95%, 2 × 100% ethanol, and apply coverslip (see Chapter 1, *Protocol 6*).

Protocol 7. Visualization of alkaline phosphatase labelled probes

Materials

- buffer 1: pH 7.5

2 M Tris-HCl pH 7.5	25 ml
NaCl	4.38 g
distilled H_2O	to 500 ml

- buffer 2: pH 9.5

2 M Tris-HCl pH 9.5	25 ml
NaCl	2.92 g
$MgCl_2$	5.07 g
distilled H_2O	to 500 ml

- stop buffer: pH 7.5

2 M Tris-HCl pH 7.5	2.5 ml
NaCl	4.38 g
EDTA	0.19 g
distilled H_2O	to 500 ml

- NBT stock solution (nitroblue tetrazolium): 75 mg NBT in 1 ml 70% dimethyl formamide (prepared in glass tube only), store at −20°C

- BCIP stock solution (5-bromo-4-chloro-3-indolyl phosphate toluidinium salt)
  50 mg BCIP in 1 ml 100% dimethyl formamide

Method

1. Carry out *in situ* hybridization on sections according to *Protocol 5*.
2. Wash slides in buffer 1 for 20 min.
3. Incubate in buffer 2 (pH 9.5) for 5–20 min.
4. Incubate for 24–48 h in dark with substrate solution prepared by mixing 20 ml buffer 2, 90 μl NBT stock solution, and 70 μl BCIP stock solution. Either immerse slides completely in substrate solution or use 0.5–1.0 ml per slide.
5. Wash in stop buffer, pH 7.5 for 5–12 h.
6. Apply coverslip to slides with glycerin, or process for emulsion dipping according to *Protocol 6*.

5. Combined radiolabelled and alkaline phosphatase labelled probes

When both radiolabelled and alkaline phosphatase labelled probes are combined for the purposes of double labelling, *Protocol 5* is followed with both probes being added to the same hybridization buffer. The further processing is followed as described for each individual probe, with *Protocol 7*, providing visualization of the alkaline phosphatase labelled probes being followed first, followed by *Protocol 6*, for autoradiographic visualization of the radiolabelled probes.

6. Limitations of the method

In considering the limitations of the oligonucleotide ISHH it is best to state what this method demonstrates. *In situ* hybridization histochemistry provides a means of labelling neurones on the basis of their containing a mRNA transcript encoding a particular gene product. Labelling is of neurone perikarya, as this is the location of the vast majority of mRNA along with the bulk of the cellular machinery involved in peptide/protein translation. Thus, ISHH does not directly provide information concerning the axonal projections of neurones that are labelled. Moreover, because ISHH labels mRNA transcripts, it does not provide information concerning post-translational processing of gene products. These are inherent limitations of the method. Limitations of the method that are somewhat variable have to do with the specificity and sensitivity of the procedures. As stated earlier, the specificity of the labelling

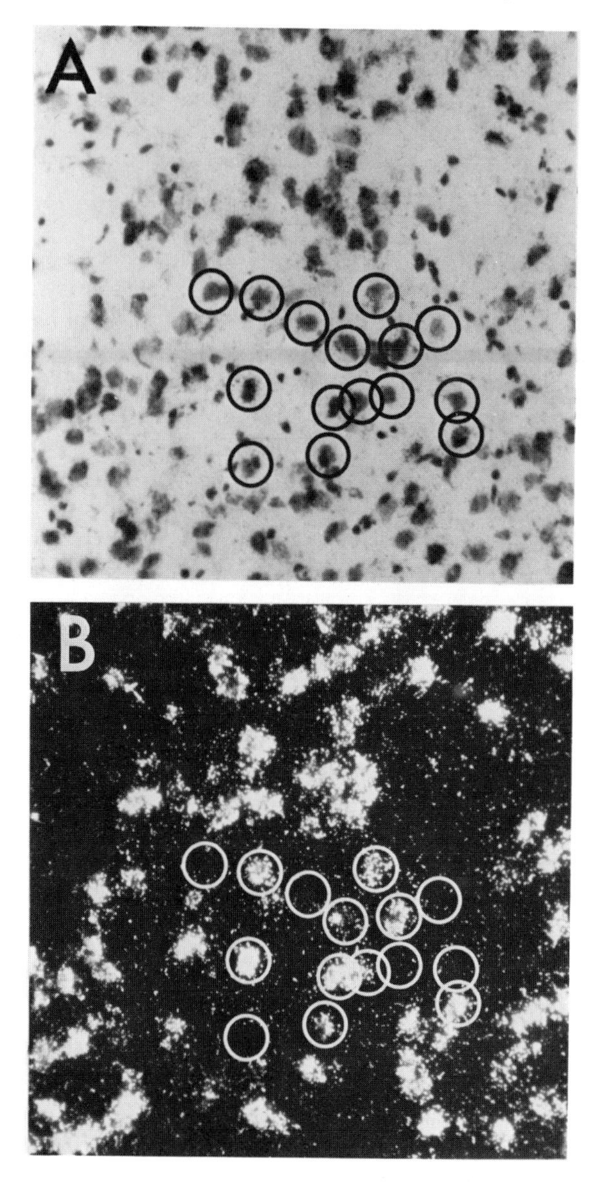

Figure 1. Photomicrographs of a field in the striatum viewed with bright-field (A) and dark-field (B) illumination. Thionin stained cells are identified under bright-field illumination (A), and cells labelled with an enkephalin oligonucleotide probe are visualized by the accumulation of white grains under dark-field illumination (B). Examples of selected neurones (circles in (A)) and the corresponding area in the dark-field image (circles in (B)), show that some of the neurones are labelled by the autoradiographic oligonucleotide procedure, whereas others are not. (From Gerfen *et al.* (5).)

is dependent on the use of oligonucleotides that are complementary to a portion of the mRNA to be targeted that is unique. The degree of specific binding is dependent in part on the stringency of the hybridization parameters, including the ionic content and temperature of the hybridization solutions. The sensitivity of the method is dependent on many factors, and as discussed above there are more sensitive procedures. Thus, in using oligonucleotide probes the absence of labelling is necessarily considered in the context of the relative sensitivity of the procedure. This being said, for many applications the abundance of certain messenger RNAs in neurones is sufficient for the oligonucleotide procedures to be more than adequate.

Figure 1 shows photomicrographs of ISHH labelling of neurones in the striatum of a rat using radioactively labelled probes directed against preproenkephalin mRNA. While enkephalin mRNA is relatively abundant in striatal neurones, this set of photomicrographs illustrates several aspects of ISHH labelling. First, the specificity of labelling with this probe is suggested by two facts; one, that labelling is concentrated over cell bodies and two, some cells show clear labelling whereas others do not. This latter point is a critical aspect of specificity, the demonstration of the absence of labelling in the presence of clearly labelled cells. Specific labelling may be seen by the regional distribution of labelling, such as labelling of the striatum but not the cortex, or as seen in *Figure 1* by the labelling of a subpopulation of cells in a given region. Such patterns of labelling provide definitive evidence of the specificity of the oligonucleotide probe. Second, the sensitivity of the labelling using a particular probe may be questioned in the following manner. In *Figure 1* approximately half of the cells that are neurones show levels of labelling that are sufficiently above background to allow them to be distinguished. The question then may be asked as to whether unlabelled neurones do not contain the mRNA to which the probe is directed, or whether they contain insufficient amounts of the transcript to be detected with this particular method. This question may never be completely answered as there is always the possibility that a neurone may express a very few copies of a particular transcript, which might be detectable with some methods but not with others. However, a way of estimating the relationship between the sensitivity of the method and the ability to detect labelled cells is provided by using radiolabelled probes diluted with unlabelled probes (see *Protocol 3*). Determining how the percentage of neurones labelled in a given brain area varies as a function of diluted probe provides such an estimate. As with any neuroanatomical technique, its utility is dependent in large part on the understanding of its limitations.

References

1. Young III, W. S. (1990). In *Handbook of Chemical Neuroanatomy, Analysis of Neuronal Microcircuits and Synaptic Interactions* (ed. A. Björklund, T. Hökfelt, F. G. Wouterlood, and A. N. van den Pol), Vol. 8, p. 481. Elsevier, Amsterdam.

2. Young III, W. S., Bonner, T. I., and Brann, M. R. (1986). *Proc. Natl Acad. Sci. USA,* **83,** 9827.
3. Lewis, M. E., Sherman, T. G., and Watson, S. J. (1985). *Peptides,* **6** (suppl. 2), 75.
4. Kiyama, H., Emson, P. C., Ruth, J., and Morgan, C. (1990). *Mol. Brain Res.,* **7,** 213.
5. Gerfen, C. R., McGinty, J. F., and Young III, W. S. (1991). *J. Neurosci.,* **11,** 1016.

9

Intracellular Lucifer Yellow injection in fixed brain slices

EBERHARD H. BUHL

1. Introduction

Intracellular filling of neurones with Lucifer Yellow (LY) in fixed brain slices is a relatively novel anatomical tool to determine neuronal geometry (1, 2). In the absence of electrical activity, the procedure is based on direct visual guidance of the dye injections, therefore providing an inherently high degree of staining selectivity. Moreover, being highly compatible with a variety of other neuroanatomical protocols, intracellular filling in fixed tissue is an attractive technique to unravel neuronal microcircuitry (3, 4).

It is the purpose of this chapter to outline initially the necessary equipment, followed by a detailed description of the injection procedure. Subsequently, several alternative protocols are provided to visualize LY at the light and electron microscopical levels, while the final sections describe the combination with retrograde and anterograde tracing methods. It is however beyond the scope of this technical overview to critically discuss the methodological value of intracellular filling in fixed slices (for review see 5).

2. Equipment

2.1 Injection set-up

In the absence of recordable neuronal activity, intracellular dye injections in fixed tissue require optical monitoring of the filling procedure (6, 7). Most conventional microscopes have the disadvantage that focusing is brought about by vertical stage movements which would also reposition the fixed-slice bath. Therefore, in order to fill neurones by intracellular injection it is necessary to employ a *fixed stage* microscope, (e.g. Zeiss ACM). Visually guided impalements of cells are undertaken by advancing the micropipettes at an angle as close to the vertical as possible. Long distance objectives, (e.g. Zeiss UD 20/0.57, UD 40/0.65, Nikon ELWD × 40) with a working distance ranging between 8–10 mm allow an electrode position of approximately 45° from the vertical (2).

Table 1. Characteristics of a useful range of Zeiss wide-bandpass filters[a]

Excitation	Exciter filter	Beam splitter	Barrier filter
UV–violet	390–420 nm	425 nm	450 nm
Blue–violet	395–440 nm	460 nm	470 nm
Blue	450–490 nm	510 nm	520 nm
Green	515–565 nm	580 nm	590 nm

[a] Most other manufacturers provide products with fairly similar specifications.

Epifluorescence illumination, (e.g. Zeiss HBO 50 W high pressure mercury lamp) is essential to view dye-filled pipettes in conjunction with a variety of fluorescent marker molecules. When choosing appropriate filter sets for fluorescence microphotography, narrow-bandpass filters with selective excitation will increase the image contrast. For injection purposes however, wide-bandpass filters (*Table 1*) prove to be advantageous by providing more intensive excitation and therefore a brighter image. Up to four different filters sets may be required to optimally visualize the available range of fluorescent dyes (for review see 8, 9).

(a) UV–violet: fast blue (10), diamidino yellow (11), nuclear yellow (10, 12), DAPI (4,6-diamidino-2-phenylindole; 13), true blue (14), Primuline (13), bisbenzimide (12, 15), fluoro-gold (16), LY (17, 18).

(b) Blue–violet: fast blue, diamidino yellow, nuclear yellow, DAPI, LY (bright).

(c) Blue: acridine orange, FITC (fluorescein isothyocyanate), green latex beads (19), LY (less intense).

(d) Green: rhodamine latex beads (20, 21) DiI (22), TRITC (tetramethyl-rhodamine isothiocyanate), Evans blue (13), propidium iodide (15).

2.2 Micromanipulator

For targeting and impaling neurones it is necessary to employ a micromanipulator with three planes of movement and a minimum 1 μm spatial resolution. Mechanical, motor-driven, and hydraulic (electrode drift may be a problem) devices are equally suitable. To enable large scale electrode manoeuvres, for instance for pipette changes, it may be advantageous to fit the micromanipulator on a coarse, three dimensional electrode positioner with a movement range exceeding 2 cm. Frequently, left and right handed versions are available. Before acquiring an appropriate manipulator it is important to determine whether and how the instrument can be fitted to the injection microscope. Major manufacturers, such as Narashige, (e.g. hydraulic models

MO-303, MO-302, MO-203), or Märzhäuser, (e.g. models HS 6/3, motorized DC 3 with control unit MS 314), offer a broad range of suitable equipment. Usually these products are available through a net of distributors, less frequently from the manufacturers.

2.3 Pipette puller and iontophoretic pump

For intracellular dye injections in fixed tissue it is crucial to make ultrafine micropipettes with tip diameters in the range of 0.1–0.2 μm. In principle, most electrode pullers should fulfil these requirements. By adjusting the heat and the strength of pull (solenoid) it is usually feasible to obtain suitable electrode tips with appropriate length, taper, and diameter. Although a range of modern pullers possess a variety of accessory features, these are by no means essential for the production of useful micropipettes.

A microiontophoresis system is essential to deliver constant currents in the nA range with electrode impedance consistently exceeding 100 MΩ. To prevent LY leakage into the slice-bath it may be necessary to apply a retention current of the opposite polarity. As there is no appreciable difference with respect to the mode of dye ejection, an additional pulse unit is not required. Finally, it is of practical value if the instrument can measure the electrode impedance, for instance through a bridge amplifier.

Although most microelectrode amplifiers with inbuilt current clamp facilities, (e.g. Axoclamp-2A from Axon Instruments) will fulfil these specifications, some iontophoretic current pumps, (e.g. Ionophor 3, Bio-Logic, or Neuroscience Trading) are equally suitable. Moreover, even simple, battery-driven devices may be adequate.

3. Injection procedure

3.1 Fixation

Intracellular injection procedures, regardless whether performed in living or fixed tissue, depend on the biophysical properties of neuronal membranes. Essentially they subserve an important role as a highly impermeable barrier for both ionic and lipophilic substances, and thus maintain concentration gradients across the cellular boundary. It is therefore feasible to introduce, by means of iontophoretic or pressure injection, diffusible markers that will label a neurone and its processes in its entirety. Hence it is a pre-requisite for intracellular work in fixed tissue to preserve the structural integrity of the cell membrane, thereby preventing the marker from leaking into the extracellular space (6). Fortuitously a large variety of aldehyde containing fixatives appear to be suitable (4). To date, all available recipes contain either phosphate-buffered formaldehyde as the basic recipe and, depending on the experimental requirements, up to 15% saturated picric acid (v/v), and/or up to 1% of glutaraldehyde (v/v) may be added to the fixative (see Chapter 1, *Protocol 2* for preparation of fixatives).

3.1.1 Perfusion–fixation

A detailed protocol for perfusion–fixation is provided in Chapter 1, *Protocol 3*. However, it should be stressed here that following the perfusion particular care should be taken when dissecting the brain. Avoid squashing or damaging the region of interest. As a rule of thumb, stronger fixation will increase the fragility of membranes. If the brain consistency appears to be too soft for subsequent vibrating microtome sectioning, immerse it for several hours in fixative. Alternatively, store the brain in 0.1 M phosphate buffer (PB, pH 7.4) at 4°C until sectioning.

3.1.2 Immersion-fixation

For several reasons it is preferable to employ perfusion rather than immersion fixation. First, when immersing tissue in fixative the progress of diffusion is considerably delayed towards the centre of the block. Second, as a consequence this diffusion gradient may also result in greatly varying degrees of fixation. Finally, red blood cells that remain in the vasculature provide a potential obstacle for subsequent experimental steps that require a minimum of endogenous peroxidase activity in the tissue.

If immersion fixation is however unavoidable, e.g. with human biopsy or autopsy material (23, 24), keep the tissue sample as small as possible, not exceeding 0.5 cm in thickness. After minimally 2–5 h in fixative transfer the tissue into 0.1 M PB. Prolonged storage in fixative is detrimental for subsequent use, e.g. increase in background fluorescence, excessive dye leakage. If not required immediately, store the material in the refrigerator.

3.2 Preparation of slices

To obtain viable slices it is imperative to avoid all procedures that would be detrimental to membrane preservation, such as freezing, use of detergents, exposure to lipophilic solvents, and hyper- as well as hypotonic solutions.

Protocol 1. Preparation of slices (see also Chapter 1, *Protocol 4*)

1. Dissect and trim the region of interest from the brain. Preferably leave pia mater attached to avoid mechanical stress.
2. Blot off excess liquid.
3. Attach the tissue sample to vibrating microtome chuck with quick setting cyanaocrylate glue ('superglue').
4. Fix the block in holder and fill the microtome bath with 0.1 M PB. Preferably use the same buffer at 4°C for electron microscopic experiments.
5. After removing grease with acetone, insert a new, high quality (razor) blade.

6. Start cutting at very low speed using maximal frequency of vibration.
7. Adjust the section thickness, depending on how much of the neurone's dendritic and axonal arbor is required. Slices exceeding 150 μm in thickness may however require re-sectioning at a later stage.
8. If sections come off easily, the cutting speed may be increased. Avoid however pushing or squeezing the tissue with too much forward thrust of the blade.
9. Pick up sections by gently rolling them around a soft brush. Transfer them into 0.1 M PB. For serial sections, tissue culture wells prove to be advantageous.
10. Store the sections at 4°C. If the material is initially suitable for injection purposes it should remain viable for at least one week.

3.3 Preparation of micropipettes

Micropipettes for intracellular recording and filling in living tissue are invariably a compromise of two opposing requirements. To improve the quality of recording, the tip size should be as large as possible, thus reducing electrode resistance and noise, whereas smaller and sharper tips generally have less detrimental effects on the cell when impaled. In fixed tissue however, since electrical activity is absent it is possible to minimize electrode tip sizes; the electrodes however should be able to pass a constant hyperpolarizing current in the range of 1 nA.

Appropriate pulling parameters to obtain adequate micropipettes have to be empirically determined for every individual electrode puller in conjunction with the chosen brand of capillaries. Even minute changes in the puller's filament position may be sufficient to substantially alter the shape and therefore also properties of electrode tips. Despite the obvious impracticability of recommending absolute values there are however a few governing principles for the intentional manipulation of pulling parameters (for review see 25).

(a) Increasing the width of the heating filament will increase tip length and, to some extent, decrease tip diameter.
(b) A higher airflow setting (not available on many pullers) will result in shorter tips without altering the tip diameter.
(c) Higher heat settings will give longer and finer tips.
(d) Larger values of pull strength (solenoid) will decrease the tip size.

For the choice of suitable glass capillaries the following considerations should be taken into account. Those containing a glass filament are preferable, since capillary forces allow solutions to spread almost instantaneously to the electrode tip. With identical pulling parameters thick wall capillaries and/or borosilicate tubing provide thinner tips than conventional tubing.

Protocol 2. Preparation of micropipettes

1. Prepare a 5–10% aqueous stock solution of Lucifer Yellow (17, 18). The salt should dissolve very readily. Filtering is usually not required. Keep the stock in the refrigerator, where it should remain viable for many months. If dried out, LY may be reconstituted without detrimental effects.
2. Pull pipette (for strategy see above). Tip shape and taper may be assessed in the light microscope, however tip diameters range between 0.1–0.2 μm, which is well below the resolution level.
3. Use a microsyringe to fill pipette shank with approximately 1–2 μl LY. If tubing containing a filament is used, the dye will rapidly spread to the electrode tip.
4. Insert metal wire, e.g. copper, silver, tungsten, into capillary. It should be in contact with the filling solution.
5. Determine electrode DC resistance which, when measured in PB, should range between 150 and 300 MΩ. The electrode impedance provides a relative measure, although not linear, for the tip diameter. Note, however, that variations in the molarity of filling solutions will also result in resistance changes.
6. If several micropipettes are prepared in advance, store them in a moisturized container to prevent the tips from drying out.

3.4 Injection technique

The following description of the injection protocol is largely based on the author's own experience. A number of parameters may therefore slightly differ from the procedure utilized by other laboratories (24, 26–30).

Protocol 3. Intracellular injection of neurones in fixed slices

1. In the absence of pre-labelled neurones, targeting may be facilitated by visualizing cells after immersion in a fluorescent counterstain, e.g. 5 min in a 1 μM solution of acridine orange in 0.1 M PB (7), or 10^{-7} M DAPI in 0.1 M PB (31). Depending on tissue, fixation, type of filter, and degree of background fluorescence the optimal incubation time and concentration range of any dye may require empirical adjustment.
2. Transfer slice into a dish filled with 0.1 M PB.
3. Float the tissue on a glass slide.
4. Cover the section with a fenestrated Millipore filter leaving the region of interest uncovered. Prevent material from drying out.
5. Place small weights on top of the filter to prevent the preparation from floating in the bath.

6. Place slide into injection chamber and submerge in 0.1 M PB. Adding 2 mM ascorbic acid to chamber fluid may be useful to reduce the induction of an autofluorescent background (6). Otherwise change the medium at regular intervals, thus removing leaking LY from the bath.
7. Transfer the chamber to the stage of the microscope. Ground the preparation bath to the iontophoresis pump.
8. Attach a dye-filled electrode to the micromanipulator and connect to the iontophoresis pump.
9. Advance electrode towards tissue at an angle of at least 40–45° from the vertical. Employ the epifluorescence illumination to visually guide pipette movements.
10. When the tip is immersed in the bathing solution, test the suitability of the pipette by applying 1–2 nA negative constant current. Provided the background is sufficiently low, a diffuse yellow cloud should be seen to emerge from the pipette tip. With ultrafine tips, the use of higher currents harbours the risk of clogging the tip with dye. This is readily recognized by the tip turning bright orange and a concomitant increase in electrode impedance.
11. Excessive dye leakage in the absence of applied current may be prevented by a holding current with positive polarity.
12. Adjust the microscope stage to centre the labelled cell in the field of view. Avoid cells located at the surface of the slice since many processes may have been truncated during sectioning.
13. Align the electrode with appropriate micromanipulator movements and advance towards target.
14. When direct contact with neuronal cell membrane is suspected, intracellular penetration may be facilitated by either gently tapping the micromanipulator or by, if available, briefly (1–2 msec) oscillating the capacitance compensation circuit ('buzzing').
15. Ascertain whether the impalement is successful by applying a brief current pulse which should result in rapid dye filling of the soma and proximal dendrites. If the LY spreads in a diffuse cloud, the electrode is probably still located in the extracellular space. Bear in mind that fixed membranes have a very limited capacity to reseal after injury. Therefore it is recommended to abandon the target when membrane damage is suspected after an unsuccessful penetration manoeuvre. Depending on soma size, depth in tissue, and the experimenter's skill, the rate of satisfactory impalements may vary between 30–70%.
16. Continue the filling with negative constant current (0.5–3 nA) until terminal dendrites appear brightly fluorescent. Adjust the current according to cell size. Large cells with an extensive dendritic arbor can withstand higher current intensities and may require substantially longer

Protocol 3. *Continued*

injection periods, occasionally exceeding 15 min. Avoid prolonged fluorescence illumination during dye injection. This will lead to fading of the fluorescence and may also cause ultrastructural damage (G. Meredith and F. G. Wouterlood, personal communication). When filling neurones with long, thin-diameter processes, it appears that a reduction of the current amplitude in conjunction with an appropriate increase of the duration will improve the dye equilibration.

17. After the dye injection has been completed, withdraw the pipette. Several neurones may be filled in a single preparation. If not required immediately, the slice should be kept in 0.1 M PB at 4°C. However, prolonged storage will result in a gradual loss of staining intensity and a concomitant increase in background fluorescence.

---

4. Visualization of Lucifer Yellow injected neurones in the fluorescence and light microscope

4.1 Embedding for fluorescence microscopy

A plethora of different mounting media is available for embedding fluorescent specimens (*Figure 1*). All of them share the common property of being essentially free from undesired autofluorescence. Several non-permanent mounting media prove to be advantageous because dehydration and clearing steps are not required.

(a) Glycerol, (e.g. 50% glycerol and 50% 0.1 M PB pH 7.4). Note that glycerol appears to be incompatible with rhodamine latex beads.

(b) Dimethyl sulphoxide (DMSO; 100%) has the advantage of minimizing shrinkage artefacts (32). Incompatible with latex microspheres.

(c) Methyl salicylate (100%).

To prevent sections from drying out, seal the edges of coverslip with nail varnish. Note that variations in pH of the mounting medium may have an effect on photostability and fluorescence yield of dyes. A number of additives has been suggested to retard the fading of fluorescent markers, although their efficacy remains controversial (33):

- sodium azide (25 g/l) (34)
- sodium iodide (25 g/l) (34)
- *p*-phenylendiamine (1 g/l) (35)
- *n*-propyl-gallate (50 g/l) (36)

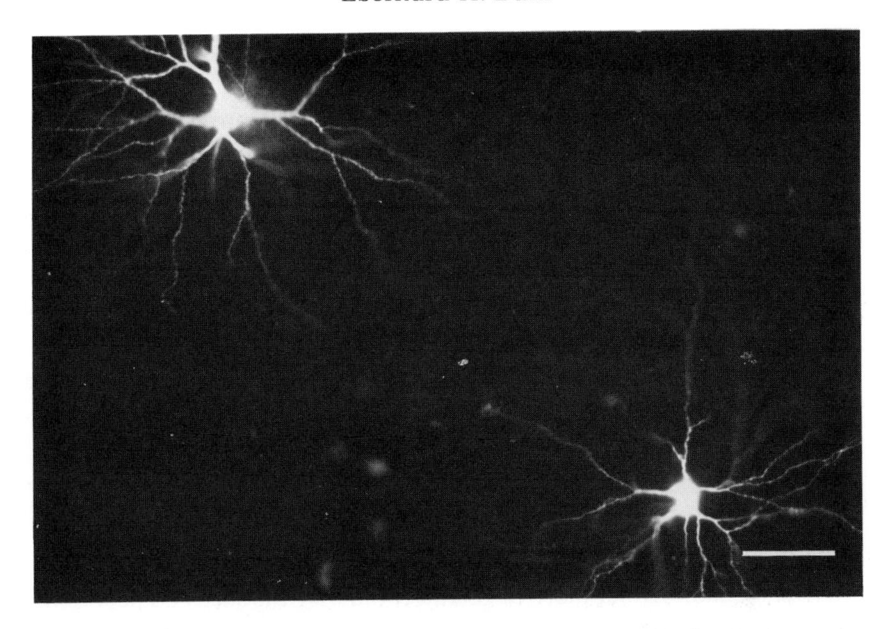

Figure 1. Two pyramidal cells in cat visual cortex, visualized in the fluorescence microscope after intracellular injection with LY. Scale bar = 50 μm.

Embedding protocols providing more permanent specimens often require prolonged exposure to ethanol and/or xylene, which may result in quenching the fluorescence of various tracers, e.g. rhodamine coupled latex beads, green latex microspheres. Fortuitously, LY is compatible with most histological procedures, although it loses its fluorescence after treatment with osmium tetroxide (18). For embedding protocol see Section 4.1.1.

4.1.1 Sectioning of thick slices

It is an inherent problem of fluorescence microscopy that background intensity increases linearly with section thickness, while the signal intensity remains approximately constant. Moreover, thinner specimens may be also required for subsequent methodological steps, such as immunocytochemistry. Several different strategies may be used.

(a) Avoid sectioning by using confocal microscopy, which is ideally suited for 3-D reconstructions.

(b) Cut frozen sections (29). Technically easy, but careful cryoprotection is necessary to prevent freezing artifacts. The lower limit of section thickness with this method is approximately 25 μm.

(c) Polyethylene glycol embedding is the most sophisticated approach, but sections well below 10 μm may be obtained. Highly suitable for dual immunocytochemistry ('mirror technique') of identified neurones (for detailed description see 37).

(d) Vibrating microtome sectioning after agar or gelatin embedding. Note however, that gelatin embedding may be detrimental for subsequent immunoreactions (Meredith, personal communication).

Protocol 4. Gelatin embedding and re-sectioning of slices

1. Make a solution of 10% gelatin in distilled water. Heat to dissolve, but avoid boiling.
2. Cool down the gelatin but maintain the temperature above melting point.
3. Blot excess liquid off the slice and carefully flatten on the bottom of a Petri dish. Cool on ice.
4. Submerge the slice to a depth of 3–4 mm in gelatin solution. Prevent from floating, while gelatin sets.
5. Transfer to refrigerator until firm.
6. Trim a quadrangular piece of gelatin containing the slice and peel it from the bottom of the Petri dish.
7. Immerse the block for approximately 2 h in 4% paraformaldehyde in 0.1 M PB (hardens gelatin and facilitates cutting).
8. Rinse in 0.1 M PB.
9. Section on vibrating microtome (see *Protocol 1*).
10. Wash the sections 3 × 15 min in 0.1 M PB.
11. Mount the sections on coated slide (see Chapter 1, *Protocol 5*).
12. Allow the tissue to dry vertically for several hours.
13. Dehydrate in ethanol: 50%, 70%, 90%, 95%, 2 × 100%—10 min each. Skip, if ethanol quenches the fluorescence.
14. Clear for 2 × 10 min in xylene. If xylene attenuates the staining intensity, reduce the exposure time to minimum 1 min each.
15. Apply coverslip with non-fluorescent resin, e.g. Fluoromount (Gurr), Entellan (Merck), Krystalon (Harleco).
16. Store sections in a cool, dark place.

4.2 Photoconversion

Despite differences in their stability, more or less all fluorescent dyes are susceptible to gradual fading during prolonged exposure to their respective excitation wavelength. Hence fluorescence material is not ideally suited for quantitative analysis or time consuming camera lucida reconstructions. Photoconversion in the presence of diaminobenzidine (DAB) (the suitability of other chromogens, such as tetramethylbenzidine or benzidine dihydrochloride, remains to be determined) provides a convenient method to obtain permanent preparations for light microscopy purposes (*Figure 2A*) (2, 38–40).

Protocol 5. Photoconversion of Lucifer Yellow-filled neurones

1. Dissolve 15 mg DAB[a] in 5 ml distilled water.
2. Dissolve 10 mg potassium cyanide[b] in 5 ml 0.2 M PB. Potassium cyanide suppresses the endogenous peroxidase activity in the tissue, and thus reduces the background intensity (41, 42).
3. Mix both solutions. For convenience the author uses a 10 ml syringe. To avoid the DAB precipitating, store the syringe in darkness at 4°C. The mixture remains viable for several hours. Filter before use, e.g. with a disposable membrane filter that may be attached to the syringe.
4. Transfer the slice to a small disposable Petri dish and submerge it in the photoconversion mixture. Allow 5–10 min to equilibrate.
5. Replace on the microscope stage and expose the injected neurone(s) to LY excitation wavelength until all visible fluorescence has faded. High power lenses will result in shorter conversion times and therefore less background. Use objectives with long working distance to avoid accidental contact with the DAB solution. Employ transmission illumination to monitor the concomitant appearance of dark brown precipitate. Note that the developing reaction product may quench some of the remaining fluorescence, which can result in prematurely terminating the conversion reaction. If well-filled neurones are poorly converted, increase the illumination time to determine the point of optimal signal:noise (background) ratio.
6. Rinse the slice 3 × 10 min in 0.1 M PB.
7. Mount the photoconverted slice on a coated slide (see Chapter 1, *Protocol 5*).
8. Allow the tissue to dry vertically for several hours.
9. Dehydrate in ethanol: 50%, 70%, 90%, 95%, 2 × 100%—10 min each, clear with 2 × 10 min changes in xylene, and apply a coverslip (see Chapter 1, *Protocol 6*).

[a] DAB is a suspect carcinogen, see *Safety note 3* in Chapter 5 (p. 119) for precautions in handling.
[b] Potassium cyanide is extremely toxic, all manipulations before it is dissolved should be carried out with appropriate protective clothing and in a fume cupboard.

4.2.1 Osmium intensification

After photoconversion injected neurones usually have a dark brown appearance (*Figure 2A*). Several intensification protocols exist that take advantage

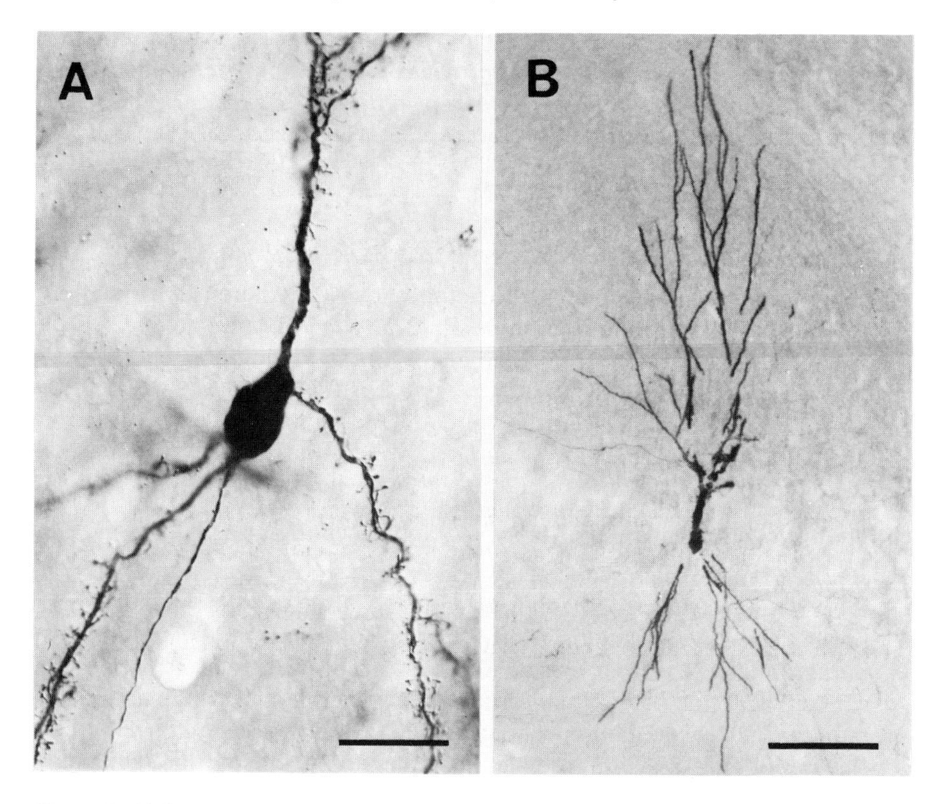

Figure 2. Light microscopic appearance of LY injected neurones following photoconversion (A), and immunocytochemical visualization with an antiserum directed against LY (B). Scale bars = (A) 20 μm, (B) 100 μm.

of the affinity of the DAB polymer for heavy metal ions thus increasing the opacity of the reaction product for light microscopy. Osmium intensification appeals mainly due to its methodological simplicity (43, 44).

Protocol 6. Osmium intensification

1. Mount the slice on a coated slide (Chapter 1, *Protocol 5*). Avoid using sections exceeding 100–150 μm in thickness (opaque background).
2. Allow the preparation to dry vertically for several hours.
3. In a fume hood, cover the tissue for several minutes with 0.2–0.5% osmium tetroxide[a] (prepare freshly from stock—2% or 4% in distilled water; see Chapter 1, *Protocol 7*) in 0.1 M PB. Empirically determine the optimal concentration range and incubation times.

4. Briefly dip the sections in distilled water.
5. For embedding procedure, follow *Protocol 5*.

[a] Note that phosphate may cause a higher degree of unspecific precipitation in the osmium step. If the background appears unacceptably high, substitute PB with 0.1 M Tris-buffer.

4.3 Employing antisera against Lucifer Yellow

Although it is technically simple, the photoconversion procedure has the disadvantage that only one field of view may be converted at one time. As an alternative, large numbers of injected neurones can be simultaneously visualized by utilizing antisera against LY (*Figure 2B*) (24, 45, 46). The following protocol has been established employing a polyclonal antiserum raised in rabbit (kindly provided by J. McIlhinney, MRC Anatomical Neuropharmacology Unit, Oxford). Note that different antibodies may require substantial modification of fixation prameters, incubation periods, and the concentration of the primary antiserum. Often a minimal amount of glutaraldehyde is required in the fixative. It appears that several antisera recognize LY in its bleached form. It is therefore worthwhile processing material depleted of most of the visible fluorescence after prolonged exposure times.

Protocol 7. Immunocytochemical visualization of LY at the light microscopical level[a]

1. Post-fix the slice in fixative (2% glutaraldehyde, 4% paraformaldehyde in 0.1 M PB) for several hours (see Chapter 1, *Protocol 2*).
2. Wash 2 × 15 min in 0.1 M PB.
3. Infiltrate the slice for 15 min with 10% sucrose in PB.
4. Infiltrate the slice for 30 min with 20% sucrose in PB.
5. Blot off excess liquid, transfer to an Eppendorf tube, and freeze in liquid nitrogen.
6. Thaw at room temperature and transfer slice to 0.1 M PB.
7. Section the slice with vibrating microtome at 40–60 μm (see *Protocol 4* and Chapter 1, *Protocol 4*). If the antiserum penetrates sufficiently well then the whole unsectioned slice may be used but increase the incubation time in the primary antiserum.
8. Wash 3 × 30 min in 0.1 M PB.
9. Wash 2 × 20 min in Tris-buffered saline (TBS; 50 mM Tris, 0.85% NaCl, pH 7.4), with 0.5% Triton X-100 added.
10. Incubate one hour with 20% normal swine serum (NS) in TBS, with 0.5% Triton X-100. Normal serum of species in which secondary anti-

Protocol 7. *Continued*

serum was raised blocks non-specific binding sites and therefore reduces background labelling (see also Chapter 5).

11. Incubate overnight in primary antiserum (rabbit anti-LY, 1:500 dilution) in TBS, with 1% NS, and 0.5% Triton X-100.
12. Wash 3 × 30 min in TBS, with 1% NS, and 0.5% Triton X-100.
13. Incubate 3–6 h in secondary antiserum (HRP conjugated swine anti-rabbit, diluted 1:100) in TBS, with 1% NS, and 0.5% Triton X-100.
14. Wash 3 × 30 min in TBS, with 1% NS, and 0.5% Triton X-100.
15. Wash 2 × 20 min in Tris-buffer (TB, 50 mM) pH 8.0.
16. Pre-incubate in darkness, 20 min in chromogen (15 mg DAB, 600 mg nickel ammonium sulphate in 100 ml TB, pH 8.0) (see *Safety note 4* in Chapter 5, p. 123).
17. For 2 ml add 20 μl of 0.5% hydrogen peroxide (final concentration of 0.005%). Monitor the progress of staining in a microscope, approximately 2–10 min.
18. Wash 3 × 30 min in TB pH 8.0.
19. Wash 2 × 15 min in 0.1 M PB.
20. For embedding procedure follow *Protocol 5*.

[a] For alternative immunocytochemical protocols see Chapter 5.

5. Correlated light and electron microscopy of photoconverted neurones

A major disadvantage of LY, i.e. the fact that it is not electron dense, is overcome by the photoconversion procedure. Due to the osmiophilic nature of the DAB precipitate these preparations may be processed for ultrastructural analysis (3, 23). Moreover, unlike other chromogens the DAB reaction product remains stable during conventional embedding procedures. Under the electron microscope, injected neurones and their processes will appear darkly contrasted. Therefore it is feasible to morphologically identify neurones and subsequently determine ultrastructural features in conjunction with their synaptic circuitry (47). However, to permit such correlated light and electron microscopic investigations it is necessary to employ one of the conventional flat-embedding procedures.

5.1 Flat-embedding

In recent years, several equally effective methods have been devised to view resin embedded specimens in the light microscope, prior to their analysis in the electron microscope (48–50). It has been suggested to sandwich the material between either acetate sheets or, alternatively, between a Teflon-coated slide and coverslip. However, our laboratory routinely uses plain glass which proves to be both convenient and satisfactory (51). A detailed methodological description of the procedure is provided elsewhere in this volume (see Chapter 1). After flat-embedding, injected neurones may be graphically reconstructed with the aid of a camera lucida. Note however that specimens exceeding 100 μm in thickness may be too opaque for transillumination in the light microscope.

5.2 Visualization in the electron microscope

At the ultrastructural level, photoconverted neurones and their processes appear opaque due to their content of electron dense reaction product (*Figure 3*) (4). The precipitate is finely dispersed throughout karyo- and cytoplasm of the cell without obscuring morphological details, such as synaptic vesicles in labelled axon terminals (47). Frequently the DAB polymer tends to aggregate on the surface of the plasmalemma and organelles. At higher magnification, the degree of tissue preservation is usually sufficient to clearly resolve synaptic contacts (4). However, if the quality of sections is poor this may be the result of:

- inadequate perfusion, no glutaraldehyde in fixative, poor quality fixative, for instance, no electron microscopic-grade glutaraldehyde.
- osmolality changes during processing
- prolonged exposure to buffer solutions; dendrites attain a 'washed-out' appearance
- improper resin formulation or mixing, incomplete infiltration
- poor section quality, for instance too thick
- section contamination, for instance 'fixation pepper'
- staining procedure artefacts

Depending on the quality of the injection, the concentration of reaction product may diminish somewhat towards distal processes. However, as a rule of thumb, light microscopically discernible contrast differences between labelled and unlabelled structures are normally resolved in the electron microscope. Occasionally, depending on the amount of non-specific DAB precipitate in the tissue, the neuropil surrounding labelled processes may appear too dark. If so, try reducing the concentration of osmium tetroxide (not below 0.5%) and/or of any other contrasting agent, such as uranyl acetate and lead citrate (Chapter 1, *Protocol 11*).

6. Combination with retrograde tracing

The majority of neuroanatomical staining methods, although providing good morphological details of neurones, render only very limited information with

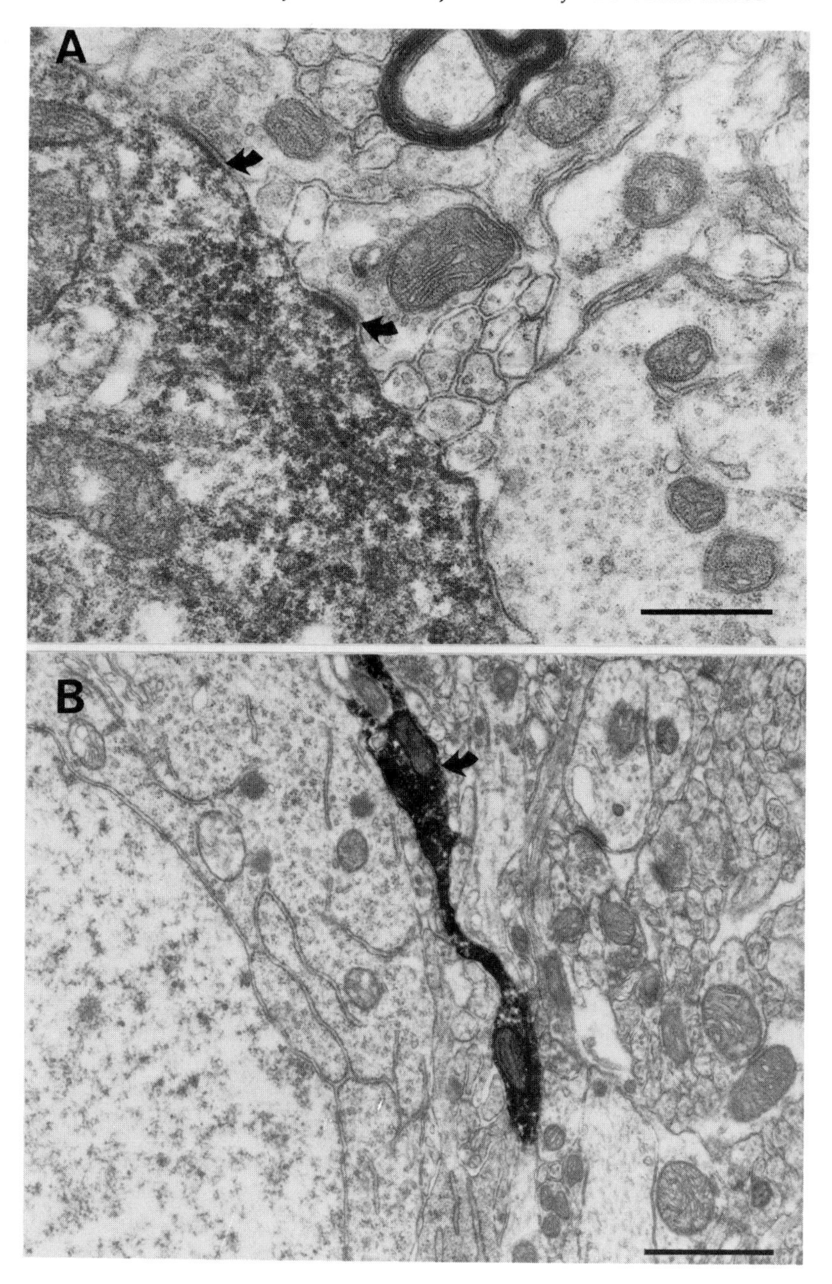

Figure 3. Ultrastructural details of photoconverted spiny stellate neurones in rat entorhinal cortex. Labelled profiles such as the cell body (A) or axon collaterals (B) contain copious amounts of dark, electron-dense reaction product. Arrows denote axo-somatic synapses (A), and a varicose swelling containing synaptic vesicles (B), respectively. Scale bars = (A) 0.5 μm, (B) 1 μm.

respect to the efferent connectivity. In contrast, retrograde tracing methods are rarely sensitive enough to properly assess the detailed morphology of neurones with identified projection sites. A combination of both methods is therefore desirable, especially because it is becoming increasingly evident that morphologically distinct subsets of neurones may share a particular innervation site (21). Since optical monitoring is a pre-requisite of intracellular filling in fixed tissue, it is therefore feasible to visibly label nerve cells, prior to their injection, by means of a retrogradely-transported fluorescent tracer (2, 52, 53).

6.1 Choice of marker

In general, fluoresecnt tracers are characterized by several favourable properties, such as their simple visualization and their excellent suitability for double and triple label experiments (54). However, amongst the almost bewildering variety of available compounds individual markers differ substantially with respect to:

- absorption and emission characteristics, i.e. their visibility in individual filter combinations
- stability during illumination, i.e. the rate of fading
- uptake mechanism, e.g. zone of effective uptake
- direction of transport (retrograde and/or anterograde)
- permanence of labelling, e.g. speed of diffusion into adjoining cells
- sensitivity

Obviously, the choice of an appropriate marker is largely determined by the experimental requirements, and it is therefore advantageous to differentiate fluorescent tracers according to their characteristics. From the available compounds a choice selection is provided here of several well characterized and widely used tracers. Each marker is followed by a brief description of its properties.

(a) *Fast blue* (FB) (10): fluoresces in blue–violet and UV–violet filter, retrogradely transported, intense cytoplasmic labelling, suitable for iontophoretic injections, fades fairly fast, marked loss of labelling during immunocytochemistry (9).

(b) *Rodamine beads* (20): fluoresce in green filter, weakly in blue filter where also LY-pipette is visible, highly localized uptake site, retrogradely transported, granular cytoplasmic labelling, fades very slowly, ideal for long-term labelling, compatible with most immunocytochemistry protocols. Caution: do not reconstitute when dried out.

(c) *Fluoro-gold* (16): fluoresces in UV–violet filter, retrogradely transported, strong cytoplasmic labelling and extensive dendritic filling, suitable for iontophoretic injections (55), compatible with other histochemical procedures (9).

(d) *DiI* (56): fluoresces in green filter, strong membrane and/or cytoplasmic labelling, anterogradely and retrogradely transported, ideal for long-term labelling (57), slow rate of fading, since highly lipophilic, poor compatibility with most embedding procedures and media (ethanol, xylene, glycerol).

(e) *Diamidino yellow* (11): fluoresces in UV–violet and blue–violet filter, distinct yellow nuclear labelling, highly suitable for double and triple-labelling studies.

In principle, any of these tracers may be used in conjunction with intracellular LY-injection. However, dyes that are visible in the same filter combination(s) as LY may facilitate targeting, but the intense fluorescence of LY quickly renders them undetectable, once filling is initiated. If the presence of the retrograde label needs to be documented, it is essential to choose a marker that remains discernible after the LY injection (5). Fortuitously, several tracers, such as rhodamine beads (58) and DiI (2), retain their visibility, when switching to the green excitation filter because LY appears rather dull. Conversely, targeting any of these labels with a dye filled pipette is facilitated under the blue filter, where they may shine through as reddish yellow. Alternatively, the favourable properties of two different markers, such as FB and DiI, may be combined by simply mixing them and selecting those neurones that contain both tracers (52).

6.2 Tracer injection and survival time

Fluorescent dyes may be administered using a variety of methods, such as injection with a microsyringe, pressure ejection through a micropipette, iontophoresis, and the implantation of crystals. For pressure injections through either pipette or syringe, most tracers are delivered as 1–5% (w/v) aqueous solutions (8, 9). Suspensions of rhodamine coupled latex beads may be diluted up to 1:4 with phosphate-buffered saline. Cacodylic acid seems to be a suitable vehicle to iontophorese a number of dyes such as propidium iodide, fast blue and fluoro-gold (55).

Protocol 8. Iontophoretic injection of fluoro-gold (55)

1. Prepare a 2% solution of fluoro-gold in 0.1 M cacodylic acid (sodium cacodylate-trihydrate; see *Safety note 2* in Chapter 5, p. 108). The resulting solution is of approximately neutral pH.
2. Prepare glass pipettes with tips broken at approximately 20 μm.
3. Fill the pipettes by either capillary action or suction.
4. Perform craniotomy, and stereotaxically lower electrode into desired location.

5. Start iontophoresis with 5–10 μA pulsed positive current for 5–10 min. Decreasing the current intensity and time will result in injection sites as small as 500 μm in diameter.
6. For smaller injection sites in the range of 100–150 μm, use pressure injections of rhodamine beads (50–200 nl).
7. Withdraw pipette and allow the animal to recover.

The optimal survival time may vary considerably, depending on the rate of transport, speed of intracellular breakdown, as well as the species and particular systems investigated. In general, the optimal period is in the range of two to four days. Although longer survival times may result in better labelling, several tracers (notable exceptions: rhodamine beads and DiI) may start migrating into adjoining glial cells (12).

7. Visualization of afferents

When progressing further towards the analysis of neuronal microcircuits it may prove necessary to investigate the source and termination pattern of synaptic inputs to morphologically identified neurones (59, 60). To visualize termination sites of an afferent pathway, several anterograde tracing methods may be used in conjunction with intracellular dye injections.

7.1 Anterograde fluorescent tracing

While the majority of fluorescent dyes are solely transported in the retrograde direction, a number of tracers has been successfully employed for anterograde tracing purposes. These compounds have the unique advantage that afferents, e.g. thalamic axons delineating ocular dominance columns (61), may be visualized during the injection procedure. However, their universal applicability appears to be limited due to their unsuitability for electron microscopy purposes.

(a) *DiI* (62). Pressure injections of 0.005–0.01 μl of a 25% solution/suspension of DiI in dimethylformamide. Optimal survival time may vary between 8 to 90 hours. Longer survival periods result in no appreciable loss of labelling.
(b) *Tetramethylrhodamine isothiocyanate* (*TRITC*) (61). Approximately 0.5 μl pressure injections of 5% TRITC, isomer *R* (Sigma), dissolved in dimethyl sulphoxide. At least two weeks transport are necessary to label cat geniculo-cortical axons.
(c) *Fluorescent dextrans* (63, 64). Dextrans with a molecular weight of approximately 10 000 Daltons are usually conjugated to a fluorescent dye, such as cascade blue, fluorescein, Lucifer Yellow, tetramethylrhodamine,

texas red (all available from Molecular Probes, Eugene, OR). Prepare 2–20% solution in distilled water. For pressure injection, volumes can range between 0.01–2 μl. Survival periods may vary between 3 to 14 days.

7.2 Lesion induced anterograde degeneration

In vertebrates, axotomy will invariably result in the anterograde degeneration of the distal part of the axon. After an appropriate survival period, when viewed in the electron microscope, such severed axon terminals have several distinctive morphological features, such as loss of synaptic vesicles and dark electron-dense cytoplasm. A consequence of this is that lesion techniques have been successfully employed to label synaptic boutons from an identified source (59, 65). The main appeal of this approach is in the technical simplicity, as the electron microscopic identification of degenerating terminals requires no further visualization procedures that are invariably detrimental for the ultrastructural preservation (5). However, lesion methods have at least three obvious disadvantages. First, they are not suitable for quantitative studies, due to the protracted course of the degeneration process. Secondly, without employing silver impregnation methods, degenerating terminals are not visible in the light microscope. Thirdly, combination with immunocytochemical techniques to identify the transmitter of the terminals is not advisable because the boutons will undergo changes in their transmitter content.

Several different approaches may be utilized to induce anterograde degeneration (reviewed in 66).

(a) *Aspiration and knife cuts*. Technically simple, but may result in significant damage of ancillary structures as well as fibres of passage. Depending on the neural target the optimal survival time may vary considerably, usually between one to five days.

(b) *Electrolytic lesions*. Based on passing anodal or cathodal current from the tip of an insulated electrode. The approach is readily combined with stereotaxic procedures. Lesion size is determined by variation in the current amplitude. Damage of fibres of passage.

(c) *Excitotoxins*. Pressure injections of microlitre amounts of glutamate receptor agonists, such as kainic acid (1–2 μg/μl), ibotenic acid (10 μg/μl), or domoic acid (0.5 μg/μl). These have the advantage of sparing fibres of passage. Various factors, such as the system under investigation, may require adjustment of the injected amount and concentration of the drug.

7.3 Combination of the anterograde transport of *Phaseolus vulgaris*–leucoagglutinin with intracellular LY-injection in fixed slices

Anterograde tracing with the lectin *Phaseolus vulgaris*–leucoagglutinin (PHA-L) is a highly sensitive approach to label afferent pathways (see

Chapter 3) (reviewed in 67). Although requiring a considerable number of technical steps, which may be detrimental to the ultrastructural preservation, this method has the distinct advantage that prior to electron microscopy labelled axons may be fully analysed at the light microscopic level. The following protocol is taken from a pioneering study of Wouterlood and colleagues (29) in which PHA-L tracing was combined with fixed-slice LY-injection, visualizing both tracers with a dual immunocytochemistry procedure (*Figure 4*).

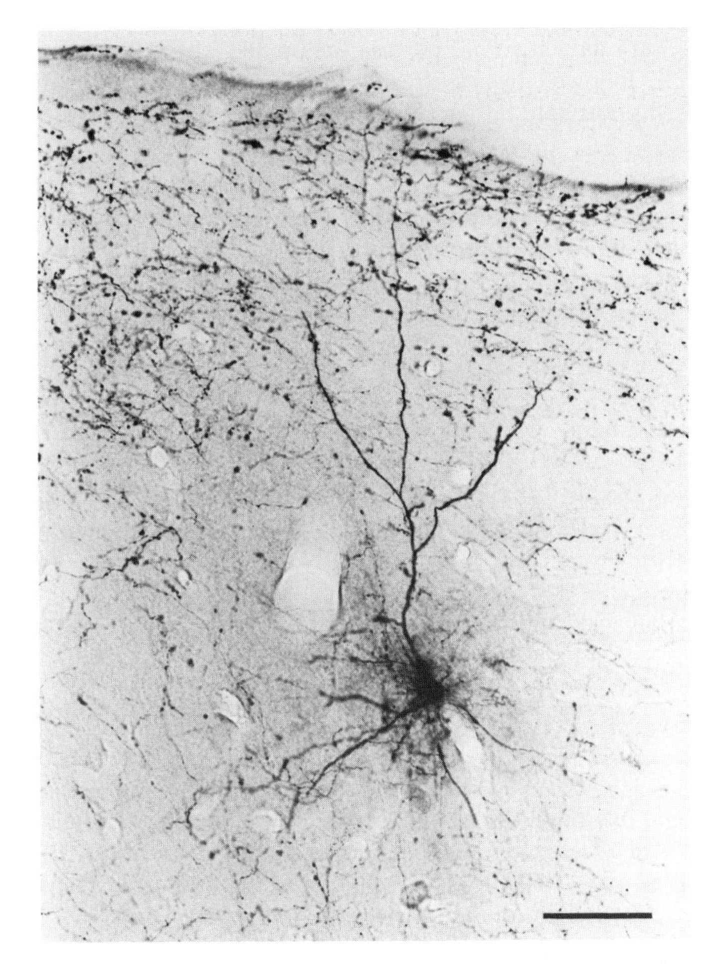

Figure 4. Light micrograph showing LY-injected neurone in the lateral entorhinal cortex of the rat surrounded by PHA-L labelled afferents from the nucleus reuniens. Both marker substances were revealed with a dual immunocytochemistry procedure. (Courtesy of Prof. F. G. Wouterlood.) Scale bar = 50 μm.

Protocol 9. Light microscopic visualization of LY-filled neurones and PHA-L[a] labelled afferents using dual immunocytochemistry[b] (29, 68)

1. Prepare PHA-L (Vector, Burlingame, USA): 25 μg/μl in 0.05 M Tris-buffered saline (TBS) pH 7.4.
2. Anaesthetize the animal and perform craniotomy.
3. Iontophorese PHA-L through a glass micropipette (tip diameter 10–20 μm). Injection parameters: 6 μA positive DC current (7 sec on/7 sec off, 20 min).
4. After 7–14 days survival, perfuse the animal with 0.9% saline at 38°C, pH 6.9, followed by 4% freshly depolymerized paraformaldehyde in 0.125 M phosphate buffer (PB) pH 7.4 (see Chapter 1, *Protocols 2* and *3*).
5. Following perfusion, remove the brain and prepare 200 μm vibrating microtome sections. Cut alternate 40 μm sections to examine the injection site and transport of PHA-L.
6. Store sections in vials on ice containing 0.1 M PB, with 50 μl of 0.1 M NaN_3 solution/ml of medium.
7. Intracellularly inject, for instance, retrogradely pre-labelled neurones (see *Protocol 3*).
8. After dye filling, store slices overnight in cold 0.1% glutaraldehyde in 0.1 M PB.
9. Rinse the slices several times in PB, and cryoprotect by immersion in a solution consisting of 20% glycerine and 2% dimethyl sulphoxide in 0.1 M PB.
10. On the stage of a freezing microtome, mount the slice on flat-trimmed surface of a solidly frozen block of 30% sucrose in 0.1 M PB. Cut at 30 μm thickness.
11. For incubations and rinsing, use a buffer composed of 0.05 M Tris, 0.85% NaCl, 0.5% Triton X-100 (TBS-TX).
12. Wash 3 × 10 min in TBS-TX.
13. Incubate overnight (16 h) under continuous gentle agitation in a cocktail composed of goat anti-PHA-L antiserum (Vector Labs., Burlingame, USA; diluted 1:8000), and rabbit anti-LY antiserum (developed by Taghert *et al.* (45); diluted 1:3000) in TBS-TX.
14. Wash 3 × 10 min in TBS-TX.
15. Incubate the sections for 90 min in donkey anti-goat IgG (diluted 1:100) in TBS-TX at room temperature.
16. Wash 3 × 10 min in TBS-TX.

17. Incubate the sections for 90 min in goat peroxidase anti-peroxidase complex (goat-PAP; 1:2000) at room temperature.
18. Wash 3 × 10 min in TBS-TX.
19. Transfer the sections to 0.05 M Tris-HCl buffer, pH 8.0.
20. Visualize the transported PHA-L by first pre-incubating sections 5–10 min with the chromogen, nickel-enhanced diaminobenzidine (Ni-DAB; 200 mg nickel ammonium sulphate and 7.5 mg 3,3′-diaminobenzidine in 50 ml 0.05 M Tris, pH 8.0).
21. Add 10 μl of 25% H_2O_2 and monitor the progress of the reaction under a microscope. A *deep-blue to black* precipitate should develop in labelled structures.
22. Rinse in 0.05 M Tris-HCl pH 7.4.
23. Wash 3 × 10 min in TBS-TX.
24. Incubate sections for 2 h in biotinylated goat anti-rabbit IgG (diluted 1:250 in TBS-TX) at room temperature.
25. Wash 3 × 10 min in TBS-TX.
26. Incubate for 90 min in avidin–biotin–peroxidase complex (Vectastain kit, Vector, Burlingame, USA) with continuous gentle agitation.
27. Wash 3 × 10 min in TBS-TX, followed by 0.05 M Tris-HCl buffer, pH 7.6.
28. Visualize LY by reacting sections in 0.04% DAB and 0.015% H_2O_2 in 0.05 M Tris-HCl buffer, pH 7.6. A *brown* precipitate should form in LY-containing processes.
29. Mount sections on coated slides, leave to dry, dehydrate, and apply a coverslip with resin (see *Protocol 4*).

[a] For further details on the preparation, use, and visualization of PHA-L see Chapter 3.
[b] For further details on immunocytochemical protocols see Chapter 5, and on double immunocytochemical protocols see Chapter 11.

Acknowledgements

The author gratefully acknowledges his colleagues J. F. Dann, P. Germroth, J. Lübke, G. E. Meredith, L. Peichl, J. D. Pettigrew, W. Schlote, W. K. Schwerdtfeger, P. Somogyi, W. Singer, D. I. Vaney, H. Wässle, and F. G. Wouterlood for their invaluable contributions to this review.

References

1. Schwerdtfeger, W. K. and Buhl, E. (1986). *Brain Res.,* **386,** 146.
2. Buhl, E. H. and Lübke, J. (1989). *Neurosci.,* **28,** 3.

3. Buhl, E. H., Schwerdtfeger, W. K., and Germroth, P. (1989). In *The Hippocampus—New Vistas* (ed. V. Chan-Palay and C. Köhler), p. 71. Alan R. Liss, New York.
4. Buhl, E. H., Schwerdtfeger, W. K., and Germroth, P. (1990). In *Handbook of Chemical Neuroanatomy* (ed. A. Björklund, T. Hökfelt, F. G. Wouterlood, and A. N. van den Pol), Vol. VIII, p. 273. Elsevier, Amsterdam.
5. Buhl, E. H. (1993). *J. Microsc. Tech.* In press.
6. Tauchi, M. and Masland, R. H. (1984). *Proc. R. Soc. Lond. (B),* **223,** 101.
7. Tauchi, M. and Masland, R. H. (1985). *J. Neurosci.,* **5,** 2494.
8. Skirboll, L., Hökfelt, T., Norell, G., Phillipson, O., Kuypers, H. G. J. M., Bentivoglio, M., Catsman-Berrevoets, C. E., Visser, T. J., Steinbusch, H., Verhofstad, A., Cuello, A. C., Goldstein, M., and Brownstein, M. (1984). *Brain Res. Rev.,* **8,** 99.
9. Skirboll, L. R., Thor, K., Helke, C., Hökfelt, T., Robertson, B., and Long, R. (1989). In *Neuroanatomical Tract-Tracing Methods 2: Recent Progress* (ed. L. Heimer and L. Zaborszki), p. 5. Plenum Press, New York and London.
10. Bentivoglio, M., Kuypers, H. G. J. M., Catsman-Berrevoets, C. E., Loewe, H., and Dann, O. (1980). *Neurosci. Lett.,* **18,** 25.
11. Keizer, K., Kuypers, H. G. J. M., Huisman, A. M., and Dann, O. (1983). *Exp. Brain Res.,* **51,** 179.
12. Bentivoglio, M., Kuypers, H. G. J. M., and Catsman-Berrevoets, C. E. (1980). *Neurosci. Lett.,* **18,** 19.
13. Kuypers, H. G. J. M., Catsman-Berrevoets, C. E., and Padt, R. E. (1977). *Neurosci. Lett.,* **6,** 127.
14. Bentivoglio, M., Kuypers, H. G. J. M., Catsman-Berrevoets, C. E., and Dann, O. (1979). *Neurosci. Lett.,* **12,** 235.
15. Kuypers, H. G. J. M., Bentivoglio, M., van der Kooy, D., and Catsman-Berrevoets, C. E. (1979). *Neurosci. Lett.,* **12,** 1.
16. Schmued, L. C. and Fallon, J. H. (1986). *Brain Res.,* **377,** 147.
17. Stewart, W. W. (1978). *Cell,* **14,** 741.
18. Stewart, W. W. (1981). *Nature,* **292,** 17.
19. Katz, L. C. and Iarovici, D. M. (1990). *Neurosci.,* **34,** 511.
20. Katz, L. C., Burkhalter, A., and Dreyer, W. J. (1984). *Nature,* **310,** 498.
21. Katz, L. C. (1987). *J. Neurosci.,* **7,** 1223.
22. Honig, M. G. and Hume, R. I. (1989). *Trends Neurosci.,* **12,** 333.
23. Buhl, E. H. and Schlote, W. (1987). *Acta Neuropathol. (Berl.),* **75,** 140.
24. Einstein, G. (1988). *J. Neurosci. Meth.,* **26,** 95.
25. Brown, K. T. and Flaming, D. G. (1986). *Advanced Micropipette Techniques for Cell Physiology.* Wiley, Chichester.
26. Rho, J.-H. and Sidman, R. L. (1986). *Neurosci. Lett.,* **72,** 21.
27. Rho, J.-H. and Swanson, L. W. (1987). *Brain Res.,* **436,** 143.
28. Felthauser, A. M. and Claiborne, B. J. (1990). *Brain Res.,* **118,** 249.
29. Wouterlood, F. G., Jorritsma-Byham, B., and Goede, P. H. (1990). *J. Neurosci. Meth.,* **33,** 207.
30. Wyss, J. M., Van Groen, T., and Sripanidkulchai, K. (1990). *J. Comp. Neurol.,* **295,** 33.
31. Dann, J. F., Buhl, E. H., and Peichl, L. (1988). *J. Neurosci.,* **8,** 1485.
32. Grace, A. A. and Llinás, R. (1985). *Neurosci.,* **16,** 461.

33. Böck, G., Hilchenbach, M., Schauenstein, K., and Wick, G. (1985). *J. Histochem. Cytochem.*, **33,** 699.
34. Johnson, G. D., Davidson, R. S., McNamee, K. C., Russel, G., Goodwin, D., and Holborow, E. J. (1982). *J. Immunol. Meth.*, **55,** 231.
35. Platt, J. L. and Michael, A. F. (1983). *J. Histochem. Cytochem.*, **31,** 840.
36. Giloh, H. and Sedat, J. W. (1982). *Science,* **217,** 1252.
37. Smithson, K. G. and Hatton, G. I. (1990). In *Handbook of Chemical Neuroanatomy* (ed. A. Björklund, T. Hökfelt, F. G. Wouterlood, and A. N. van den Pol), Vol. VIII, p. 305. Elsevier, Amsterdam.
38. Maranto, A. R. (1982). *Science,* **217,** 953.
39. Sandell, J. H. and Masland, R. H. (1988). *J. Histochem. Cytochem.*, **36,** 555.
40. Bentivoglio, M. and Su, H.-S. (1990). *Neurosci. Lett.*, **113,** 127.
41. Buhl, E. H. and Dann, J. F. (1990). *Neurosci. Lett.*, **116,** 263.
42. Buhl, E. H. and Dann, J. F. (1991). *Hippocampus,* **1,** 131.
43. Johansson, O. and Backman, J. (1983). *J. Neurosci. Meth.*, **7,** 185.
44. Lübke, J. and Albus, K. (1989). *Dev. Brain Res.*, **45,** 29.
45. Taghert, P. H., Bastiani, M. J., Ho, R. K., and Goodman, C. S. (1982). *Dev. Biol.*, **94,** 391.
46. Meredith, G. E. and Wouterlood, F. G. (1993). *J. Micr. Res. Techn.* In press.
47. Germroth, P., Schwerdtfeger, W. K., and Buhl, E. H. (1991). *J. Comp. Neurol.*, **305,** 215.
48. Holländer, H. (1970). *Brain Res.*, **20,** 39.
49. Wilson, C. J. and Groves, P. M. (1979). *J. Neurosci. Meth.*, **1,** 383.
50. Carson, K. A. and Mesulam, M.-M. (1982). In *Tracing Neural Connections with Horseradish Peroxidase* (ed. M.-M. Mesulam), p. 153. Wiley, Chichester.
51. Somogyi, P. and Freund, T. F. (1989). In *Neuroanatomical Tract-Tracing Methods 2: Recent Progress* (ed. L. Heimer and L. Zaborszky), p. 239. Plenum Press, New York and London.
52. Buhl, E. H. and Singer, W. (1989). *Exp. Brain Res.*, **75,** 470.
53. Germroth, P., Schwerdtfeger, W. K., and Buhl, E. H. (1989). *Neurosci.*, **30,** 683.
54. Kuypers, H. G. J. M., Bentivoglio, M., Catsman-Berrevoets, C. E., and Bharos, A. T. (1980). *Exp. Brain Res.*, **40,** 383.
55. Schmued, L. C. and Heimer, L. (1990). *J. Histochem. Cytochem.*, **38,** 721.
56. Honig, M. G. and Hume, R. I. (1986). *J. Cell Biol.*, **103,** 171.
57. Vidal-Sanz, M., Villegas-Pérez, M. P., Bray, G. M., and Aguayo, A. J. (1988). *Exp. Neurol.*, **102,** 92.
58. Einstein, G. and Fitzpatrick, D. (1991). *J. Comp. Neurol.*, **303,** 132.
59. Buhl, E. H., Schwerdtfeger, W. K., Germroth, P., and Singer, W. (1989). *J. Neurosci. Meth.*, **29,** 241.
60. Somogyi, P. (1990). *J. Elec. Micros. Tech.*, **15,** 332.
61. Katz, L. C., Gilbert, C. D., and Wiesel, T. N. (1989). *J. Neurosci.*, **9,** 1389.
62. O'Leary, D. D. M. and Terashima, T. (1988). *Neuron.*, **1,** 901.
63. Glover, J. C., Petursdottir, G., and Jansen, J. K. S. (1986). *J. Neurosci. Meth.*, **18,** 243.
64. Nance, D. M. and Burns, J. (1990). *Brain Res. Bull.*, **25,** 139.
65. Schwerdtfeger, W. K., Buhl, E. H., and Germroth, P. (1990). *J. Comp. Neurol.*, **292,** 163.

66. Jonsson, G. (1981). In *Techniques in Neuroanatomical Research* (ed. Ch. Heym and W.-G. Forssmann), p. 71. Springer-Verlag, Berlin and Heidelberg.
67. Groenewegen, H. J. and Wouterlood, F. G. (1990). In *Handbook of Chemical Neuroanatomy* (ed. A. Björklund, T. Hökfelt, F. G. Wouterlood, and A. N. van den Pol), Vol. VIII, p. 47. Elsevier, Amsterdam.
68. Wouterlood, F. G. (1991). *Eur. J. Neurosci.*, **3**, 641.

10

Intracellular staining *in vivo*

D. J. MAXWELL

1. Introduction

Intracellular staining techniques are unique because they provide *anatomical and physiological* data about individual neurones or axons. A number of staining techniques have been developed, but they all depend upon the use of recording micropipettes which contain marker substances such as horseradish peroxidase (HRP) (1, 2), Lucifer Yellow (3), or biocytin (4, 5). In this chapter it is intended to provide a detailed account of the use of HRP in intracellular staining which is arguably still the method of choice for *in vivo* staining in mammals, especially if the analysis is to be taken to the ultrastructural level. Methods compatible with light microscopy (LM) and combined light and electron microscopy (EM) are described.

It has been the experience of the author that some neuroanatomists shy away from the intracellular staining technique and often feel intimidated by the complexity of the equipment required for the successful implementation of it. Conversely, electrophysiologists are often daunted by the various procedures available for processing tissue and the difficulties of combining ultrastructural and light microscopic analysis on the same material. Although the technique undoubtedly requires skill, the presumed difficulties are to some extent illusory; there is no reason why intracellular staining cannot be performed in a reasonably well equipped electrophysiological laboratory which has some history of intracellular recording. The technique brings together the expertise of the electrophysiologist and experimental neuroanatomist and provides an opportunity for collaboration between those trained in the two disciplines.

2. Intracellular staining with HRP

2.1 Uses and advantages of HRP as an intracellular marker

Intracellular staining with HRP may be used to reveal the morphology and synaptic organization of physiologically characterized neurones and axon terminations (*Figure 1*). The principal advantages of the technique are listed below.

(a) It provides a unique opportunity to correlate electrophysiological, morphological, and ultrastructural properties of the same cell or axon.

(b) Neurones or axons are labelled with a Golgi-like fill but, unlike the Golgi method, only single structures are labelled and they can be identified with ease even when processes are distributed throughout series of sections.

(c) It is non-toxic. Electrophysiological recordings may be made for some time after the introduction of HRP into a cell.

(d) The reaction product is electron dense and no additional steps are required to make the technique compatible with electron microscopy.

(e) It may be successfully combined with a number of neuroanatomical techniques such as anterograde degeneration (see Chapter 3) (6), retrograde tract-tracing (see Chapter 2) (7), and pre- (8, 9) and post-embedding (10, 11) immunocytochemistry (see Chapters 5 and 6).

2.2 Disadvantages of intracellular staining with HRP

(a) It is of limited use if thick slices of tissue or wholemounts are required. If sections are too thick, penetration problems may be encountered during the HRP reaction. It is usual to reconstruct neurones from series of sections that do not exceed 100 μm in thickness. Lucifer Yellow is better for thick slices or wholemount preparations (3).

(b) It is difficult to label very small neurones and unmyelinated axons. Electrodes which pass HRP are generally too crude to impale such structures. Biocytin (or Neurobiotin: see *Appendix 1*) can be used in electrodes with fine tips and is better for labelling very small structures (5).

(c) Axons are labelled for up to a centimetre only. When HRP is introduced into an axon, anterograde movement is probably by passive diffusion. Biocytin may be superior to HRP in this respect (12).

(d) Ultrastructural preservation may be compromised. The region of CNS under study is often exposed for 18 hours or more and is invariably subjected to multiple electrode tracks; this often results in a diminution of vascular perfusion in the exposed region and, consequently, poor perfusion with fixative. In addition, heavy reaction products may obscure subcellular details of labelled structures.

3. Intracellular recording and staining

There are three essential requirements for successful intracellular recording and staining.

(a) The animal preparation must be in good physiological condition.

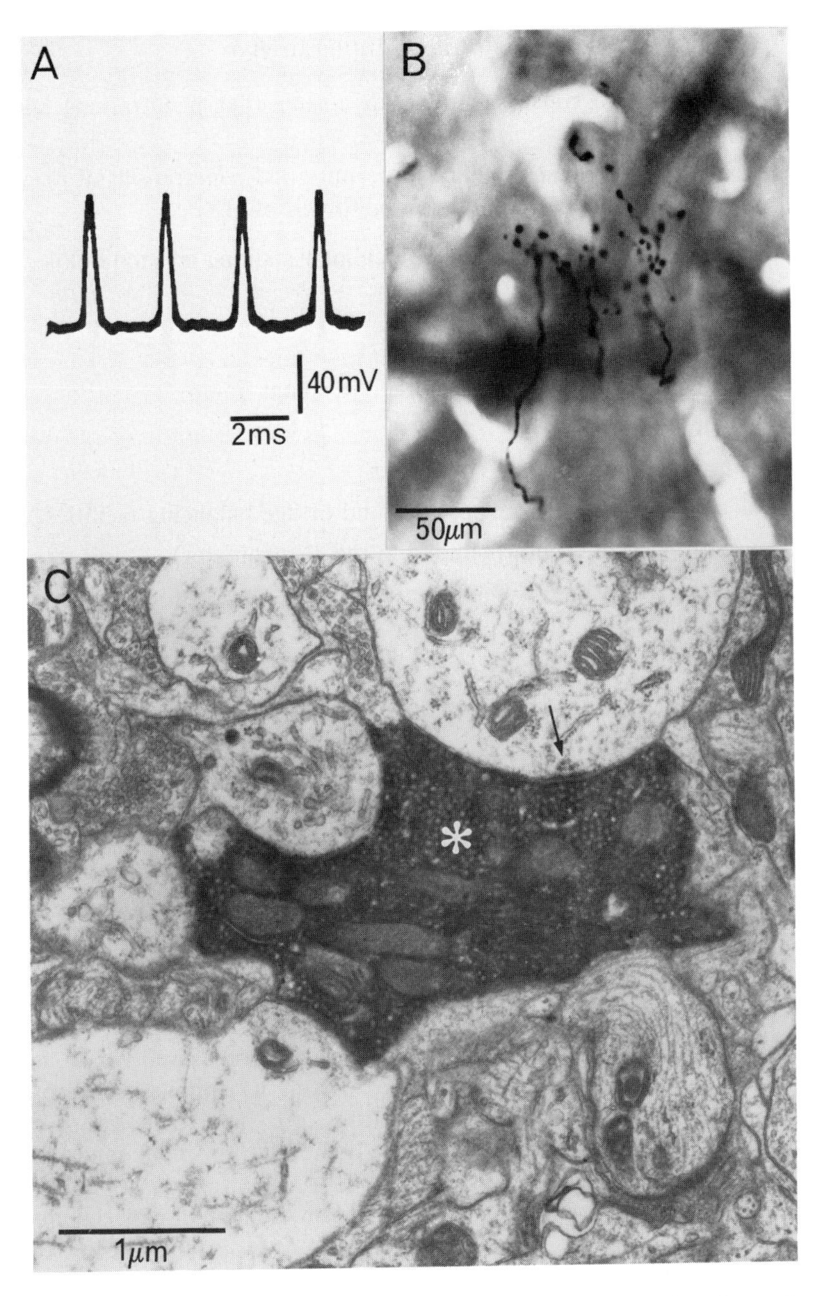

Figure 1. The staining technique with horseradish peroxidase provides electrophysiological, light microscopic, and ultrastructural data on individual neurones or their axons. The example illustrated shows a recording from a primary afferent fibre in the spinal cord (A) which was labelled intra-axonally. Its fine ramifications in the cord were examined with a light microscope (B). Axonal swellings observed with the light microscope were revealed to be synaptic boutons (asterisk) when examined with the electron microscope (C). The arrow indicates a synapse formed by the bouton with a large dendrite.

(b) The preparation must be stable to ensure that penetrations last for several minutes.

(c) Microelectrodes must be sharp to permit good penetrations of neurones but of low resistance to allow iontophoresis of HRP.

The basic equipment required for intracellular staining is listed below:

- a microelectrode puller
- an anti-vibration table
- an animal frame (either a head-holder or spinal frame)
- a micromanipulator
- an operating microscope
- an electrometer with current passing and bridge balancing facilities
- a source of current (if not included in the electrometer)
- a timing device such as a Digitimer or Hi-Med stimulator programmer to generate pulses
- an oscilloscope
- a blood pressure transducer and pen recorder
- a homeothermic blanket

3.1 Preparation of the animal

The choice of anaesthetic should be determined by consulting the literaure as this will vary depending upon the species used and the type of experiment to be undertaken. In some experiments, neuromuscular blocking agents may be required to limit movement during recording. It is important to monitor physiological parameters to assess the condition of the animal and to determine the depth of anaesthesia. We routinely monitor arterial blood pressure, end-tidal CO_2, and temperature. Blood pressure is measured via an arterial cannula attached to a pressure transducer. A venous cannula is also inserted for the administration of anaesthetic, drugs, etc. The temperature of the animal should be kept constant by using a homeothermic blanket and control unit.

Surgical procedures will vary depending upon the type of experiment to be performed. The most serious problem that can occur during surgery is uncontrolled blood loss; this should be immediately checked with artery forceps, a cautery, or bone wax. A suitable head holder or spinal frame (13) mounted on an anti-vibration table is necessary to achieve stable recordings. Greater stability may be attained by performing a pneumothorax and artificially ventilating the animal through a tracheal cannula attached to respiratory pump. The dura mater is removed to expose the recording site which is flooded with liquid paraffin at body temperature.

3.2 Preparation of microelectrodes

Good microelectrodes are the *sine qua non* of intracellular recording and staining experiments. However a good microelectrode is by definition one which performs well in the animal; it is not possible to manufacture electrodes according to rigid rules, and experimentation is necessary to create an electrode which works under a particular set of experimental conditions. The difficulty with electrodes for HRP intracellular staining experiments is that a compromise has to be made; the electrode has to have a tip which is fine enough to impale a cell or axon cleanly, but it has to have a resistance which is low enough to permit iontophoretic ejection of HRP. We routinely prepare electrodes with tips which are smaller than 1 μm and DC resistances which range from 20–40 MΩ. These are suitable for labelling all but the smallest axons and cells.

An essential piece of equipment for the manufacture of electrodes is an electrode puller. A number of electrode pullers are commercially available and the majority of them produce electrodes suitable for intracellular staining. Electrode pullers are described in detail in the books by Thomas (14), Purves (15), and Brown and Fyffe (1). Features of a good electrode (*Figure 2*) should include the following:

(a) A fine tip which is less than 0.2 μm. It is a good idea to examine electrodes with a microscope. Mount them on slides with Plasticine. You should not be able to see the tip with a × 40 objective lens.
(b) The shank should be relatively short (10–14 mm) and should taper gradually. The tip should taper more abruptly and resemble the sharpened end of a pencil.
(c) The shank should not be so narrow that it bends. A rigid electrode with a fairly wide shank is best for bevelling (see below) and intracellular recording

It is advisable to make electrodes the day before an experiment. The most suitable type of tubing for micropipettes contains a glass filament which enables the electrode to be filled easily with electrolyte solution. GC150F-15 tubing from Clark Electromedical Instruments is most satisfactory. The HRP solution for injection should be prepared according to *Protocol 1*.

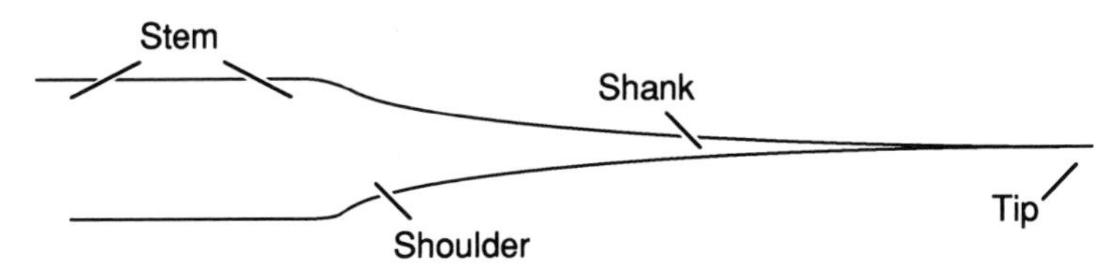

Figure 2. The principal parts of a microelectrode.

Protocol 1. Preparation of HRP solution for intracellular staining (16)

1. Place 8 mg quantities of Sigma type VI HRP in small glass vials with plastic stoppers (Bio-Rad). These can be placed in a container with silica gel and stored for several months in a freezer (−20°C).
2. Prepare stock solution of electrode buffer, 0.05 M Tris-HCl buffer containing 0.2 M KCl at pH 8.6 as follows.
   (a) Dissolve 3.03 g Tris (Tris(hydroxymethyl)methylamine) and 7.47 g KCl in 450 ml distilled water.
   (b) Bring to pH 8.6 with 1 M HCl.
   (c) Make up to 500 ml with distilled water and store at 4°C. This can be kept for 3–4 weeks.
3. Make 8% w/v solution of HRP by dissolving 8 mg HRP in 0.1 ml electrode buffer. Allow the vial containing the HRP and some of the electrode buffer to equilibrate to room temperature before mixing.

Electrodes are stored vertically with their tips down in a 250 ml beaker with a ring of Plasticine arranged inside it about 2 cm below the rim. The HRP solution is slowly drawn back into a 1 ml syringe with a 30 gauge needle (Hamilton). Each electrode is filled to the shoulder by inserting the needle into the stem until it reaches the shoulder and injecting a small volume of solution. A few millilitres of distilled water are placed in the bottom of the beaker to provide a moist atmosphere (the tips should not be in contact with the water) and the beaker is covered with a Petri dish. Electrodes are stored overnight at 4°C.

The presence of HRP increases the resistance of an electrode tip by a factor of three to four times when compared with conventional KCl electrodes, therefore most electrodes will have resistances which are too high to allow current to flow and it is necessary to take further steps such as bevelling or a controlled break to reduce the resistance. We make electrodes which have an initial resistance of 120–160 MΩ and bevel them to produce final resistances of 20–40 MΩ. Suitable machines for bevelling are discussed in the book by Brown and Fyffe (1); at present we use a K. T. Brown type bevelling apparatus which is manufactured by Sutter Instrument Co. During bevelling the resistance should come down slowly and in a controlled manner; if the resistance comes down suddenly the tip of the electrode has broken and it may be too crude for intracellular work. If a bevelling machine is not available, it may be possible to produce electrodes which will break back to suitable resistances; the success of this will depend upon the geometry of the electrode tip. Tips are broken by bringing them gently into contact with a lens tissue. After bevelling or breaking it is important to examine the electrode tip under a microscope with a × 40 objective. The tip should still be sharp (less than 1 μm) and no HRP solution should leak from it. Bubbles in the tips of electrodes may increase resistance; if this is a problem then place the electrodes in a vacuum jar at approximately −700 mm Hg for a few minutes before bevelling or breaking. Electrodes are topped-up with electrode buffer just before bevelling or recording.

Resistances may be tested by dipping the electrode tip in 0.9% NaCl solution (saline) to complete the recording circuit (see Section 3.3), and passing a current pulse of 1 nA; the resultant voltage (in millivolts) observed on the oscilloscope screen will equal the resistance in MΩ. It should be borne in mind however, that the resistance of an electrode is always higher in the animal itself.

3.3 The recording circuit

An experimental circuit for intracellular recording and iontophoresis of HRP is shown in *Figure 3A*. An electrometer with a current passing facility and bridge balance control (resistance compensation) which enables simultaneous recording of voltage and current passing is essential for intracellular staining. At present we use an Axoprobe-1A amplifier (Axon Instruments, Inc.) which is ideal for this task. A timing device such as a Digitimer or Hi-Med stimulator programmer is required to generate the iontophoretic cycle and a dual beam oscilloscope, (e.g. as supplied by Tectronix Ltd. or Gould Inc.) is used to monitor DC voltage and current. It is also useful to monitor extracellular field potentials; an additional high gain AC amplifier, (e.g. Palmer Bioscience) is required for this.

3.4 Making an impalement

An electrode is connected to the recording circuit by means of a chamber or cell and is driven into the preparation by a micromanipulator. A mechanical stepping-motor or hydraulic drive which will advance the electrode in large (10 μm) and small (2 μm) steps is best, but impalements of larger neurones can be made with a manual micromanipulator. Before driving the electrode into the CNS it is necessary to make a small hole in the pia mater. Holes are made by gently prising the pia apart with two pairs of watchmaker's forceps; this should be done with the aid of an operating microscope. The electrode is driven through the hole in large steps initially. When the electrode enters the tissue its resistance should be measured by passing a 1 nA current pulse; if the resistance is too high the electrode will not pass current. It is sometimes possible to clear a blocked electrode by withdrawing it for several tens of microns, or passing current briefly (hyperpolarizing pulses only—depolarizing pulses may eject HRP), or tweaking the capacitance compensation control, but if the electrode does not clear it should be discarded. If the structure to be impaled has a large field potential, it can be tracked extracellularly until the tip of the electrodes comes close to the cell membrane. It is usually best at this

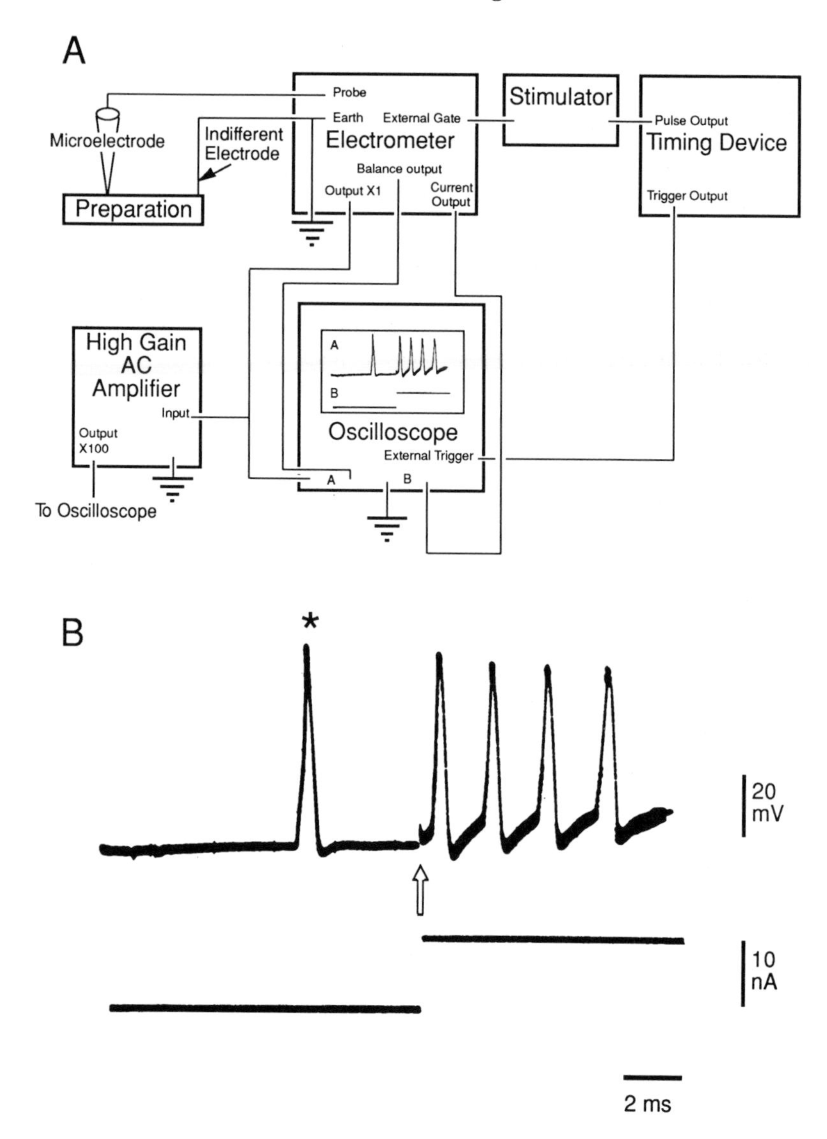

stage to gather as much electrophysiological data as possible and the unit should be characterized according to its orthodromic response properties and, if appropriate, identified antidromically by the collision test. If the structure does not have a large field potential it will be necessary to collect similar data once a successful impalement has been achieved. For small neurones and axons it is best to drive the electrode in small steps (2 μm) during the final stages of an impalement. A good electrode should penetrate a cell or axon 'cleanly', that is, the DC trace on the oscilloscope should suddenly become

Figure 3. (A) A schematic diagram illustrating a recording circuit suitable for intracellular staining. The preparation is connected to an electrometer via a microelectrode and an indifferent electrode (made of silver chloride) which goes to earth. A timing device provides a trigger pulse for the cycle and a pulse for current injection. If the electrometer does not have a current source, a stimulator must be included in the circuit. The output and balance output from the electrometer are recorded differentially on one channel of an oscilloscope (A), and the current output is monitored with the other channel (B). If extracellular recordings are required a high gain AC amplifier is necessary and is connected to a free channel of the oscilloscope, (e.g. the current monitoring channel when it is not in use). (B) An intracellular recording from a neurone (upper trace) and a current pulse (lower trace) viewed on the oscilloscope screen during recording and current passing. The recording is balanced to compensate for the current flow (indicated by the arrow) and several potentials are evoked by the current pulse. An electrically evoked antidromic potential (asterisk) is also present. (Taken and modified from reference 1 with permission.)

negative. Obviously the closer the membrane potential is to −70 mV the better, but successful labelling can be achieved with resting potentials of −50 mV. When a cell is penetrated it is usual to observe injury potentials; these will normally dissipate as the membrane seals around the electrode. The resting potential should be examined for a minute or so to ensure that it remains stable. Another indicator of a good penetration is the presence of action potentials which overshoot the zero potential mark. Further electrophysiological data may be collected at this stage before introducing HRP into a cell or axon. If extracellular recordings were made the investigator should determine that the same unit has been penetrated.

3.5 Iontophoresis of HRP

Once a stable impalement has been made and the unit has been characterized and identified electrophysiologically, HRP is ejected from the electrode tip by iontophoresis. This is achieved by delivering depolarizing pulses at relatively low frequencies rather than by using continuous current which tends to cause electrodes to block. High frequency pulses have been used by some investigators (17) to pass current through microelectrodes with very high resistances, but a modified form of electrometer (18) is necessary for this approach. We use a Hi-Med 100 series stimulator programmer (Hi-Med Instruments Ltd.) to deliver a triggering pulse every 600 ms, and a rectangular pulse of 450 ms duration which drives the current source for iontophoresis. The iontophoretic pulse begins 20 ms after the beginning of the cycle; this facilitates continuous monitoring of the resting potential and electrically evoked potentials (if present) during iontophoresis. Current should be increased gradually and the bridge should be balanced as the intensity is increased (*Figure 3B*). Eventually it will not be possible to balance the bridge and the current should be reduced until this is possible again. We have successfully labelled cells and axons by passing current pulses in the range of 5–20 nA, but small cells can be labelled with current pulses of 2–3 nA (19). It is usual for the current to fire the neurone or axon, and a helpful indication of the health of an impaled structure is the presence of potentials evoked by the depolarizing pulse (*Figure 3B*). It may be necessary to reduce the intensity of the current during the injection if blocking occurs. The amount of current required for successful filling will vary considerably depending upon the type and size of structure under investigation. The amount is calculated in arbitrary units of nA minutes, by multiplying the total time of injection in minutes by three quarters (because the cycle is 450 out of 600 ms) of the level of current in nA. Approximately 60 nA.min are adequate for medium and large cells (25–60 μm in diameter) but small cells may require considerably less than this. Axons usually require more current than cells; large axons such as Ia muscle spindle afferents may require over 200 nA.min. It is normal to observe some reduction of the membrane potential during filling; this occurs because depolarizing current is used. Once iontophoresis is complete further electrophysiological data may be gathered if the impalement is still stable. The electrode is withdrawn and the membrane potential is noted at the end of the injection; anything better than −30 mV is likely to be successful. The next injection should be made at least 4 mm away from previous injection sites to avoid overlap of labelled structures.

The location of the injection site should be recorded to facilitate preparation of histological blocks after fixation. Landmarks such as blood vessels are helpful in preparing a map of injection sites. A useful tip is to take a photograph of the region to be recorded from at the commencement of the experiment. Holes, where injections are made, can be drawn on the photograph. At the end of experiments, marker electrodes are placed at strategic locations (not in the holes themselves) to aid identification of injection sites. Marker electrodes are made with empty glass micropipettes; these are driven into the brain or spinal cord until 3–4 mm of the shank is left exposed. They are cut with an old pair of scissors just below the shoulder so that approximately 2 mm of the electrode shank remains sticking out of the CNS. These will remain in place during perfusion. Animals should be allowed to survive for at least one hour after the final injection, and it is desirable to fix the tissue not more than nine hours after the first injection was made.

4. Fixation

Fixation is performed by perfusion for light and electron microscopic studies of HRP labelled structures (*Protocol 2*). It is important to clear the tissue of blood prior to fixation because red cells possess natural peroxidase which will catalyse the HRP reaction and obscure details of labelled structures. Perfusion results in rapid fixation of tissue; the quality of labelled structures is greatly diminished in poorly fixed material, and artifacts such as ‘beading’ of dendrites may be observed if fixation is inadequate.

4.1 Perfusion (see also Chapter 1)

At present we use a perfusion apparatus which is operated by an air pump (*Figure 4A*). The animal is held in a cradle and fixative is introduced into it through an aortic cannula (*Figure 4B*). Perfusions can also be performed using a peristaltic pump or a gravity feed with a modified drip apparatus (Chapter 1, *Protocol 3*). Fixatives contain aldehydes and therefore perfusion should be performed in a fume cupboard. The procedure described is for a 2.5 Kg cat but it is essentially the same for all mammalian species and the volumes should be adjusted accordingly for other species. The recommended fixative is suitable for light and combined light and electron microscopic studies. If other techniques are to be combined with intracellular staining, (e.g. immunocytochemistry), it may be necessary to use a different fixative (8, 9) (see Chapter 5).

Protocol 2. Perfusion (2.5 Kg cat) (see Chapter 1, *Protocol 3* for perfusion of rat)

1. Prepare rinsing solution: 0.9% w/v sodium chloride, 0.1% w/v sodium nitrite and 100 U/ml heparin.
   For 5 litres stock solution add the following to 5 litres distilled water:
   - 45 g NaCl
   - 5 g $NaNO_2$
   - 3 g heparin (Sigma)

   This can be stored at room temperature for several weeks.
2. Prepare 3 litres of fixative: 2.5% v/v glutaraldehyde, 1% w/v paraformaldehyde in 0.1 M phosphate buffer, pH 7.4 (see Chapter 1, *Protocol 2*).
3. Place 500 ml of rinsing solution and 900 ml of fixative in separate containers and warm to body heat in a water bath. Cool 2 litres of fixative to 4°C in an ice bucket. Keep 100 ml of fixative for post-fixation of blocks and place in 4°C refrigerator.
4. Place rinsing solution, warm, and cold fixative in containers for perfusion. Ensure that all connections to the perfusion apparatus are tight, and test the apparatus to determine that there is a suitable flow of fixative. Make sure that connecting tubes are free from air bubbles and clear the cannula of fixative with rinsing solution.
5. Ensure that the animal is deeply anaesthetized. If a pneumothorax has not been performed, insert a cannula into the trachea and place a respiratory pump close to the perfusion apparatus. If the animal has received a pneumothorax, both animal and pump must be moved to the perfusion apparatus. Place the animal on its back in the cradle and identify the sternum. Cut through the sternum with large scissors until the heart is

Protocol 2. *Continued*

visible. Keep the points of the scissors parallel with the sternum to avoid damaging thoracic organs. Connect the animal to the respiratory pump as soon as the thorax is opened if it is not already being artificially ventilated. Bleeding may occur from the internal mammary arteries; this can be checked with artery forceps. Open the rib cage with a retractor and identify the pericardium. Remove the pericardium carefully and identify the left and right ventricles, the right atrium, and aorta. Grasp the right ventricle just above the apex of the heart with a set of artery forceps and make a small cut in the left ventricle about one third of its length up from the apex with small sharp scissors. Arterial blood should ensue from the incision. Place the aortic cannula in the left ventricle and direct it towards the aorta. Some resistance should be felt as the cannula passes through the aortic valve. Clamp the cannula in place with artery forceps and introduce the rinsing solution. Cut the right atrium with small scissors; venous blood should flow freely from the cut.

6. The blood should clear after 60–90 sec. It is best to introduce the rinsing solution at high pressure (approximately 120 mm Hg). This is followed by warm fixative at the same pressure. The musculature should begin to fix and the animal will twitch. Cold fixative is introduced at a lower pressure (approximately 80 mm Hg) and the animal is perfused slowly over a period of about 20 min until all the fixative is used up.

4.2 Making histological blocks and post-fixation

When perfusion is complete the brain or spinal cord is removed carefully and placed on a cork dissection board and examined with a dissecting microscope. Tissue should be kept moist with fixative during inspection. Marker electrodes are identified and locations of injection sites determined with the help of the photographs; it should be possible to identify the empty blood vessels. Blocks are made with a scalpel blade; the blocks should not exceed 6 mm^3. Any remaining pia and arachnoid membranes are removed from the block with watchmaker's forceps and a small oblique slice should be cut off one corner to facilitate orientation of sections during mounting (see Section 5.3). Blocks are stored for eight hours in fixative at 4°C. If the blocks are to be sectioned with a freezing microtome (see Section 5.1) and prepared for light microscopy only then they should be stored in fixative with 10% w/v sucrose added.

5. Preparation for light microscopic analysis

Different strategies are required for preparing tissue for light microscopic examination alone and for combined light and electron microscopy. This section explains how to prepare sections for LM analysis only; in the follow-

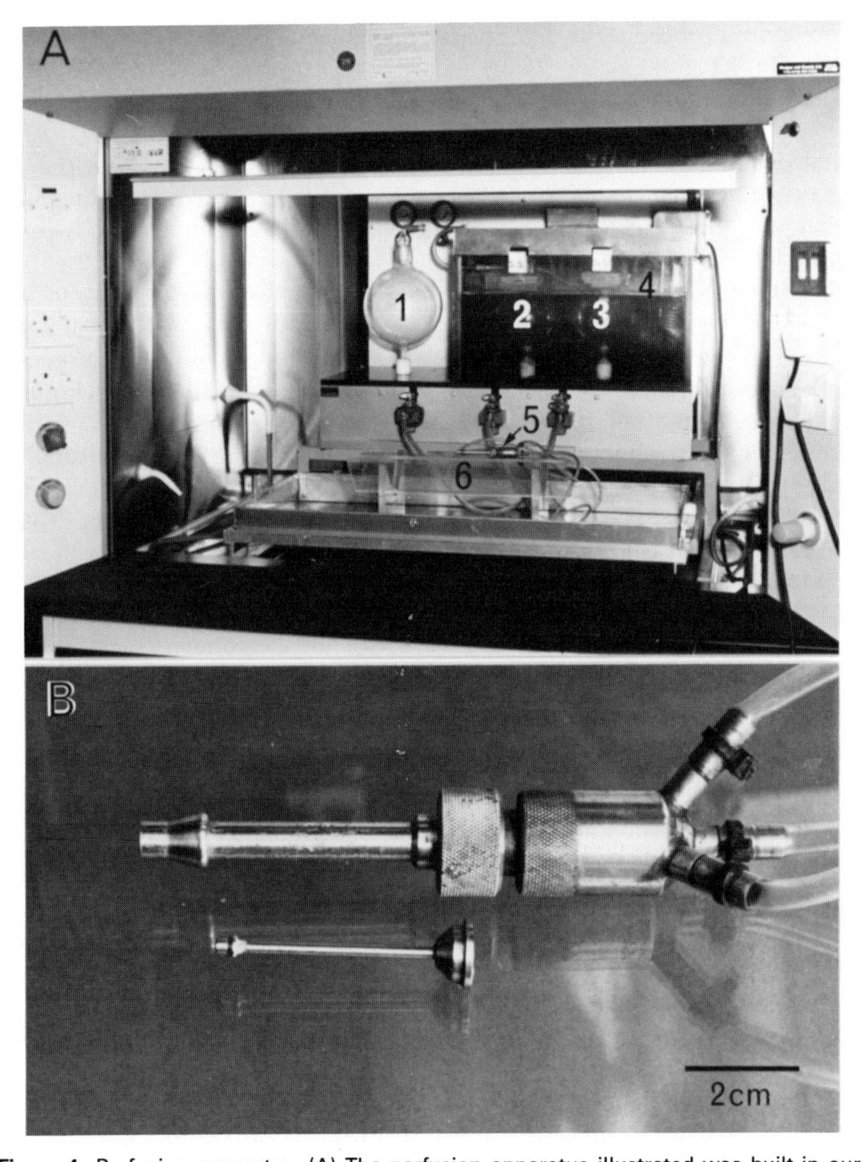

Figure 4. Perfusion apparatus. (A) The perfusion apparatus illustrated was built in our workshop and is suitable for a variety of mammalian species. The apparatus, which is housed in a fume cupboard, consists of containers for cold fixative (1), warm fixative (2), and rinsing solution (3). Containers (2) and (3) are kept at body temperature in a thermostatically controlled water bath (4). The apparatus is operated by an air pump, and the flow of solution is controlled by pressure valves and taps connected to each of the containers. Solutions are introduced into the animal via an aortic cannula which is attached to a three-way connector (5). The animal lies in a cradle (6) and perfusate collects in a stainless steel tray which drains into a sink. (B) Aortic cannulae. The cannula shown in the upper part of the illustration is suitable for a cat and is attached to the three-way connector. A rat cannula is shown for comparison.

ing section a procedure is described for combined light and electron microscopy.

5.1 Sectioning

Serial sections (60–90 μm thick) are cut with a freezing microtome (Leitz) and gathered in collection trays (*Figure 5A*) in photographic dishes containing 0.1 M phosphate buffer, pH 7.4. Sections are handled with an artist's paint brush.

5.2 HRP histochemistry

In order to reveal the presence of HRP in tissue it is necessary to perform a peroxidase reaction in the presence of a chromogen. A number of chromogens are available but the Hanker–Yates reagent (pyrocatechol/*p*-phenylenediamine) (20) combined with cobalt intensification (21) is most suitable for light microscopic studies (*Protocol 3*). This chromogen is not recommended for tissue to be taken to the ultrastructural level. The Hanker–Yates reagent is said to be non-carcinogenic and therefore it is not necessary to take the same stringent precautions as those required for diaminobenzidine (see below). However, it is wise to treat the reagent with respect and the reaction should be performed in a fume cupboard. Some background coloration may occur with this method.

Protocol 3. The Hanker–Yates method for HRP histochemistry with cobalt intensification

1. Changes of solution are made by transferring collection trays to reaction dishes containing the new solution. Make sure that the sections do not float after transfer; if they float push them down with an artist's paint brush.
2. Wash sections in two changes of 0.1 M phosphate buffer (pH 7.4) (Chapter 1, *Protocol 1*).
3. Wash sections in two changes of 0.1 M sodium cacodylate buffer (pH 7.4). (Dissolve 21.4 g sodium cacodylate in 1 litre distilled water and pH to 7.4 with 1 M HCl.)
4. Prepare the pre-incubation medium just before use. Mix the following in 225 ml of 0.1 M sodium cacodylate buffer (pH 5.1; make as in step **3** except pH to 5.1 with 1 M HCl) with a magnetic stirrer:
   - 0.338 g Hanker–Yates reagent (Sigma)
   - 1.35 g cobalt chloride
   - 0.9 g nickel sulphate

   Introduce sections into the pre-incubation medium for 15–20 min.
5. Wash sections in two changes of 0.1 M sodium cacodylate buffer (pH 7.4).

6. Prepare incubation medium. Mix 0.338 g of Hanker–Yates reagent in 225 ml 0.1 M sodium cacodylate buffer (pH 5.1) and add four drops of 30% hydrogen peroxide just before use. Incubate for 15–20 min.
7. Wash twice in 0.1 M sodium cacodylate buffer (pH 7.4).
8. Wash twice in 0.1 M phosphate buffer (pH 7.4).

5.3 Dehydration and mounting

Sections are handled individually with an artist's paint brush and dipped briefly in distilled water before mounting in serial order on gelatin-coated microscope slides (Chapter 1, *Protocol 5*). They are air-dried and placed in a jar of formalin vapour overnight. The following day they are dehydrated through a standard series of alcohol solutions, cleared in xylene, mounted in DPX, and a coverslip applied (see Chapter 1, *Protocol 6*). It is often useful to counterstain the sections; cresyl fast violet and methyl green are recommended.

6. Preparation for combined light and electron microscopic analysis

The HRP intracellular staining technique is well suited for combined light and electron microscopic analysis; a correlated study should always be performed.

6.1 Sectioning (see also Chapter 1, *Protocol 4*)

Sections for EM are cut with a Vibratome (Horwell) or other type of vibrating microtome. Blocks are attached to the cutting stage of the Vibratome with a small droplet of cyanoacrylic glue. The stability of blocks can be improved by making an agar matrix; drop a few millilitres of warm 3% w/v agar dissolved in distilled water on the block when it is attached to the cutting stage. Once the agar sets, trim it with a razor blade to form a supporting matrix around the tissue. Serial sections are gathered in collection trays (see Section 5.1) containing 0.1 M phosphate buffer (pH 7.4). Sections should be 40–70 μm thick. Thicker sections must be avoided as subsequent osmium treatment will render them too dense and obscure light microscopic details.

6.2 HRP histochemistry

The chromogen of choice in electron microscopic studies is 3,3′-diaminobenzidine tetrahydrochloride (DAB; see *Protocol 4*) (22). This compound is a suspect carcinogen and must be treated with the utmost care. DAB is handled in a specially designated area of a fume cupboard and protective clothing, gloves, and a mask must be worn. All items of equipment contaminated with DAB are immersed in a bucket of bleach (two Surgikos tablets per litre of

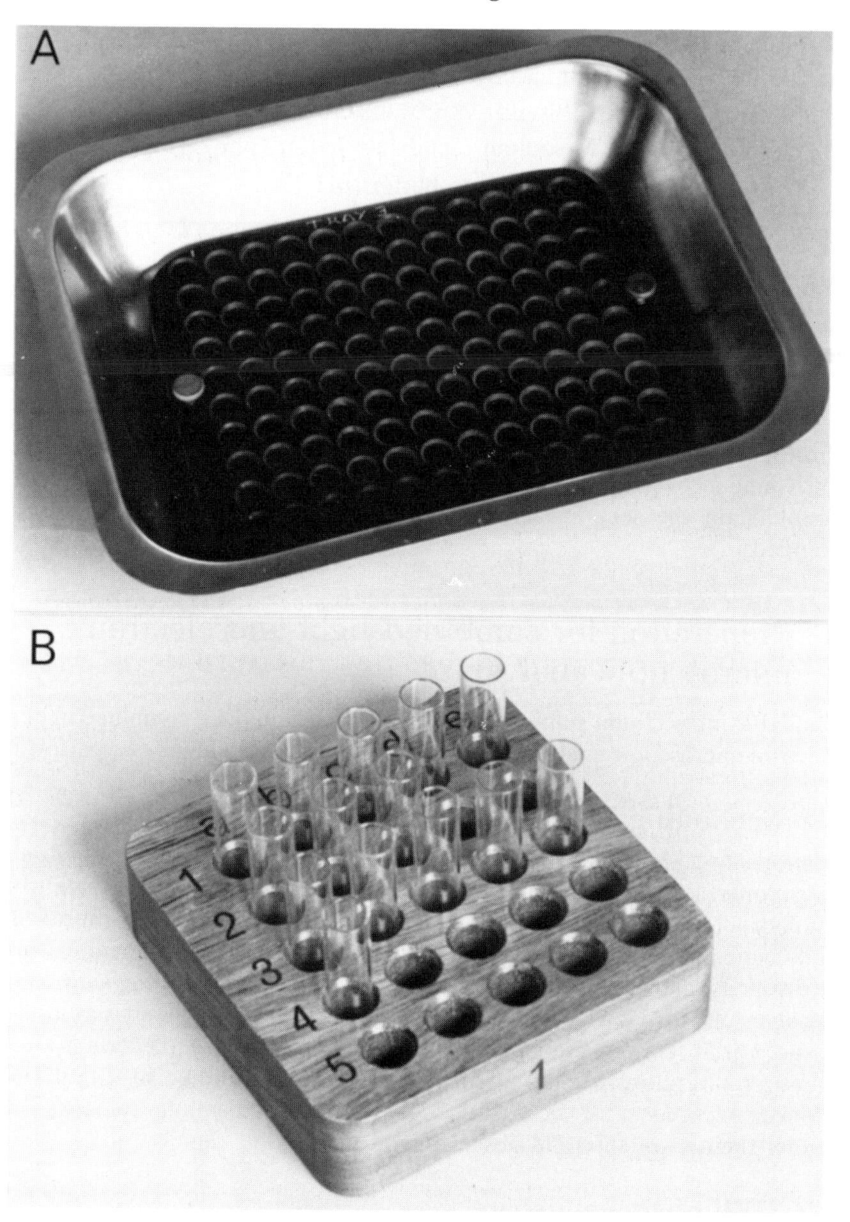

Figure 5. (A) The collection tray for serial sections. The collection tray is made of perspex and has a stainless steel mesh attached to its lower surface. It is placed in stainless steel photographic dishes which contain appropriate buffers and reagents. (B) The matrix block for serial sections to be processed for electron microscopy. Glass vials are placed in the block which enables sections to be kept in serial order. Solutions of osmium tetroxide and ethanol are introduced into the tubes and removed from them with Pasteur pipettes. Resin is introduced with a syringe.

water) for several hours after the reaction is complete (see *Safety note 4* in Chapter 5, p. 123).

Protocol 4. HRP histochemistry using DAB as the chromogen (see also Chapters 2 and 11)

1. Changes of solution are made by transferring collection trays into reaction dishes containing the new solution.
2. Wash sections twice in 0.1 M phosphate buffer (pH 7.4).
3. Wash sections twice in 0.5 M Tris-HCl buffer (pH 7.6).
4. Pre-incubate sections in 0.05% w/v DAB (Sigma) in 0.05 M Tris-HCl buffer (pH 7.6) for 15 min.
5. Incubate sections in 0.05% w/v DAB and 0.01% v/v hydrogen peroxide in 0.05 M Tris-HCl buffer (pH 7.6) for 15 min.
6. Wash sections twice in 0.05 M Tris-HCl buffer (pH 7.6).
7. Wash sections twice in 0.1 M phosphate buffer (pH 7.4).

6.3 Further processing for electron microscopy

Following HRP histochemistry sections are scanned. Place three or four in serial order on an unsubbed or uncoated slide, add a drop of phosphate buffer, and place a coverslip over them. Sections are viewed with a light microscope and those containing labelled structures are selected to be processed for electron microscopy. It may be difficult to visualize fine processes at this stage and it is advisable to over-compensate and select extra sections at each end of the series. The coverslip is removed by gently easing a razor blade under one edge and raising it carefully from the slide. Sections for EM are collected in serial order in glass vials containing 0.1 M phosphate buffer (pH 7.4). A matrix block with holes drilled in it is useful to keep the vials upright and in serial order (*Figure 5B*). Sections should be processed according to *Protocols 7* and *8* in Chapter 1. Those not selected for EM analysis are mounted on glass slides and processed for LM analysis (see Section 5.3).

6.4 Section embedding

Sections are removed from glass vials with the aid of a flame-polished glass rod and embedded in Durcupan. Sections are brittle at this stage and should be handled with care. Several section embedding techniques have been devised (23) (see Chapter 1, *Protocol 8*). We use acetate foils (24) (see *Figure 6*) which do not bind to cured resin and can easily be removed when access is required to sections. The foils (British Celanese Ltd.) are cut to the size of a glass slide (we prefer the large size: 76 × 51 mm). The base foil is 250 μm thick and the cover foil is 100 μm thick. The base foil is positioned over a glass

A

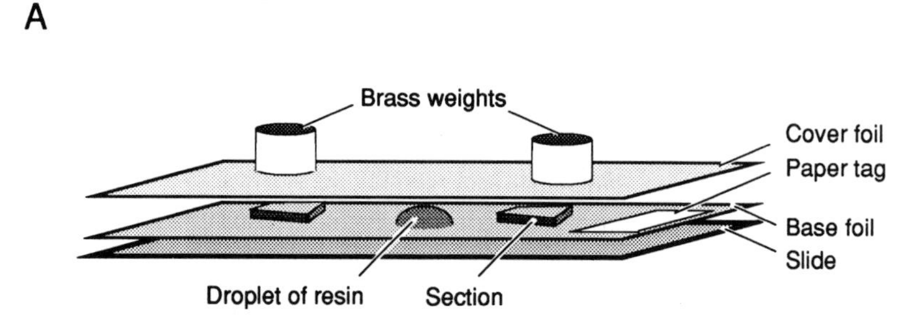

B

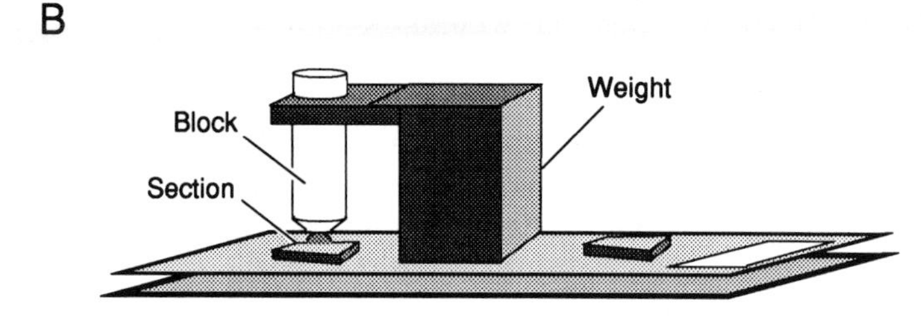

C

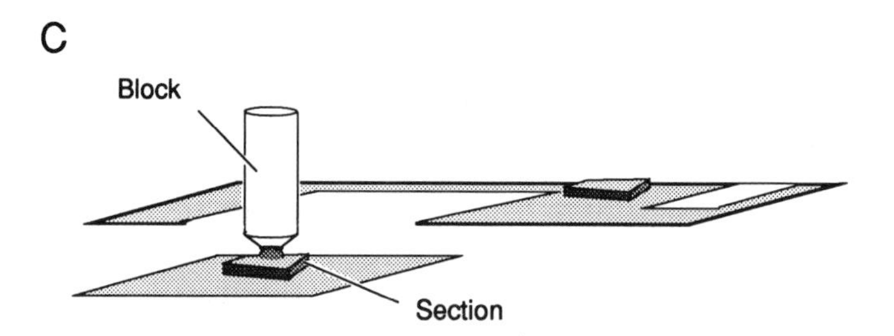

Figure 6. Flat embedding of sections with acetate foils. (A) Sections are placed between a base foil and a cover foil with a droplet of resin. A paper tag is used to record experimental information. The foils are positioned on a glass slide and kept flat with two brass weights. (B) Once the resin is cured, sections can be examined with a light microscope. Parts of sections for examination with the electron microscope are attached to a blank block with a small droplet of resin. The block is held upright with a brass weight which has an arm with a hole drilled through it. (C) When the resin has polymerized the block, which is now attached to the section, is cut out of the base foil with scissors. The remaining base foil is peeled away from the section after scoring the surface of the resin with a razor blade.

slide and six sections are mounted in serial order on it. Experimental information is written on a strip of paper (in pencil) which is placed across one side of the foil and is held in place with a droplet of Durcupan. The cover foil is placed over the sections and is held in position with a small weight. Durcupan will flow between the foils. Bubbles are expelled by gently depressing the cover foil above them with a glass rod. Excess Durcupan at edges of foils should be mopped up with strips of filter paper. The foil assembly is polymerized in an oven at 60°C for 48 hours. When polymerization is complete, the foil is taped on to its supporting glass slide and is examined with a light microscope. Sections may be stored for several years in this form.

7. Light microscopic analysis

Sections embedded between acetate foils or on glass slides are examined with a light microscope. It is usually necessary to reconstruct structures from serial sections. Reconstructions (*Figure 7A*) are made on large sheets (A2) of artist's drawing paper with the aid of a drawing tube attachment on the microscope. Reconstruction should always begin in the middle, i.e. if the reconstruction is of a neurone then start with the section containing the soma. The most difficult aspect of reconstruction is aligning structures from one section to the next. It is best to mark 'cut ends' on the drawing and match them up with cut processes in neighbouring sections by focusing on the consecutive surface of an adjacent section. A fine copy of the reconstruction is made on tracing paper with ink and captions and scales are added.

Drawings should be made of structures from individual sections prepared for combined electron microscopic analysis; this will facilitate identification of labelled structures when viewed with the electron microscope (see Section 8 and Chapter 1).

Photographs are taken of labelled structures with a standard photomicroscope (*Figure 7B*). Few difficulties are encountered with sections mounted on glass slides, but problems may arise with plastic embedded sections. It may be difficult to photograph structures if osmium staining is heavy. If this is a persistent problem it will be necessary to cut thinner vibrating microtome sections (see Section 6.1). When an oil immersion lens is used it may be difficult to focus on labelled structures. If this occurs, remove cover foils (see below) and place immersion oil directly on embedded sections. The oil can be wiped off with a lens tissue soaked in absolute ethanol but care should be taken not to damage the section. At high magnifications labelled structures should be photographed through several focal planes and photomontages constructed.

8. Electron microscopic analysis

When light microscopic analysis is complete, plastic embedded sections are prepared for EM analysis. Areas of interest should be re-examined with the light microscope. A small spot is made with a marker pen on the surface of the cover foil to indicate the location of the structures for EM analysis. The foils are removed from the supporting slide and a corresponding mark is made on the base foil. The cover foil is peeled off; start at one corner and the entire foil should come off easily. The base foil and sections are placed on the supporting slide again and examined under a dissecting microscope. Marks are identified and small drops of Durcupan are placed on sections over them.

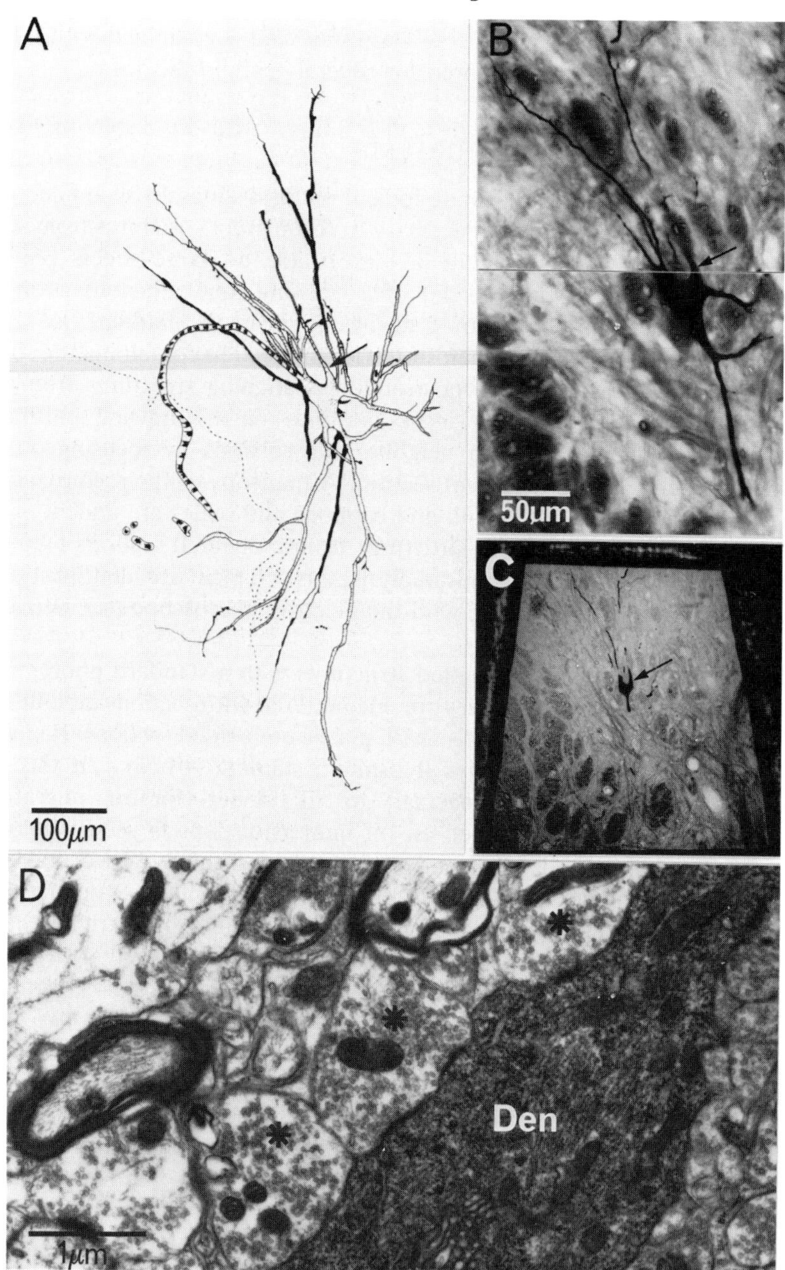

Figure 7. Correlated light and electron microscopic analysis. (A) A reconstruction of a cell made from several serial sections. (B) A photomicrograph of the same cell. (C) The cell viewed in a block face after sectioning with an ultramicrotome. (D) A dendrite (Den) of the cell viewed with an electron microscope. This dendrite is indicated with an arrow in (A–C). Several synaptic boutons (asterisks) are associated with it.

A cured plastic block with a flat bottom is held in place over a section by using a metal weight with an arm which has a hole drilled through it (*Figure 6B*). The block is placed in the hole and held upright. It is aligned with the mark by viewing the underlying section through the block with the dissecting microscope. The Durcupan is cured for 48 hours at 60°C. After polymerization the weight is removed, and the section along with the base foil and the attached block is cut out with scissors (*Figure 6C*). The Durcupan on the surface of the base foil is scored with a razor blade close to the block, and the base foil is peeled off leaving the exposed section attached to the block. The section is examined again with the light microscope; the block is placed upright on a slide (it may be held in position by placing a ring of Plasticine around its base) and viewed. It should be possible to illuminate the section through the block. A drawing is made at low magnification with the drawing tube to aid trimming of the block face. This should illustrate the positions of structures for EM analysis and suitable landmarks such as blood vessels, bundles of myelinated fibres, or cell bodies. The block face is trimmed by placing the block in a chuck with a hole drilled through it which enables the section to be trans-illuminated and examined with the optics of the ultramicrotome or a dissecting microscope. Landmarks are identified and the block face is trimmed manually with a clean razor blade (see Chapter 1, *Protocol 9* for alternative method of re-embedding).

The block face is examined with a light microscope (the block is mounted on a glass slide with Plasticine as described above) and photographed (*Figure 7C*). Labelled structures may also be redrawn to illustrate their positions in the block. Serial ultrathin sections are cut with an ultramicrotome and collected on Formvar-coated single-slot copper grids (2 × 1 mm slots; Bio-Rad) (see Chapter 1, *Protocol 10*). It is useful to have a diamond knife for this purpose but in skilled hands, a glass knife will suffice. When a series has been cut (about 40 sections) the block face is examined again with the light microscope and is compared with the drawing made before cutting. It should be possible to determine which structures are missing and hence are included in the series of thin sections. This process may be repeated several times until the structures desired for EM analysis are present in the series.

Sections are contrasted with Reynolds' lead citrate (25) (Chapter 1, *Protocol 11*) prior to viewing with the EM. Labelled structures usually contain obvious electron-dense reaction product (*Figure 7D*), and are identified with the aid of landmarks which can be recognized from the drawings and photographs made with the light microscope.

9. Concluding remarks

The development of intracellular staining represents a major turning point in the history of neuroscience. The HRP intracellular labelling technique described in this chapter equips the neuroscientist with a unique and powerful analytical tool. When used in isolation the technique provides electrophysiological, morphological, and ultrastructural data on single identified neurones or axons. When used in combination with other anatomical techniques, such as immunocytochemistry or retrograde tract-tracing, the technique enables us to examine the neurochemistry or circuit organization of identified neurones. Alternatives and variations exist for most of the processing steps detailed above. The methods described have been developed over many years in this laboratory and this chapter provides a personal account of approaches that have proved to be successful in our hands.

Acknowledgements

I wish to thank H. A. Anderson, A. G. Brown, W. M. Christie, C. A. Ingham, and A. D. Short for useful discussions and comments on this chapter. The illustrations were prepared by W. M. Christie and C. M. Warwick.

References

1. Brown, A. G. and Fyffe, R. E. W. (1984). *Intracellular staining in mammalian neurons.* Academic Press, London.
2. Bishop, G. A. and King, J. S. (1982). In *Tracing neural connections with horseradish peroxidase* (ed. M.-M. Mesulam), pp. 153–247. John Wiley and Sons, New York.
3. Stewart, W. W. (1981). *Nature,* **292,** 17.
4. Horikawa, K. and Armstrong, W. E. (1988). *J. Neurosci. Methods,* **11,** 1.
5. Wilson, C. J., Chang, H. T., and Kitai, S. T. (1990). *J. Neurosci.,* **10,** 508.
6. Maxwell, D. J., Fyffe, R. E. W., and Brown, A. G. (1984). *Neurosci.,* **12,** 151.
7. Maxwell, D. J., Koerber, H. R., and Bannatyne, B. A. (1985). *Neurosci.,* **16,** 375.
8. Miletic, V., Hoffert, M. J., Ruda, M. A., Dubner, R., and Shigenaga, Y. (1984). *J. Comp. Neurol.,* **228,** 129.
9. Maxwell, D. J. and Noble, R. (1987). *Brain Res.,* **408,** 308.
10. Somogyi, P. and Soltész, I. (1986). *Neurosci.,* **19,** 1051.
11. Maxwell, D. J., Christie, W. M., Short, A. D., and Brown, A. G. (1991). *J. Comp. Neurol.,* **307,** 375.
12. Kawaguchi, Y., Wilson, C. J., and Emson, P. C. (1990). *J. Neurosci.,* **10,** 3421.
13. Clark, R. and Ramsey, R. L. (1975). *J. Physiol.,* **244,** 5p.
14. Thomas, R. C. (1978). *Ion-sensitive Intracellular Microelectrodes.* Academic Press, London.
15. Purves, R. D. (1981). *Microelectrode Methods for Intracellular Recording and Ionophoresis.* Academic Press, London.
16. Snow, P. J., Rose, P. K., and Brown, A. G. (1976). *Science,* **191,** 312.
17. Light, A. R. and Perl, E. R. (1979). *J. Comp. Neurol.,* **186,** 133.
18. Jochem, W. J., Light, A. R., and Perl, E. R. (1981). *J. Neurosci. Methods,* **3,** 261.
19. Chang, H. T. and Wilson, C. J. (1990). In *Handbook of Chemical Neuroanatomy* (ed. A. Björklund, T. Hökfelt, F. G. Wouterlood, and A. N. van den Pol), Vol. 8, pp. 351–402. Elsevier, Amsterdam.

20. Hanker, J. S., Yates, P. E., Metz, C. B., and Rustioni, A. (1977). *Histochem. J.*, **9,** 789.
21. Adams, J. C. (1977). *Neurosci.,* **2,** 141.
22. Graham, R. C. and Karnovsky, M. J. (1966). *J. Histochem. Cytochem.,* **14,** 291.
23. Metz, C. B., Kavookjian, A. M., and Light, A. R. (1982). *J. Electrophysiol. Tech.,* **9,** 151.
24. Holländer, H. (1970). *Brain Res.,* **20,** 39.
25. Reynolds, E. S. (1963). *J. Cell Biol.,* **17,** 208.
26. Kita, H. and Armstrong, W. (1991). *J. Neurosci. Methods,* **37,** 141.

Appendix: A note on the use of biocytin and Neurobiotin

Advantages and disadvantages of biocytin and Neurobiotin

Recently two biotin-containing compounds (biocytin (4) and Neurobiotin (26)) have been introduced as intracellular markers for use with light and electron microscopy (*Figure 8*). These compounds have a high affinity to avidin and their presence in tissue is detected by using an avidin–HRP reagent. The principal advantages of these two markers over HRP are as follows.

(a) They both have low molecular weights, and their presence in an electrolyte solution does not significantly increase the resistance of micropipettes. Therefore they may be used in electrodes with very fine tips which will penetrate small structures.

(b) Axons are labelled for considerable distances.

(c) At the ultrastructural level, the reaction product is concentrated mainly around microtubules therefore post-synaptic densities are not obscured and can be examined with ease (*Figure 8D*).

However there are some considerable disadvantages in using these compounds in ultrastructural studies.

(a) It is advisable to include Triton X-100 in the incubation solution to ensure complete penetration of the avidin–HRP reagent; this results in poor ultrastructural preservation.

(b) If Triton X-100 is omitted, ultrastructural preservation is good but the reaction product is weak and may be absent in the centre of a section.

Biocytin (a complex formed between biotin and lysine) has two major disadvantages when compared with Neurobiotin (N-(2-aminoethyl)biotinamide).

(a) It is not particularly soluble and may precipitate in solution if left for any length of time.

(b) It may be ejected from electrodes by hyperpolarizing and depolarizing pulses. This is a disadvantage if hyperpolarizing pulses are used to stabilize impalements.

Method of injection for biocytin and Neurobiotin

The injection procedure for biocytin or Neurobiotin is similar to that for HRP but there are some differences.

(a) Electrodes with finer tips may be used and it is often not necessary to bevel or break the tips. We find that bevelling can still be useful and use electrodes with resistances which range from 20–60 MΩ. Other workers use electrodes with resistances in excess of 80 MΩ (5).

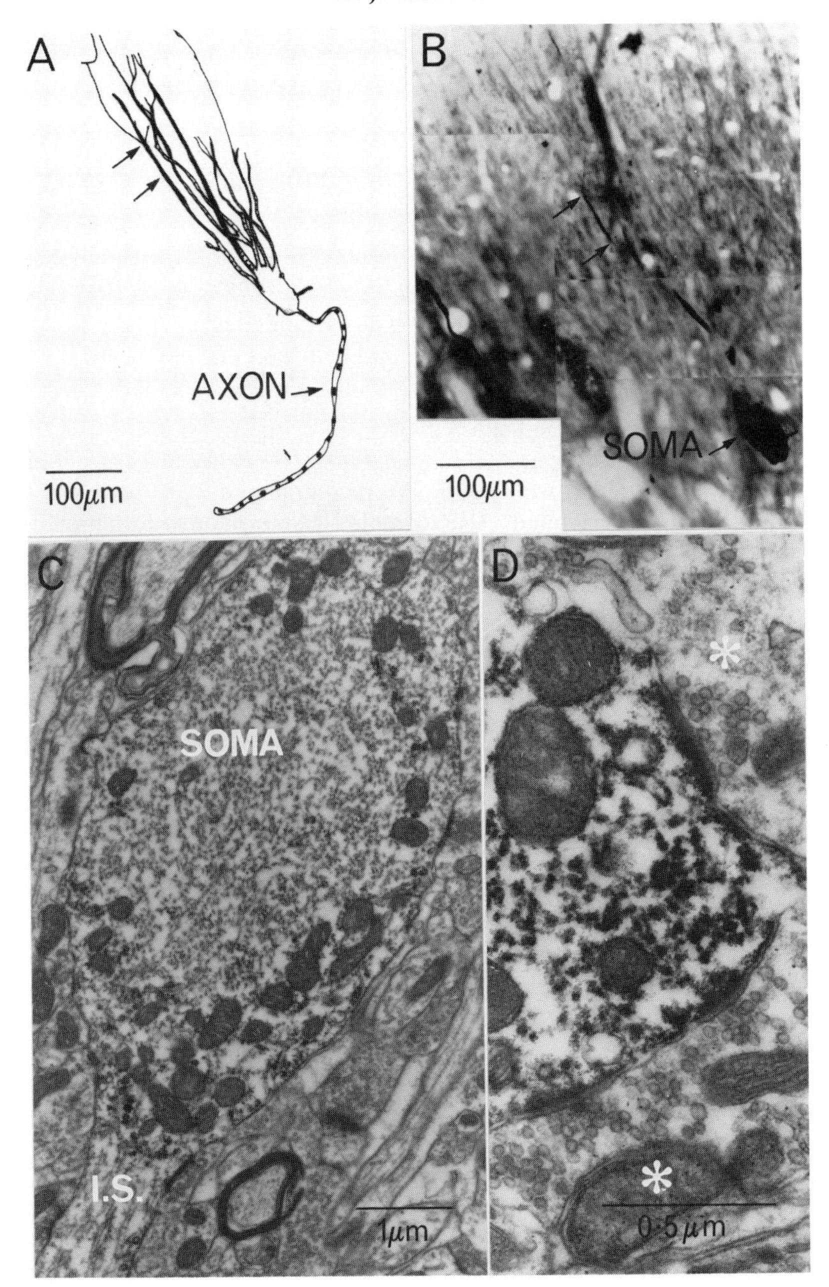

Figure 8. Correlated light and electron microscopic analysis of a neurone labelled with Neurobiotin. (A) A reconstruction of the cell. (B) A photomontage of the cell. The double arrows indicate part of a dendrite similarly indicated in (A). (C) An electron micrograph illustrating the cell body of the neurone. (I.S. = initial axon segment.) (D) An electron micrograph illustrating a dendrite which receives several synaptic boutons (asterisks).

(b) Electrodes are filled with a 1% (w/v) solution of biocytin (Sigma) or Neurobiotin (Vector Laboratories) in 0.05 M Tris-buffer, with 0.5 M KCl at pH 7.4, or 1.0 M potassium acetate.

(c) Cells may be labelled by passing depolarizing pulses ranging over 1–12 nA as described in Section 3.5 above. Cells require from 8–30 nA.min, and axons may require up to 60 nA.min.

(d) Animals are fixed with 3 litres (for adult cat) of 1% glutaraldehyde (v/v) and 1% paraformaldehyde (w/v) in 0.1 M phosphate buffer (pH 7.4) (4).

(e) Blocks should be washed in phosphate-buffered saline (PBS) at pH 7.4. Sections are cut with a Vibratome and collected in a collection tray (see Section 6.1) containing PBS. They should be washed six times for 15 mins in PBS before reacting with an avidin–HRP reagent.

(f) Sections should be incubated in an avidin–HRP reagent for two hours in PBS before reacting with DAB. We recommend a 0.5% v/v solution of streptavidin–biotinylated HRP complex (Amersham International plc: RPN 1051) which is particularly sensitive. Triton X-100 (0.05% v/v) should be added if the material is to be prepared for LM analysis only. Sections are washed several times in PBS before reacting with DAB (see Section 6.2). Sections are then prepared for LM (see Section 5.3) or combined LM and EM (see Sections 6.3 and 6.4) as described above.

11

Combined approaches to experimental neuroanatomy: combined tracing and immunocytochemical techniques for the study of neuronal microcircuits

YOLAND SMITH and J. P. BOLAM

1. Introduction

Most of the chapters in this volume have so far dealt with individual techniques in experimental neuroanatomy at the electron microscopic level. From these techniques we can identify projection neurones and examine the morphology of their afferent terminals. Moreover, the structural characteristics of the post-synaptic target of a set of anterogradely labelled terminals can be analysed from material containing immunostained structures, or intracellularly labelled neurones. These approaches in themselves produce valuable information concerning neuronal elements within the microcircuits and networks of the brain. However, the amount of data obtained using such approaches is limited in the sense that the identified structure is examined 'in isolation'. In order to establish the position of an identified neurone, or population of terminals within the neural network in relation to other neuronal elements, it is necessary to know the *nature* of the terminals afferent to a labelled neurone, or the *nature* of the post-synaptic targets of identified terminals. By this we mean that it is necessary to know the origin, neurochemical nature, and pattern of innervation of the synaptic terminals afferent to an identified neurone. Similarly, it is important to know the morphology, the chemical nature and the synaptic output of the neurones that are post-synaptic to a specific population of labelled terminals. Thus, to establish the microcircuitry or neuronal networks of a particular area of the brain it is necessary to *combine* the individual experimental approaches in a single experimental animal.

In several of the chapters, points at which individual experimental or histological techniques can be combined have already been described. The object of this chapter is to describe in detail some of the ways in which individual experimental approaches can be combined. The combinations of individual techniques will not be dealt with in an exhaustive manner since they are virtually limitless, often the only limitation being the ingenuity of the experimenter. The main emphasis will be on combinations of different tract-tracing techniques (anterograde and retrograde), and combinations of tract-tracing techniques with immunocytochemistry.

2. Combination of retrograde labelling with pre-embedding immunocytochemistry

The main objectives of this combination are two-fold.

(a) The identification of some chemical characteristic (usually relating to the nature of the transmitter) of a population of projection neurones.

(b) The identification of the transmitter characteristics of terminals *afferent* to a population of projection neurones.

The approach to this combination is first to administer the retrograde tracer to the animal and after the appropriate survival time the animal is perfuse–fixed. Sections containing the injection site and transport sites are cut and reacted to reveal the transported marker, and then subjected to immunocytochemistry (*Protocol 1*). Although various retrograde tracers (gold-labelled markers and cholera toxin conjugated to various markers) can readily be combined with pre-embedding immunocytochemistry (see Chapter 2), the most commonly used retrograde tracer and the easiest to combine with immunocytochemical techniques is horseradish peroxidase conjugated to wheatgerm agglutinin (WGA-HRP).

The choice of fixative for animals to be used for combined retrograde labelling and immunocytochemistry depends almost entirely on the sensitivity to fixation of the antigen that is to be localized by immunocytochemical means, since most retrograde markers are fairly robust and in particular, horseradish peroxidase activity is preserved in the tissue exposed to a wide variety of fixatives. The reader is therefore referred to Chapter 5 and should refer to both the manufacturers' recommendations and publications in which the same antiserum or antibody preparation has been used. In practise, it is generally the case that low concentrations of glutaraldehyde and relatively high concentrations of paraformaldehyde are required. The chromogen used in the immunoperoxidase reaction is usually diaminobenzidine (DAB) and the chromogen used to reveal the retrogradely-transported WGA-HRP is tetramethylbenzidine (TMB) (*Figure 1A*). The combined procedure may also be applied using DAB as the chromogen for both of the peroxidase reactions (*Figure 1B*).

Protocol 1. Combination of retrograde labelling with pre-embedding immunocytochemistry

1. Prepare and inject by pressure or iontophoresis WGA-HRP solution. Use a 0.5–7% solution in 0.9% NaCl solution (see Chapter 2).
2. Allow the animal to survive for 24–48 h.
3. Perfuse–fix the animal (see Chapter 1, *Protocol 3*) with a mixture of paraformaldehyde and glutaraldehyde (see Chapter 1, *Protocol 2*).
4. Perfuse the animal with cold phosphate buffer (0.1 M, pH 7.4), same volume as the fixative (see Chapter 1, *Protocol 2*).
5. Dissect the brain from the skull. Cut areas of interest, (i.e. injection sites and transport sites) into 5 mm-thick blocks and store in PBS at 4°C (see Chapter 1, *Protocol 1*) until sectioning.
6. Section areas containing the injection sites and the transport sites at 50–70 μm on a vibrating microtome (see Chapter 1, *Protocol 4*), and collect the sections in cold PBS.
7. *Optional.* Treat the sections for 15–20 min with 1% sodium borohydride (see Chapter 5, *Protocol 6*).
8. Wash several times in PBS, and then 0.1 M phosphate buffer at pH 6.2.
9. Incubate the sections to reveal the injected and transported WGA-HRP using TMB as the chromogen in the peroxidase reaction.[a] Prepare the TMB reaction mixture in the following manner:
   - dissolve 10 mg TMB in 5 ml of ethanol
   - dissolve 250 mg of ammonium molybdate (VI) tetrahydrate in 100 ml 0.1 M phosphate buffer pH 6.2
   - mix 2.5 ml of the TMB solution with 97.5 ml of the ammonium molybdate solution
10. Incubate the sections in this mixture for up to 40 min adding sufficient of 0.3% H_2O_2 every 5–10 min to give a final concentration of 0.003% (200 μl per 20 ml).
11. Wash sections 3 × 5 min in 0.1 M phosphate buffer at pH 6.2.
12. Stabilize the TMB reaction product by incubating for 5–8 min in an ice-cold solution consisting of:
    - 50 mg DAB[b] in 50 ml phosphate buffer (0.1 M, pH 7.4)
    - 2 ml of a 1% aqueous solution of cobalt chloride
    - 333 μl of a 0.3% solution of hydrogen peroxide per 10 ml of the mixture
13. Wash the sections for 3 × 5 min in PBS.
14. Separate the sections that will be prepared for light microscopy alone from those for electron microscopy.

Protocol 1. *Continued*

15. *Optional.* Freeze–thaw the sections that will be prepared for electron microscopy in liquid nitrogen (see Chapter 5, *Protocol 4*). Treat sections for light microscopy with Triton X-100, and include Triton in the primary antibody solution (Chapter 5, *Protocol 5*).

16. Stain the sections immunocytochemically to reveal the antigen of interest using the peroxidase anti-peroxidase method (see Chapter 5, *Protocol 8*), or the avidin–biotin–peroxidase method (see Chapter 5, *Protocol 9*).

17. Mount the sections prepared for light microscopy on gelatin-coated slides (see Chapter 1, *Protocol 5*), dehydrate, and apply coverslips (see Chapter 1, *Protocol 6*).

18. Post-fix the sections prepared for electron microscopy in osmium tetroxide (see Chapter 1, *Protocol 7*), dehydrate, and mount on microscope slides in an electron microscope resin (see Chapter 1, *Protocol 8*).

[a] See Chapter 2 for alternative protocols to reveal WGA-HRP.
[b] See *Safety note 3* in Chapter 5 (p. 119).

2.1 Appearance of the staining

The outcome of this combination are sections that contain both retrogradely labelled neurones and immunostained structures. At the light microscopic level, the retrogradely labelled neurones are recognized by the large dark blue granules of the TMB reaction product (*Figure 1A*). The immunostained structures will contain the typical DAB peroxidase reaction product, i.e. a brown, amorphous substance. After treatment with osmium tetroxide the characteristic location and the texture difference between the two reaction

Figure 1. Combination of retrograde labelling and pre-embedding immunocytochemistry (*Protocol 1*). (A) is a light micrograph of a section of the rat globus pallidus that contains a retrogradely labelled neurone (1), an immunostained neurone (2), and a neurone that is both retrogradely labelled and immunostained (3). The retrogradely labelled neurone contains the large granules of TMB reaction product and has a relatively clear cytoplasm, the immunostained neurone contains the amorphous DAB reaction product, and the double stained neurone has both the granules of TMB reaction product and the amorphous DAB reaction product. (Substantia nigra of rat injected with WGA-HRP; globus pallidus incubated to reveal transported HRP and then immunostained by the ABC method to reveal parvalbumin.) (B) is an electron micrograph of a neurone retrogradely labelled with WGA-HRP. It contains DAB reaction product that is present in multi-vesicular bodies (arrowheads). The neurone has a bouton apposed to it (arrow and inset) that is immunostained by the PAP method and revealed using DAB. It contains the typical amorphous, DAB immunoreaction product (see also Chapter 5). (Substantia nigra of rat injected with WGA-HRP, striatum incubated to reveal retrogradely-transported HRP using DAB as the chromogen, and then immunostained by the PAP method for substance P immunoreactivity, also using DAB as the chromogen.) Scale markers: (A) 10 μm, (B) 1 μm, inset, 0.1 μm.

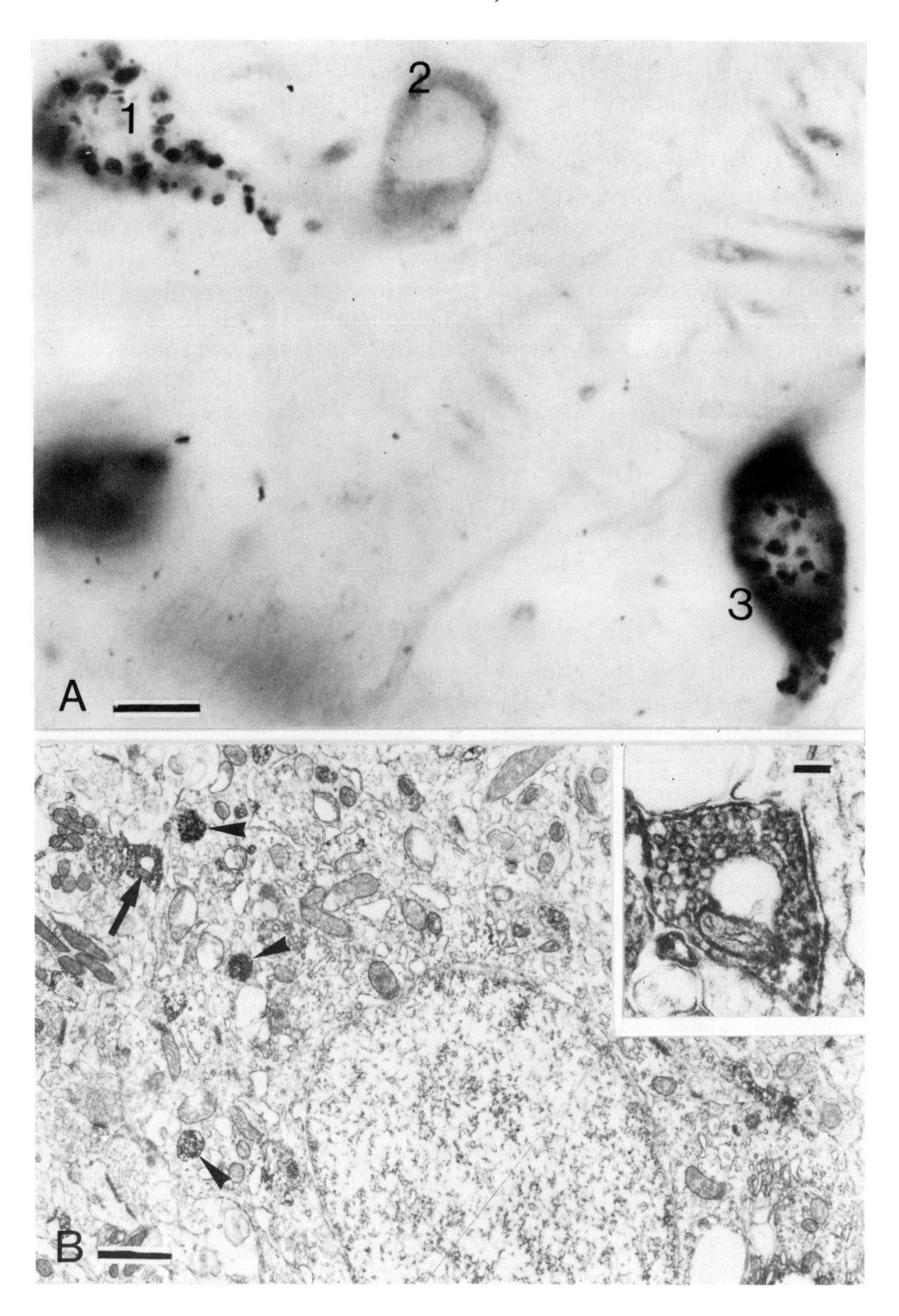
1
2
3
A
B

products is maintained. Thus, it is possible to identify immunostained perikarya that contain the retrogradely-transported WGA-HRP on the basis of the colour and location of the reaction products; the perikaryon will have an overall brown appearance and contain the granules of the TMB reaction product (see *Figure 1*). Similarly it will be possible to identify immunostained terminals that are apposed to retrogradely labelled neurones. The sections may also contain, if the connection is reciprocal, terminals anterogradely labelled with the TMB reaction product.

At the electron microscopic level the two reaction products are distinguishable. The DAB reaction product is an amorphous floccular precipitate associated with the internal plasma membrane and external membrane of subcellular organelles, whereas the TMB reaction is crystalline, more electron dense, and in the form of clumps dispersed in the cytoplasm (see *Figure 2*). When DAB is used as the chromogen for *both* peroxidase reactions the two are distinguished on the basis of location (*Figure 1B*). Thus the DAB reaction product in retrogradely labelled structures is present in secondary lysosomes or multivesicular bodies and appear at low magnification as round granules (*Figure 1B*).

2.2 Analysis of the material

The examination of the afferent synaptic input to retrogradely labelled, immunostained neurones, or the examination of immunostained terminals that form synapses with retrogradely labelled neurones can be carried out in two ways. First, areas that are dense in labelled structures can be re-embedded (see Chapter 1, *Protocol 9*), and ultrathin sections scanned in the electron microscope to identify the labelled structures. The second approach is to examine individual retrogradely labelled neurones that are themselves immunostained and/or apposed by boutons that are immunostained, by correlated light and electron microscopy. Thus a neurone is identified, first at the light microscopic level, after it has been drawn and photographed the same neurone is then re-embedded and examined in the electron microscope (see Chapter 1). In this way, the problems of sampling of relatively rare events at the electron microscopic level are overcome.

2.3 Applications

This combination of procedures using this or similar methods has been used successfully in the analysis of microcircuits in many areas of the brain. For example, the afferent synaptic input has been characterized of neurones in the basal forebrain of the rat that were themselves characterized on the basis of immunoreactivity for choline acetyltransferase and their projection to the cortex (1). Similarly, by combining immunocytochemistry with the retrograde transport of WGA-HRP from the substantia nigra, it has been demonstrated that neurones in the striatum of the rat that project to the substantia nigra

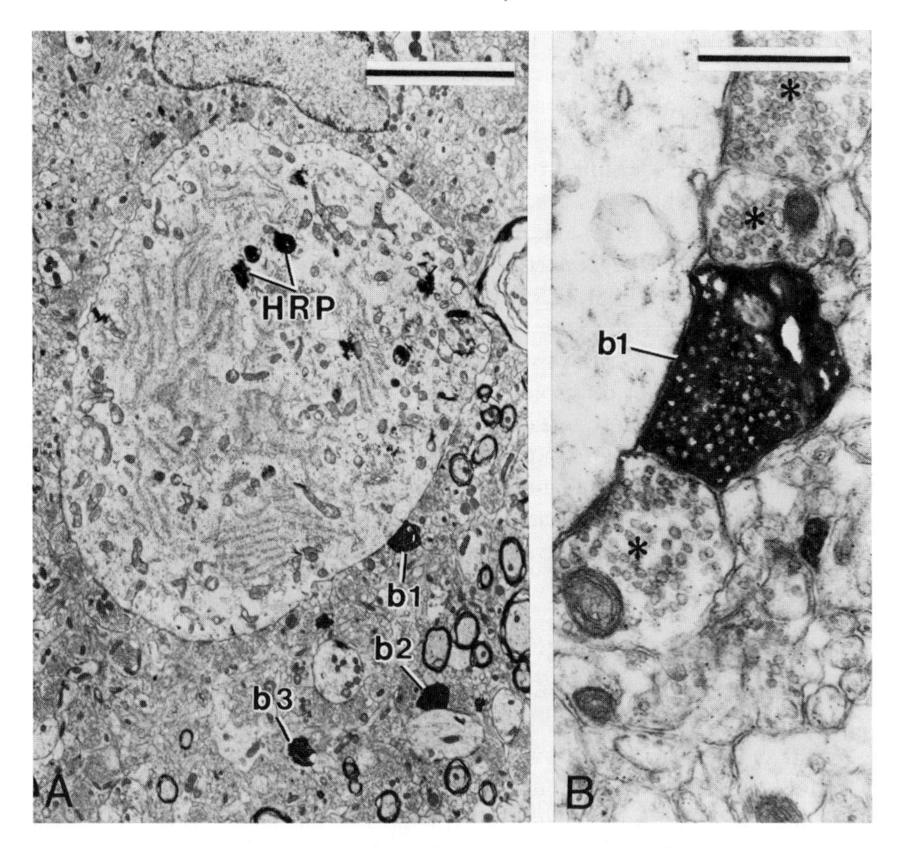

Figure 2. Anterograde transport of PHA-L combined with the retrograde transport of WGA-HRP (*Protocol 3*). (A) Electron micrograph showing a retrogradely labelled perikaryon in the rat substantia nigra after injection of WGA-HRP in the superior colliculus. The crystals of TMB reaction product are indicated by HRP. This perikaryon is contacted by a PHA-L immunoreactive bouton (b1) that has been anterogradely labelled after injection in the striatum. The association between the retrogradely labelled cell and the anterogradely labelled bouton is shown at higher magnification in (B). Note in (A) the presence of two other PHA-L positive terminals in the neuropil (b2 and b3). In (B) the asterisks indicate non-immunoreactive terminals that form contacts with the retrogradely labelled perikaryon. Scale markers: (A) 5.0 μm, (B) 1.0 μm.

receive synaptic input from terminals that are immunoreactive for choline acetyltransferase or for substance P (2, 3) (*Figure 1B*).

2.4 Limitations and controls

One limitation of this procedure is that the retrograde marker generally only labels the perikaryon and the most proximal part of the dendritic tree. Thus the synaptic input to the major part of a labelled neurone cannot be examined, and indeed it may be that it is in the distal dendritic tree that a particular class of terminals make synaptic contact. One way to overcome this is by combining the procedure with Golgi-impregnation (see Chapter 1, *Protocol 12*). The combination of Golgi-impregnation with retrograde labelling and immunocytochemistry has been successfully applied to the analysis of the chemical nature of inputs to identified projection neurones in the basal ganglia (2–4). The outcome is that *all parts* of a retrogradely labelled neurone can be examined in the electron microscope. This combination however, suffers from the drawback that we have no control over which neurones will be impregnated by the Golgi procedure. A further limitation is the problem of false-negative immunostaining, since reagents to reveal retrogradely labelled neurones penetrate into the tissue more readily than immunoreagents.

The most important control experiment in combined procedures that involve more than one peroxidase reaction is to ensure that the chromogen of the second peroxidase reaction does not become deposited at the site of the first peroxidase reaction. Thus, the first peroxidase reaction must go to completion and the peroxidase molecules should not react with the second addition of hydrogen peroxide and the second chromogen. In practise this is a rare event, the peroxidase molecules are generally obscured by the first reaction product and are no longer available to react with the second application of substrate and chromogen. Nevertheless, controls should be performed to test for this and areas should be included that will contain neurones that are *only* retrogradely labelled and neurones that are *only* immunostained (see reference 1 and *Figure 1A*). The controls should also include sections that are incubated through the whole double procedure, but with omission of the primary antiserum or the whole double procedure, but first of all inhibiting the transported peroxidase (see Chapter 5).

3. Combination of retrograde labelling with post-embedding immunocytochemistry

The main objectives of the combination of retrograde labelling with post-embedding immunocytochemistry are the same as those for the combination of retrograde labelling with pre-embedding immunocytochemistry. The advantage of this combination (*Protocol 2*) over the previous combination, is that the problems of penetration of the immunoreagents (see Chapter 6) are overcome. An outcome of this is that in optimally fixed material the analysis of immunostained terminals in contact with a retrogradely labelled neurone can be carried out in a quantitative manner (5) since the likelihood of false negative immunostaining of terminals is minimal. To analyse the chemically characterized, (i.e. immunostained) synaptic input to a population of retrogradely labelled neurones the approach is to prepare ultrathin sections of a retrogradely labelled neurone, and then immunostain the ultrathin sections by the immunogold method (see Chapter 6, *Protocol 3*).

From a theoretical point of view, the combination may also be used to identify the chemical characteristics of a population of projection neurones, although this combination has so far not been applied. The approach is to cut semi-thin sections of resin-embedded retrogradely labelled neurones and immunostain them for the antigen in question (see Chapter 6, *Protocols 1* and *2*). The remainder of the neurone that is left in the resin block can then be sectioned for electron microscopy. A similar method to this has been used extensively to chemically characterize the post-synaptic targets of intracellularly filled neurones (6, 7).

Protocol 2. Combination of retrograde labelling with post-embedding immunocytochemistry

1. Prepare tissue with retrogradely labelled neurones under study according to steps **1–13** in *Protocol 1*. The preferred chromogen for the peroxidase reaction is TMB but others may also be used.
2. Post-fix the sections in osmium tetroxide (Chapter 1, *Protocol 7*), dehydrate, and embed them on microscope slides in resin (Chapter 1, *Protocol 8*).
3. Select retrogradely labelled neurones of interest on the basis of light microscopic analysis, and re-embed in blocks of resin for ultrathin sectioning (Chapter 1, *Protocol 9*).
4. Cut ultrathin sections and collect on coated, gold, or nickel single-slot grids (see Chapter 1).
5. Immunostain the ultrathin sections by the immunogold method for the antigen under study, according to *Protocol 3* in Chapter 6.
6. Examine in the electron microscope.

3.1 Appearance of the staining

The outcome of the combined procedure are sections that contain retrogradely labelled neurones identified by the presence of peroxidase reaction product (see *Figures 1* and *2A*; see also Chapter 2), and also structures that have a high density of immunogold particles associated with them, thus identifying them as immunopositive (see *Figures 3* and *5*; see also Chapter 6). The criteria for the characterization of a structure as immunopositive in the post-embedding immunogold method are described in Chapter 6.

3.2 Analysis of the material

The retrogradely labelled neurones identified by the presence of the TMB (or other chromogen) reaction product are examined in serial sections to determine whether they receive synaptic input from axonal terminals that are immunostained. Because of the lack of problems of penetration of the immunoreagents, once it is established that the antigen is retained in the material, the immunostained input to retrogradely labelled neurones can be quantified (5). Thus the proportion of terminals in contact with a retrogradely labelled neurone that display a particular chemical characteristic can be determined. Similarly the proportion of neuronal membrane that is occupied by boutons of a particular chemical characteristic can be determined.

3.3 Applications

One example of the application of this procedure is the characterization and quantification of the afferent input to neurones in the medial globus pallidus of the rat that project to the cortex. These neurones were identified as part of the basal forebrain by virtue of their projection to the cortex, and were found to receive input from terminals that are immunoreactive for the inhibitory amino acid transmitter, GABA. This GABA-containing input was shown to account for greater than 70% of the afferent input to these cells (5).

3.4 Limitations and controls

The major limitation of this combination is that the antigen must survive the post-fixation with osmium and/or the dehydration and embedding in resin. The number of antigens to which the post-embedding procedure and hence this combined approach can be applied, is therefore limited (see Chapter 6). Embedding the tissue in resin *without* post-fixation with osmium tetroxide increases the number of antigens that can be studied in this way.

Since it is unlikely that the TMB reaction product within perikarya or dendrites will affect immunostaining in terminals that are afferent to the labelled structures, the controls that are required relate to the immunostaining procedure, and the reader is referred to Chapters 5 and 6.

4. Combination of anterograde labelling and retrograde labelling

This combination of procedures is used to determine the origin of the synaptic terminals in contact with neurones characterized on the basis of their projection site. Although various techniques have been developed over the last few years (8), the anterograde transport of PHA-L combined to the retrograde transport of WGA-HRP is the most sensitive approach to be used for such investigations (see *Protocol 3*).

Protocol 3. Anterograde transport of PHA-L[a] combined with the retrograde transport of WGA-HRP

1. Prepare and administer PHA-L (see Chapter 3, *Protocol 1*).
2. Allow the animal to survive for 7–10 days.

3. Prepare and inject WGA-HRP (see Chapter 2).
4. Allow the animal to survive for 36–48 h.
5. Perfuse–fix the animal (see Chapter 1, *Protocol 3*) with a mixture of paraformaldehyde (2–4%) and glutaraldehyde (0.1–2.5%) (see Chapter 1, *Protocol 2*).
6. Perfuse the animal with cold phosphate buffer (0.1 M, pH 7.4; same volume as the fixative) (see Chapter 1, *Protocol 1*).
7. Dissect the brain from the skull. Cut in 5 mm-thick blocks and store at 4°C in PBS (see Chapter 1, *Protocol 1*) until sectioning.
8. Cut the brain areas containing the injection sites and the transport sites at 50–70 μm on a vibrating microtome (see Chapter 1, *Protocol 4*).
9. Collect the sections in cold PBS.
10. Treat sections for 20 min with 1% sodium borohydride (see Chapter 5, *Protocol 6*).
11. Wash the sections several times in PBS.
12. Process the tissue by means of the tetramethylbenzidine method to reveal the injected and transported WGA-HRP (see *Protocol 1*, steps **8–11**).
13. Stabilize the TMB reaction product with diaminobenzidine (see *Protocol 1*, step **12**).
14. Wash the sections several times in PBS.
15. Separate the sections that are for electron microscopy from those that are for light microscopy alone.
16. Process the tissue for the immunohistochemical localization of PHA-L at the light and electron microscopic level (see Chapter 3, *Protocol 2*, steps **6–14**).
17. Post-fix sections for electron microscopy in osmium tetroxide, dehydrate, and mount on slides in resin (see Chapter 1, *Protocols 7* and *8*).
18. Mount sections prepared for light microscopy on gelatin-coated slides, dehydrate, and apply coverslips (see Chapter 1, *Protocols 5* and *6*).

[a] PHA-L can be replaced by biocytin in which case, biocytin is prepared, injected, and visualized according to *Protocols 3* and *4* in Chapter 3.

4.1 Appearance of the staining

The outcome of this method are sections containing retrogradely labelled perikarya characterized by the presence of large dark blue granules throughout the cytoplasm (see *Figure 1A*), and PHA-L immunoreactive axons and terminals that contain the brown diffuse DAB reaction product. In sections processed for electron microscopy, the colour of the DAB and the TMB reaction products is the same, but they remain easy to differentiate by their location and texture. The DAB reaction product has an amorphous texture and is associated with axonal processes and terminals, whereas the TMB reaction product has a crystalline texture and is found in perikarya and dendritic shafts (*Figure 2*).

4.2 Analysis of the material

In order to examine in the electron microscope areas containing both sets of labelled elements, the sections are analysed carefully in the light microscope for the presence of retrogradely labelled neurones apposed by PHA-L immunoreactive terminals. Once they have been photographed and drawn, these neurones are re-embedded (see Chapter 1, *Protocol 9*) and re-sectioned on the ultramicrotome. They are then examined in serial sections in the electron microscope to identify synaptic contacts between PHA-L positive terminals and the retrogradely labelled cells (*Figure 2*). The appearance of the material subjected to this combined procedure is essentially the same as in the combination of retrograde labelling and pre-embedding immunocytochemistry (*Protocol 1*), as the retrograde marker and the PHA-L or endogenous antigen are localized in the same manner in both procedures.

4.3 Applications

This approach has recently been used to test the possibility that the projection neurones in the substantia nigra pars reticulata (SNr) receive direct synaptic inputs from the globus pallidus in the rat (9) (*Figure 2*). Iontophoretic injections of PHA-L into the globus pallidus led to the anterograde labelling of a rich plexus of varicose fibres in the substantia nigra. Electron microscopic analysis revealed that these varicosities are large terminals that contain many mitochondria and form symmetric synapses predominantly with perikarya and proximal dendrites of nigrofugal neurones of the SNr (9, 10).

4.4 Limitations and controls

Although this combination of techniques is powerful for analysing the microcircuitry of neuronal systems, it is important to be aware of the limitations and technical problems that may complicate the interpretation of the data that is obtained. One of the major limitations is the fact that the granules of TMB reaction product are found only in the proximal part of the retrogradely labelled cells. Therefore, it should be kept in mind that unlabelled small dendritic shafts contacted by PHA-L immunoreactive terminals may have a parent cell body that is retrogradely labelled. In order to circumvent this problem, the retrogradely labelled cells may be Golgi-impregnated (see Chapter 1, *Protocol 12*). Another problem that may complicate the interpretation of data is the presence of WGA-HRP labelled terminals in the area of study. This will happen if the structure that has been injected with WGA-HRP is reciprocally connected with the area of study (for example the substantia nigra with the striatum), or if the retrogradely labelled cells in the area under investigation have recurrent axon collaterals. Thus, it is very important to be familiar with the texture of the TMB and the DAB reaction products in the electron microscope in order to be able to differentiate the WGA-HRP (TMB reaction product) from the PHA-L labelled (DAB reaction product) terminals. In general, the crystalline texture and the high electron density of the TMB-containing boutons make them relatively easy to differentiate from the amorphously stained DAB-containing terminals. A third limitation of this approach is the possibility that PHA-L is transported in the retrograde direction (see Chapter 3). This may complicate the interpretation of data if the brain area that received the PHA-L injection is reciprocally connected with the area under investigation and particularly, if the cells retrogradely labelled with PHA-L have recurrent axon collaterals. In such case it is not possible to determine the exact source of the PHA-L labelled terminals visualized in the area of study.

Control experiments to verify the specificity of the staining visualized with this protocol include:

- the localization of WGA-HRP alone
- the omission of the PHA-L antiserum from the incubation medium.

5. Combination of anterograde labelling and pre-embedding immunocytochemistry

The objectives of this combined approach are first, to identify the source of the terminals that form synapses on to neurones characterized by their chemical content and secondly, to study the synaptic relationships between a population of terminals characterized by its origin, and a population of terminals identified by its chemical nature on to single post-synaptic structures. The approach is to combine the anterograde transport of PHA-L or biocytin with the immunoperoxidase method. Both substances are localized by peroxidase reactions but using different chromogens (*Protocol 4*).

Protocol 4. Anterograde transport of PHA-L[a] combined with pre-embedding immunocytochemistry

1. Prepare and administer PHA-L (see Chapter 3, *Protocol 1*).
2. Allow the animal to survive for 7–10 days.
3. Perfuse–fix the animal (see Chapter 1, *Protocol 3*) with a mixture of paraformaldehyde and glutaraldehyde[b] (see Chapter 1, *Protocol 2*)

Protocol 4. *Continued*

4. Dissect the brain from the skull. Cut in 5 mm-thick blocks and store at 4°C in PBS (see Chapter 1, *Protocol 1*) until sectioning.
5. Cut the brain areas containing the injection sites and the transport sites at 50–70 μm on a vibrating microtome (see Chapter 1, *Protocol 4*).
6. Collect the sections in PBS.
7. Treat the sections for 20 min in 1% sodium borohydride (see Chapter 5, *Protocol 6*).
8. Wash the sections several times in PBS.
9. Separate the sections that are for electron microscopy from those that are for light microscopy.
10. Process the tissue for the immunohistochemical localization of PHA-L at light and electron microscopic levels (see Chapter 3, *Protocol 2*, steps **6–14**).
11. Mount the sections that include the PHA-L injection sites on gelatin-coated slides, dehydrate, and apply coverslips (see Chapter 1, *Protocols 5* and *6*).
12. Process the regions containing the PHA-L labelled terminals for the immunohistochemical localization of the antigen of interest, using the avidin–biotin–peroxidase (ABC) (see Chapter 5, *Protocol 9*), or the peroxidase anti-peroxidase (see Chapter 5, *Protocol 8*) methods.
13. In the sections processed for light microscopy, reveal the second antigen using the nickel-enhanced DAB method. Prepare the reaction mixture as follows:

    add 0.37 g of nickel ammonium sulphate ($NiSO_4 . (NH_4)_2SO_4{\cdot}6H_2O$) to 100 ml of Tris-HCl buffer (0.05 M, pH 7.6)

    add 25 mg of DAB

    add 200 μl of hydrogen peroxide (0.3% stock solution) when the DAB is completely dissolved
14. Incubate the sections in this solution for 10–12 min and then wash several times in PBS.
15. For the sections processed for electron microscopy, reveal the second antigen using benzidine dihydrochloride (BDHC) as the chromogen for the peroxidase reaction (see Chapter 5, *Protocol 11*; see also *Safety note 4* in Chapter 5, p. 123).
16. Mount the sections prepared for light microscopy on to gelatin-coated slides, dehydrate, and apply a coverslip (see Chapter 1, *Protocols 5* and *6*).
17. Post-fix the sections prepared for electron microscopy in osmium tetroxide

(see Chapter 1, *Protocol 7*; but the osmium tetroxide must be diluted in PB 0.01 M, pH 6.8), dehydrate, and embed in an electron microscope resin on microscope slides (see Chapter 1, *Protocol 8*).

[a] PHA-L can be replaced by biocytin, in which case, biocytin is prepared, injected, and visualized according to *Protocols 3* and *4* in Chapter 3.
[b] The percentage of paraformaldehyde and glutaraldehyde in the fixative is adjusted to obtain optimal labelling for the second antigen since PHA-L can tolerate a wide range of fixatives.

5.1 Appearance of the staining

The outcome of this method are sections including PHA-L labelled terminals containing the brown amorphous DAB reaction product, and the BDHC-labelled structures which appear blue prior to osmium treatment and become blue/black or grey after osmium post-fixation (see *Figure 2A* in Chapter 5). In addition to the colour, a major difference between the DAB and the BDHC reaction products is the texture; the DAB deposit is amorphous whereas the BDHC reaction product is granular. In the electron microscope, the two reaction products also show marked differences. The DAB reaction product is amorphous and is associated with subcellular organelle membranes and the internal plasma membrane, whereas the BDHC reaction product is granular or crystalline and does not appear to have any particular association with the membranes of subcellulr organelles (see *Figures 3A*, and *5*, see also *Figure 2B* in Chapter 5). Moreover, the electron-density of the BDHC deposit is often much higher than that of the DAB deposit. These structural differences between the DAB and the BDHC reaction products at both light and electron microscopic level allow this approach to be used to investigate the synaptic relationships between a population of terminals characterized by their *origin*, and a population of neurones identified by their *chemical content* (*Figure 3A*). It also allows the analysis of two populations of axon terminals, one identified on the basis of origin and the other on the basis of chemical content.

5.2 Analysis of the material

In order to avoid scanning material in the electron microscope that does not contain labelled elements, it is recommended to analyse the material in the light microscope first. At the light microscopic level, it will be possible to identify BDHC-containing cells, (i.e. immunoreactive for the antigen of interest) that are good candidates for receiving synaptic inputs from DAB-containing, (i.e. PHA-L immunoreactive) anterogradely labelled terminals. After they have been drawn and photographed, these neurones are re-embedded and sectioned for electron microscopy. The material is then examined in the electron microscope to determine whether the anterogradely labelled terminals apposed to the immunoreactive cells that were visualized at the light microscopic level, form synaptic specializations.

5.3 Applications

The application of this combination of procedures has demonstrated that tyrosine hydroxylase immunoreactive neurones, (i.e. dopaminergic neurones) in the substantia nigra of the rat receive synaptic input from terminals anterogradely labelled with PHA-L from the globus pallidus (9) (*Figure 3A*). More recently, this combination has been applied to the monkey striatum to study the organization of the synaptic afferents from the cerebral cortex on to parvalbumin-immunoreactive neurones (11). The results of this study revealed the existence of direct asymmetric synaptic contacts between the dendritic shafts of parvalbumin immunoreactive cells and the corticostriatal terminals.

5.4 Limitations and controls

Some technical problems may occur that complicate the analysis of the material obtained with this approach. One of the major problems is the poor penetration of the BDHC deposits into immunostained sections. It is important therefore, to collect the most superficial ultrathin sections of the block when cut on the ultramicrotome, since these are the sections that are most likely to contain *both* sets of labelled elements. Furthermore, the ultrastructural characteristics of the labelled elements in these superficial sections are often not as well preserved as in deeper sections. A second problem is the possibility that the BDHC has access to the peroxidase molecules associated with PHA-L, i.e. the possibility that the chromogen for the second peroxidase reaction had access to the peroxidase molecules of the first reaction. It is therefore important to carry out control experiments in which each primary antiserum is omitted in turn. When the antiserum that localizes the second antigen is omitted, the only labelling should be the PHA-L containing terminals with the DAB reaction product. When the PHA-L

Figure 3. (A) Anterograde transport of PHA-L combined with pre-embedding immunocytochemistry (*Protocol 4*). Electron micrograph of a TH-immunoreactive dendritic shaft (d) in the rat substantia nigra that is contacted (arrowheads) by two PHA-L immunoreactive terminals that have been anterogradely labelled after injection in the globus pallidus. In this experiment, the TH immunoreactivity was localized with BDHC whereas the PHA-L immunoreactivity was localized with DAB. Note that the BDHC and the DAB reaction products display different textures. (B) Anterograde transport of PHA-L combined with post-embedding immunocytochemistry (*Protocol 5*). Electron micrograph showing two PHA-L immunoreactive pallidal terminals that form synapses with a perikaryon (Per) in the rat subthalamic nucleus. The PHA-L immunoreactivity is indicated by the presence of the amorphous DAB reaction product in these boutons. This tissue has been processed by the post-embedding immunogold method to reveal GABA. The two PHA-L positive terminals are associated with a large number of gold particles (some are indicated by arrows) indicating that they display GABA immunoreactivity. Compare the density of gold particles over the PHA-L immunoreactive boutons with that over the GABA negative terminal indicated by an asterisk. Scale markers: 1.0 μm in (A) and (B).

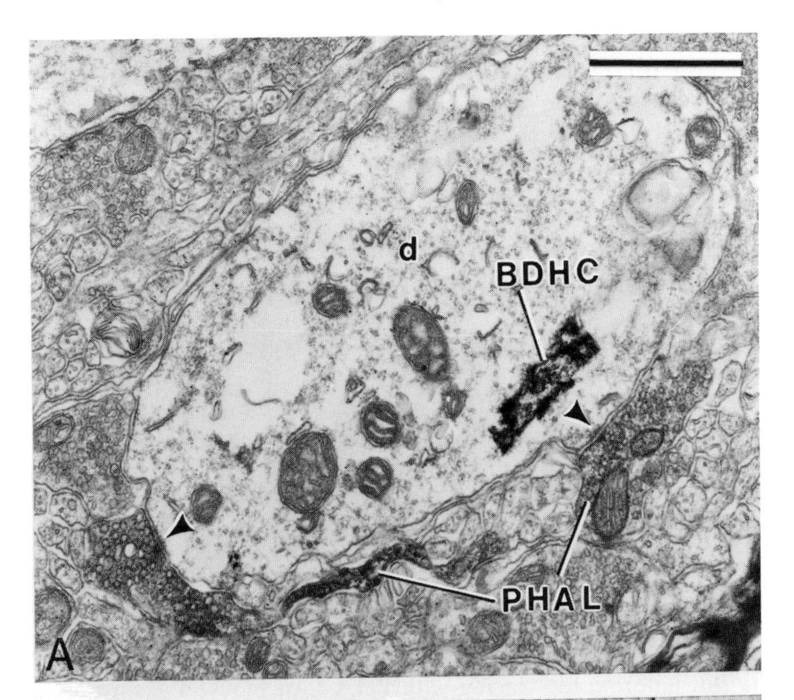
d
BDHC
PHAL
A

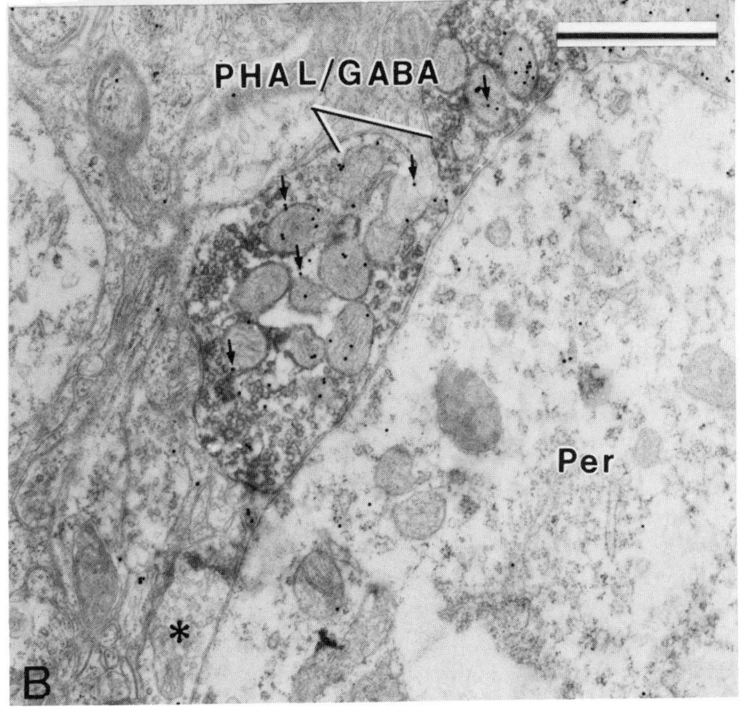
PHAL/GABA
Per
*
B

antiserum is omitted, only the BDHC-labelled immunoreactive elements should be visualized. A further control experiment that should be carried out is to reverse the order in which the antigens are revealed, i.e. localize the endogenous substance first with DAB and the PHA-L positive terminals second with BDHC.

6. Combination of anterograde labelling and post-embedding immunocytochemistry

This combination of procedures is used for studying the chemical nature of a population of terminals characterized by its origin. The anterograde tracers that have been combined with post-embedding immunocytochemistry are WGA-HRP, PHA-L, or biocytin (8). Because of the advantages of PHA-L and biocytin for anterograde labelling of terminal boutons (see Chapter 3), *Protocol 5* describes the combination of post-embedding immunogold staining with the anterograde transport of these substances.

Protocol 5. Anterograde transport of PHA-L[a] combined with post-embedding immunocytochemistry

1. Carry out anterograde tracing with PHA-L or biocytin according to *Protocols 1–4* in Chapter 3.
2. Observe sections in the light microscope.
3. Draw, photograph, and re-embed areas of interest (see Chapter 1, *Protocol 9*).
4. Cut serial ultrathin sections on an ultramicrotome and mount them on coated (see Chapter 1, *Protocol 10*) single-slot nickel or gold grids.
5. Process a series of ultrathin sections for the post-embedding immunogold method to reveal the antigen of interest (see Chapter 6, *Protocol 3*).
6. Stain ultrathin sections with lead citrate (see Chapter 1, *Protocol 11*).
7. Observe in the electron microscope.

[a] PHA-L can be replaced by biocytin, in which case, biocytin is prepared, injected, and visualized according to *Protocols 3* and *4* in Chapter 3.

6.1 Appearance of the staining

The outcome of this procedure are ultrathin sections of anterogradely labelled axonal processes and terminals that are identified as PHA-L positive by the DAB immunoreaction product. The sections also contain structures, including axonal processes, neuronal perikarya, dendritic shafts, and glial cells that have gold particles overlying them. Furthermore, some DAB-containing terminals, (i.e. PHA-L immunoreactive) may be associated with a large number of immunogold particles thus identifying as immunoreactive for the endogenous antigen (*Figure 3B*). The characterization of structures as immunopositive when using immunogold procedures has been discussed in detail in Chapter 6. In essence, a structure is considered immunopositive if the density of immunogold particles overlying it is at least five times greater than overlying the background, and that it remains constant in serial sections (*Figure 3B*).

6.2 Analysis of the material

As it has been suggested for the combined procedures described above, it is recommended to analyse the material at the light microscopic level first for the presence of anterogradely labelled terminals. Areas that are rich in PHA-L labelled structures are re-embedded and ultrathin sections cut. One grid out of two is stained with lead citrate and scanned in the electron microscope for the presence of DAB-containing (i.e. PHA-L positive) boutons. The grids adjacent to those that were found to contain PHA-L positive terminals are then processed for the immunohistochemical localization of the antigen of interest by the immunogold procedure (see Chapter 6, *Protocol 3*). The PHA-L positive boutons associated with a significant number of gold particles are photographed, and the density of gold particles is measured using a digitizing pad connected to a computer.

6.3 Applications

This approach has recently been used to demonstrate that a population of septo-hippocampal fibres, identified by the anterograde transport of PHA-L, display GABA immunoreactivity (12). It has also been used to show that terminals of neurones in the globus pallidus, anterogradely labelled with PHA-L that form symmetric synapses with neurones in the substantia nigra and the subthalamic nucleus, display GABA immunoreactivity (9, 13) (*Figure 3B*).

6.4 Limitations and controls

There are several limitations of this combined procedure.

(a) The limited number of antigens that can be localized by post-embedding procedures. Apart from small amino acids such as GABA and glutamate, the antigenicity of very few substances is preserved after osmium post-fixation, dehydration, and embedding in resin.

(b) The density of gold particles associated with anterogradely labelled terminals is often lower than that associated with non-labelled boutons. This is due to the fact that the peroxidase reaction product used to localize the first antigen (PHA-L) sometimes obscures the antigenic sites of the endogenous substance (GABA or glutamate) to be localized. It is recommended to carry out post-embedding immunostaining on lightly stained anterogradely labelled terminals. It is often necessary to quantify the density of gold particles overlying the anterogradely labelled terminals to be sure that they display immunoreactivity. Nevertheless false-negative results will commonly occur.

(c) The electron density of the DAB reaction product in anterogradely labelled terminals is significantly reduced after post-embedding immunocytochemistry. For this reason it is sometimes difficult to ensure that the GABA-immunoreactive terminals do indeed contain the DAB reaction product. It is therefore recommended to collect a series of sections adjacent to those processed for the post-embedding immunostaining to verify whether the terminals that are associated with a large number of gold particles also contain the DAB reaction product.

Control experiments should be carried out to test the specificity of both immunoreactions. Thus, the primary antibody against PHA-L and the primary antibody against the endogenous antigen, (e.g. glutamate or GABA) should be omitted in turn from the immunohistochemical reactions (see Chapters 5 and 6).

7. Double anterograde labelling combined with retrograde labelling

The objective of this approach is to test the possibility that two sets of anterogradely labelled terminals arising from different sources form convergent synaptic contacts on to single post-synaptic neurones characterized by their projection site. Furthermore, this approach can be combined with the post-embedding immunogold method (see Chapter 6, *Protocol 3*) to determine some aspects of the chemical nature of the anterogradely labelled terminals (10). The approach is to combine the anterograde transport of both PHA-L and biocytin with the retrograde transport of WGA-HRP. Each of the markers is visualized using a peroxidase reaction, but the combined method takes advantage of the fact that different chromogens used for the peroxidase reactions have different colours, form, and location (*Protocol 6*). The same protocol shown in *Protocol 6*, with the omission of the WGA-HRP injection and processing, can be used to examine two sets of anterogradely labelled terminals without characterization of the post-synaptic neurone.

Protocol 6. Anterograde transport of PHA-L and biocytin combined with the retrograde transport of WGA-HRP

1. Prepare and administer PHA-L (see Chapter 3, *Protocol 1*).
2. Allow the animal to survive for 7–10 days.

3. Prepare and administer biocytin (see Chapter 3, *Protocol 3*) and WGA-HRP (see Chapter 2).
4. Allow the animal to survive for 24–48 h.
5. Perfuse–fix the animal (see Chapter 1, *Protocol 3*) with a mixture of paraformaldehyde (2–4%) and glutaraldehyde (0.1–2.5%) (see Chapter 1, *Protocol 2*), and then with cold phosphate buffer (0.1 M, pH 7.4) (see Chapter 1, *Protocol 1*).
6. Dissect the brain from the skull, cut in 5 mm-thick blocks and store at 4°C until sectioning.
7. Section the blocks at 50–70 μm on a vibrating microtome.
8. Treat the sections with 1% sodium borohydride for 20 min (Chapter 5, *Protocol 6*).
9. Wash the sections several times in PBS.
10. Process the tissue for the histochemical localization of WGA-HRP using TMB as chromogen for the peroxidase reaction (see *Protocol 1*, steps **8–12**).
11. Process the tissue for the histochemical localization of biocytin at light and electron microscopic level, using DAB as the chromogen for the peroxidase reaction (see Chapter 3, *Protocol 4*, steps **2–4**).
12. Process the tissue for the immunohistochemical localization of PHA-L (see Chapter 3, *Protocol 2*, steps **7–12**) using the nickel-enhanced DAB method (see *Protocol 4*, steps **13–14**) to localize the injection site, and for the sections containing transported PHA-L that will be analysed at the light microscopic level only. In sections prepared for electron microscopy, reveal the transported PHA-L using the BDHC method (see Chapter 5, *Protocol 11*).
13. Mount sections prepared for light microscopy on to gelatin-coated slides, dehydrate, and apply coverslips (see Chapter 1, *Protocols 5* and *6*).
14. Post-fix the sections processed for electron microscopy in osmium tetroxide (see Chapter 1, *Protocol 7*; but the osmium tetroxide must be diluted in PB 0.01 M, pH 6.8), dehydrate, and embed in resin on microscope slides (see Chapter 1, *Protocol 8*).
15. Examine the sections in the light microscope, draw and photograph regions of interest, re-embed, and cut ultrathin sections (see Chapter 1, *Protocol 9*).
16. Examine in the electron microscope.

7.1 Appearance of the staining

The outcome of this approach are two sets of anterogradely labelled terminals that can be differentiated from each other by the texture of the peroxidase reaction product associated with them (*Figure 4*). In the sections prepared for

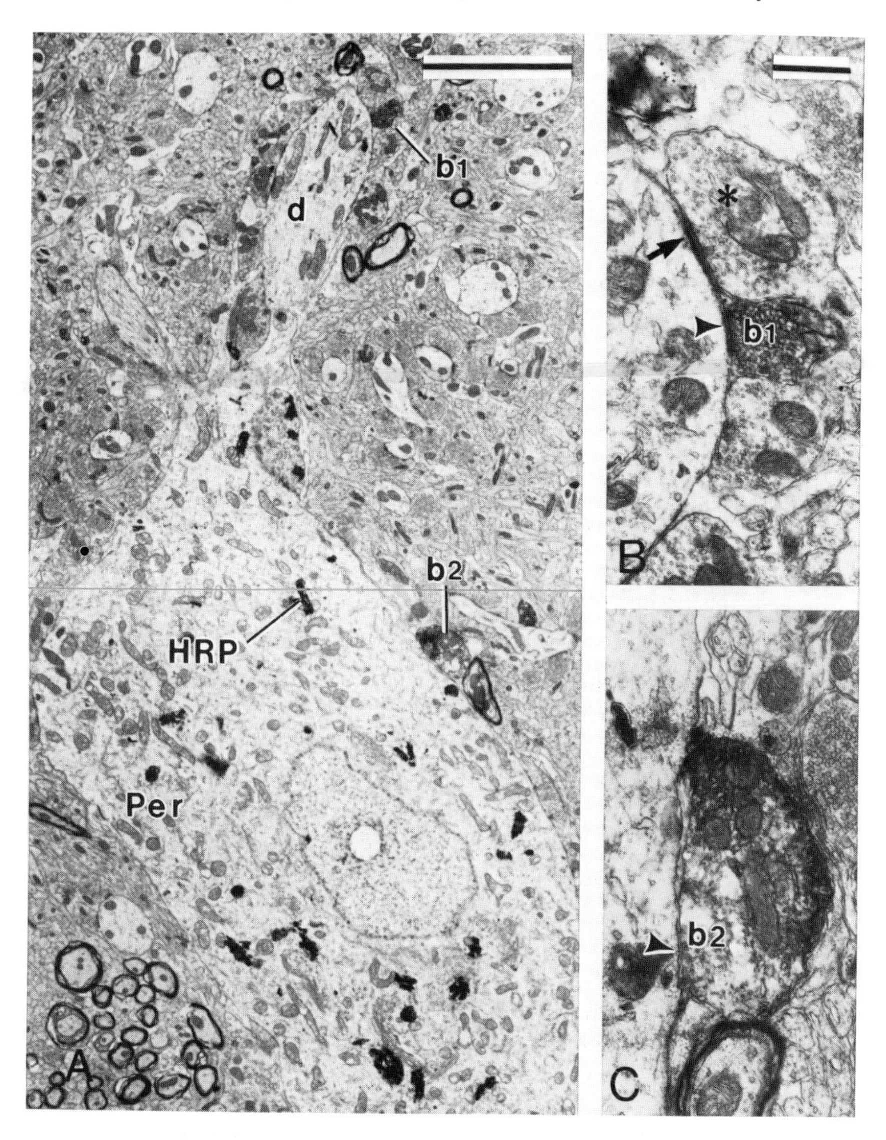

light microscopy, the two sets of anterogradely labelled fibres are easily distinguishable since the brown DAB reaction product is distinct from the blue Ni-DAB reaction product. In the sections prepared for electron microscopy, the two reaction products are also distinguishable; the biocytin labelled terminals contain the amorphous DAB reaction product, whereas the PHA-L labelled terminals contain the crystalline BDHC reaction product (*Figure 4*). In some cases, because of the size of the labelled terminals, it is difficult to distinguish at the light microscopic level, the DAB from the BDHC labelled

Figure 4. Anterograde transport of PHA-L and biocytin combined with the retrograde transport of WGA-HRP (*Protocol 6*). Electron micrographs showing a retrogradely labelled nigrocollicular cell (indicated by HRP in (A)) that receives convergent synaptic inputs from the striatum (b1) and the globus pallidus (b2) in the rat substantia nigra. In this experiment, PHA-L was injected in the globus pallidus and biocytin was injected in the striatum. In the same animals, WGA-HRP was injected in the superior colliculus. The three markers were all localized by peroxidase reactions but using different chromogens. The biocytin was revealed using DAB as the chromogen, PHA-L was localized with BDHC as the chromogen, and the retrogradely-transported WGA-HRP with TMB as the chromogen. Note in (B) and (C) the difference between the DAB reaction product associated with b1 (B) and the BDHC reaction product associated with b2 (C). Both the striatal (DAB labelled, b1) and the pallidal (BDHC labelled, b2) terminals form symmetric synapses (indicated by arrowheads in (B) and (C)) with the retrogradely labelled cell. In (B), a non-labelled terminal (indicated by an asterisk) forms a symmetric synapse (arrow) with the nigrocollicular cell. Scale markers: (A) 5.0 μm, (B) and (C) 0.5 μm.

---

terminals. Nevertheless, in the electron microscope the two sets of terminals remain easy to distinguish (compare *Figure 4B* and *4C*). In addition to these two sets of anterogradely labelled terminals, the section will contain retrogradely labelled neurones characterized by the presence of large TMB crystals randomly distributed throughout the cytoplasm of the perikaryon and the dendritic shafts of labelled cells (*Figure 4A*; see also *Figure 2A* and Chapter 2 for TMB reaction product).

7.2 Analysis of the material

The best way to analyse this material is to carry out correlated light and electron microscopy (see Chapter 1). First, the area of study is scanned for the presence of retrogradely labelled cells that are apposed by biocytin and PHA-L labelled terminals. This cell is drawn and photographed before being re-embedded and cut in serial ultrathin sections. In the electron microscope, the retrogradely labelled cell is examined through its entire extent to determine whether the biocytin and PHA-L labelled terminals identified at the light microscopic level form synapses with this neurone. If necessary, ultrathin sections adjacent to those containing both sets of terminals and the retrogradely labelled cell can be processed for the post-embedding immunogold procedure to determine the chemical nature of the anterogradely labelled terminals (10).

7.3 Applications

This approach was developed to test the possibility that synaptic terminals from two different sources converge on to single post-synaptic targets characterized by their projection sites. We have recently shown that after injection of biocytin in the striatum and PHA-L in the globus pallidus, rich plexuses of both sets of anterogradely labelled terminals overlap in the ipsilateral substantia nigra. In the electron microscope, it has been found that many projection neurones in the substantia nigra pars reticulata receive convergent synaptic inputs from the PHA-L labelled boutons arising from the globus pallidus and the biocytin positive boutons arising from the striatum (10, 14) (*Figure 4*). Moreover, we have also demonstrated, by using the post-embedding immunogold method for GABA, that both striatal and pallidal terminals, that converge on to single projection neurones in the substantia nigra, display GABA immunoreactivity (10).

7.4 Limitations and controls

The combination of three tract-tracing methods in one experiment inevitably has some technical limitations. First, the major limitation is the poor penetration of the BDHC reaction product into the tissue (see *Protocol 4*). As mentioned above, it is necessary to collect the first few micrometres of a re-embedded block to have all three sets of labelled elements on single ultrathin sections. Second, the ultrastructural features of the terminals localized with BDHC may be damaged (see *Figure 4C*). Third, it may be difficult to differentiate the BDHC reaction product from the TMB reaction product in the electron microscope. Fortunately, in many cases the location of the two deposits is largely different, i.e. the TMB deposit occurs in perikarya and proximal dendrites whereas the BDHC reaction product is found in anterogradely labelled terminals. However, the TMB reaction product may occur in terminals if the WGA-HRP is transported anterogradely to the area of study, or if the retrogradely labelled cells have recurrent axon collaterals (see *Protocol 3*). In such conditions it may be difficult to differentiate the PHA-L positive terminals (BDHC labelled) from the WGA-HRP containing terminals. It is therefore important to carry out control experiments in which the WGA-HRP only is revealed; this allows one to verify whether WGA-HRP labelled terminals occur in the material under investigation.

In addition to the localization of WGA-HRP alone, two other control experiments must be carried out to verify the specificity of the staining. First, reverse the order in which the anterograde tracers are revealed; i.e. localize PHA-L first with DAB, and biocytin second with BDHC. In such a case the PAP method must be used to localize the PHA-L immunoreactivity (see Chapter 5). Secondly, omit the ABC or the primary antibody against PHA-L in turn from the incubation medium. In the case where the ABC is omitted, localize the PHA-L immunoreactivity using the PAP method (see Chapter 5).

8. Double/triple immunocytochemistry at the electron microscopic level

The main objective of the double immunohistochemical procedure at the electron microscopic level is to determine the chemical nature of the synaptic input to chemically characterized neurones. The same approach is used when the anterograde transport of PHA-L is combined with the pre-embedding immunocytochemistry for the transmitter in the post-synaptic target neurones (see *Protocol 4*). This method involves the use of DAB and BDHC as the chromogens for the peroxidase reactions to localize the two sets of immunoreactive structures (*Protocol 7*; see Chapter 5, *Protocol 11*). Furthermore, co-localization of two chemicals within single terminals can be carried out by combining this double immunohistochemical method with the post-embedding immunogold procedure in a manner similar to that described in *Protocol 5* (see Chapter 6, *Protocol 3*).

Protocol 7. Double/triple immunocytochemical labelling at the electron microscopic level

1. Perfuse–fix the animal (see Chapter 1, *Protocols 2* and *3*).
2. Cut the brain in 50–70 μm thick sections on a vibrating microtome (see Chapter 1, *Protocol 4*).
3. Collect the sections in PBS (see Chapter 1, *Protocol 1*).
4. Process the tissue for the localization of the first antigen using the ABC (see Chapter 5, *Protocol 9*), or the PAP (see Chapter 5, *Protocol 8*) method.
5. Reveal the antigen using DAB as the chromogen in the peroxidase reaction (see Chapter 3, *Protocol 2*, step **13**).
6. Wash the sections several times in PBS.
7. Process the tissue for the immunohistochemical localization of the second antigen using the ABC or the PAP method (see Chapter 5, *Protocols 8* and *9*).
8. Reveal the second antigen using BDHC as the chromogen in the peroxidase reaction (see Chapter 5, *Protocol 11*; see also *Safety note 4* in Chapter 5, p. 123).
9. Post-fix in osmium tetroxide (see Chapter 1, *Protocol 7*, but dilute the osmium tetroxide in PB 0.01 M, pH 6.8), dehydrate, and embed the sections in resin on microscope slides (see Chapter 1, *Protocol 8*).
10. Examine the sections in the light microscope.
11. Re-embed areas of interest (see Chapter 1, *Protocol 9*).
12. Cut ultrathin sections and mount them on coated (see Chapter 1, *Protocol 10*) single-slot nickel or gold grids.
13. Process the tissue for post-embedding immunocytochemistry (see Chapter 6, *Protocol 3*).
14. Examine the sections in the electron microscope.

8.1 Appearance of the staining

The outcomes of this approach are:

- neuronal elements labelled with the DAB reaction product resulting from the first immunocytochemical reaction
- neuronal structures containing the BDHC reaction product resulting from the second immunocytochemical reaction
- neuronal structures associated with immunogold particles
- neuronal elements containing either the DAB or the BDHC peroxidase reaction products and associated with immunogold particles

The two peroxidase reaction products are distinguishable as described above (see Section 5.1). In the electron microscope, double labelling of a single neuronal structure is indicated by the presence of either the DAB or the BDHC reaction product, together with a significant number of the immunogold particles (at least five times higher than the background) (*Figure 5*) (see *Protocol 5* and Chapter 6).

8.2 Analysis of the material

The approaches to analyse such material have been described in detail in Sections 5.2 and 6.2.

8.3 Applications

This approach has recently been used to demonstrate that substance P positive/GABA terminals form symmetric synapses with tyrosine hydroxylase immunoreactive dendrites in the rat substantia nigra (15) (*Figure 5*). In this experiment, sections of the rat substantia nigra were processed for the pre-embedding immunohistochemical localization of substance P and tyrosine hydroxylase (TH). The substance P immunoreactive structures were localized using DAB as the chromogen for the peroxidase reaction, whereas the TH positive elements were revealed using BDHC. Ultrathin sections containing both sets of labelled structures were then processed to reveal GABA by the immunogold method (see Chapter 6, *Protocol 3*).

The double peroxidase method, i.e. the use of both DAB and BDHC for chromogens in the peroxidase reactions, is used in several of the other

Figure 5. Double pre-embedding immunocytochemistry combined with post-embedding immunocytochemistry (*Protocol 7*). Electron micrograph of the substantia nigra of the rat reacted to reveal three neural antigens. It was reacted first to reveal substance P immunoreactivity using DAB as the chromogen for the peroxidase reaction, an axonal bouton (SP-bouton) contains the DAB reaction product. Secondly it was reacted to reveal tyrosine hydroxylase immunoreactivity using BDHC as the chromogen; the dendrite (den), con-

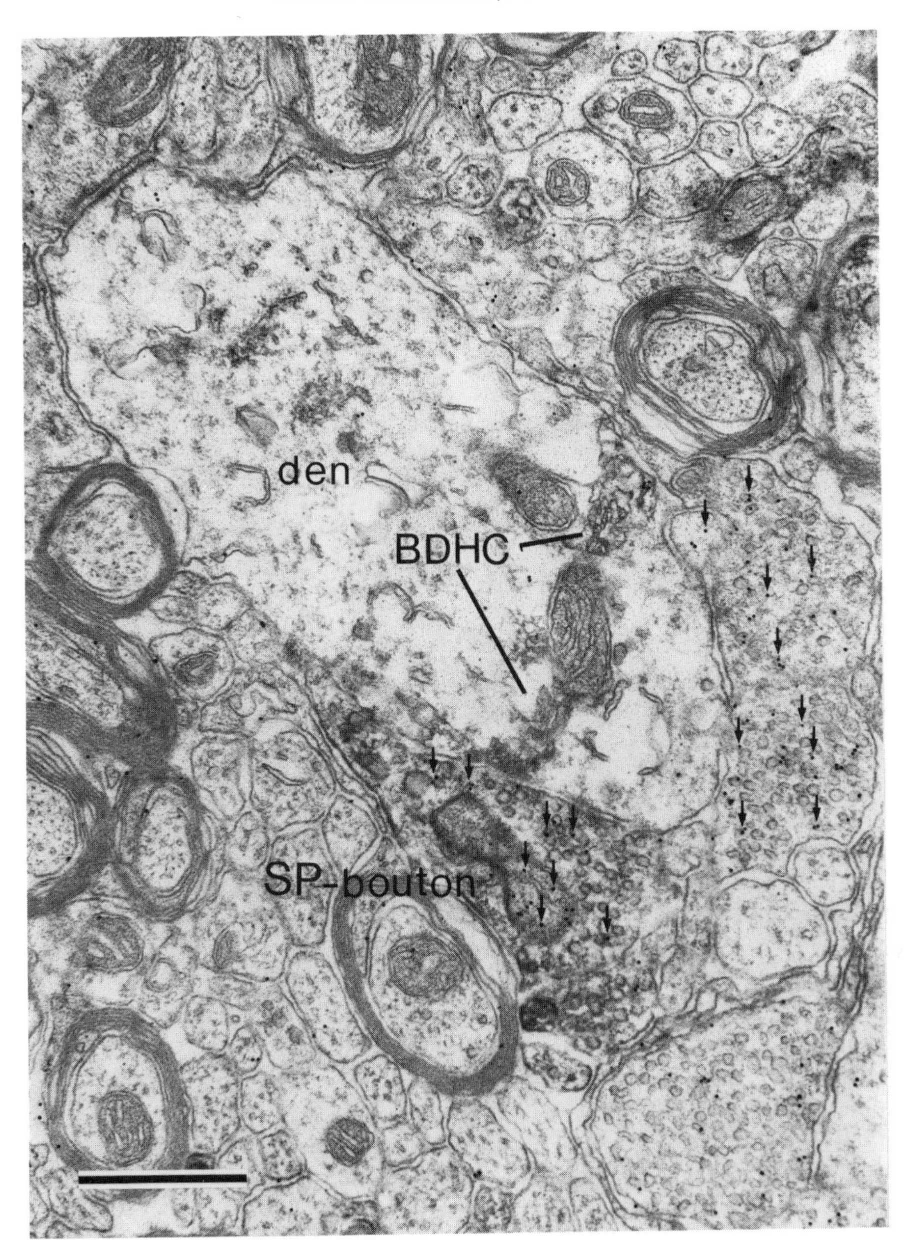

tains the reaction product (BDHC) which is partially bleached due to subsequent processing. Finally, the section was subjectd to the post-embedding immunogold method to reveal GABA; three boutons apposed to the dendrite, including the substance P immunoreactive one, contain relatively high concentrations of the immunogold particles (some of which are indicated by arrows) identifying them as GABA-immunoreactive. Scale marker: 0.5 μm.

combined procedures described in this chapter, see *Protocols 4* and *6* (see *Figures 3A* and *Figure 2B* in Chapter 5).

8.4 Limitations and controls

This combination of immunohistochemical techniques suffers from all the disadvantages mentioned above for the *Protocols 4–6*.

Control experiments including incubations in solutions from which the primary antisera to localize the first, the second, and the third antigens are omitted in turn must be carried out to ensure the specificity of the immunostaining (see Chapters 5 and 6).

References

1. Ingham, C. A., Bolam, J. P., Wainer, B. H., and Smith, A. D. (1985). *J. Comp. Neurol.,* **239,** 176.
2. Bolam, J. P. and Izzo, P. N. (1988). *Exp. Brain Res.,* **70,** 361.
3. Izzo, P. N. and Bolam, J. P. (1988). *J. Comp. Neurol.,* **269,** 219.
4. Freund, T. F., Powell, J., and Smith, A. D. (1984). *Neurosci.,* **13,** 1189.
5. Ingham, C. A., Bolam, J. P., and Smith, A. D. (1988). *J. Comp. Neurol.,* **273,** 263.
6. Somogyi, P. (1988). In *Molecular Neuroanatomy* (ed. F. W. Van Leeuwen, R. M. Buijs, C. W. Pool, and O. Pach), pp. 339–59. Elsevier Science Publishers, Amsterdam.
7. Somogyi, P. and Freund, T. F. (1989). In *Neuroanatomical Tract-tracing Methods 2* (ed. L. Heimer and L. Zaborszky), pp. 239–64. Plenum Publishing Corporation, New York.
8. Bolam, J. P. and Ingham C. A. (1990). In *Handbook of Chemical Neuroanatomy: Analysis of Neuronal Microcircuits and Synaptic Interactions* (ed. A. Björklund, T. Hökfelt, F. G. Wouterlood, and A. N. van den Pol), Vol. 8, pp. 125–98. Elsevier Science Publishers, Amsterdam.
9. Smith, Y. and Bolam, J. P. (1990). *J. Comp. Neurol.,* **296,** 47.
10. von Krosigk, M., Smith, Y., Bolam, J. P., and Smith, A. D. (1991). *Proc. 3rd IBRO Congress,* **144**.
11. Lapper, S. R., Smith, Y., Sadikot, A. F., Parent, A., and Bolam, J. P. (1992). *Brain Res.*, **580,** 215.
12. Freund, T. F. and Antal, M. (1988). *Nature,* **336,** 170.
13. Smith, Y., Bolam, J. P., and von Krosigk, M. (1990). *Eur. J. Neurosci.,* **2,** 500.
14. Smith, Y. and Bolam, J. P. (1991). *Neurosci.,* **44,** 45.
15. Bolam, J. P. and Smith, Y. (1990). *Brain Res.,* **529,** 57.

A1

Suppliers of specialist items

See also Chapter 2, *Table 1*.

Agar Scientific Ltd, 66a Cambridge Road, Stanstead, Essex, CM24 8DA, UK; Ted Pella Inc, 4595 Mountain Lakes Blvd, Redding, CA 96003, USA.

Aldrich Chemical Co., (paraformaldehyde), The Old Brickyard, New Road, Gillingham, Dorset, SP8 4JL, UK; 1001 West St. Paul Avenue, Milwaukee, Wisconsin 53233, USA.

amplifiers, Palmer Bioscience, Harbour Estate, Sheerness, Kent, UK.

Axon Instruments, 1101, Chess Drive, Foster City, CA 94404, USA.

Bevelling Machine, Clarke Electromedical Instruments, PO Box 8, Pangbourne, Reading, Berks., RG8 7HU, UK.

BDH-Merk Ltd, Broom Road, Poole, Dorset, BH12 4NN, UK; Gallard Schelesinger Industries Inc., 584 Mineloa Avenue, Carle Place, New York, NY 11514, USA.

Bio-Logic, 4 Rue Docteur Pascal, 38130 Echirolles, France.

Boehringer Manheim, Boehringer Manheim House, Bell Lane, Lewes, Sussex, BN7 1LG, UK; 9115 Hague Road, PO Box 50414, Indianapolis, IN 46250.

cellulose acetate foil, British Celanese Ltd, PO Box 5, Spondon, Derby, DE2 7BP, UK.

Dako Ltd, 16, Manor Courtyard, Hughenden Avenue, High Wycombe, Bucks., HP13 5RE, UK; (Dako Corp.) 6392 Via Real, Carpinteria, CA 93013, USA.

Digitimer Ltd, (timing devices) 37, Hydeway, Welwyn Garden City, Herts, AL7 3BE, UK.

Durcupan, Fluka Chemicals Ltd, Peakdale Road, Glossop, Derbyshire, SK13 9XE, UK; Fluka Chemical Corp. 980, South Second Street, Rokonkoma, New York 11779, USA.

electrode glass, Clark Electromedical Instruments, PO Box 8, Pangbourne, Reading, Berkshire, RG8 7HU, UK; A-M Systems Inc., WA, USA.

electron microscope equipment suppliers, Agar Scientific Ltd, 66a Cambridge Road, Stanstead, Essex, CM24 8DA, UK; EMSCOPE Labs Ltd, Kingsworth Industrial Estate, Ashford, Kent, TN23 2LW, UK; Fisons, Bishops Meadow Road, Loughborough, Leics. LE11 0RG; UK; Raymond A. Lamb, 6, Sunbeam Road, London, NW10 6JL, UK; TAAB Laboratories

Equip Ltd, 3, Minerva House, Calleva Industrial Park, Aldermaston, Reading, Berkshire, RG7 4QW, UK; Ted Pella Inc, 4595 Mountain Lakes Blvd, Redding, CA 96003. Curtin Matheson Scientific, 7383 Empire Drive, Suite B, Florence, USA; Normco Inc. Suite 209, 1751 Elton Road, Silver Spring, Maryland 20903, USA; Photometrics Inc, 6 Arrow Drive, Woburn, MA 01801, USA.

fine gauge needles, V.A. Howe & Co. Ltd, 12–14 St. Ann's Crescent, London, SW18 2LS, UK.

Fisons Scientific Equipment, Bishops Meadow Road, Loughborough, Leics. LE11 0RG, UK; Curtin Matheson Scientific, 7383 Empire Drive, Suite B, Florence, USA.

freezing microtome, Leica UK Ltd, Davy Avenue, Knowhill, Milton Keynes, MK5 8LB, UK.

grid boxes, Agar Scientific Ltd, 66a Cambridge Road, Stanstead, Essex, CM24 8DA. See also electron microscope equipment suppliers.

grid-coating apparatus, Agar Scientific Ltd, 66a Cambridge Road, Stanstead, Essex, CM24 8DA, UK; Ted Pella Inc., 4595 Mountain Lakes Blvd, Redding, CA 96003, USA.

Hi-Med Instruments, PO Box 101, Reading, Berkshire, RG1 2LB, UK.

homeothermic blanket, Harvard Apparatus, Fircroft Way, Eldenbridge, Kent, TN8 6HE, UK.

Janssen Life Sciences, Lammerdries 55, B-2430 Olen, Belgium.

Labsystems Oy, Pulttittie 9–11, 00810 Helsinki 81, Finland.

Marzhauser KG, Wetzlar, Germany.

microelectrode pullers, Clarke Electromedical Instruments, PO Box 8, Pangbourne, Reading, Berkshire, RG8 7HU, UK; D. Kopf Instruments, 7324 Elmo Street, Tujunga, CA 91042, USA.

Millipore, Millipore (U.K.) Ltd, The Boulevard, Blackmoor Lane, Watford, Herts, WD1 8YW, UK; Millipore Intertech., PO Box 255, Bedford, MA 01730, USA.

Narishige Scientific Instrument Lab, 9–28 Kasuya 4-Chome Setagaya-Ku, Tokyo 157, Japan. UK agents: Intracel Ltd, Unit 4, Station Road, Shepreth, Royston, Herts, SG8 6PZ.

Neuroscience Trading, Frankfurt, Germany.

oscilloscopes Tektronic UK Ltd, Fourth Avenue, Globe Park, Marlow, Bucks, SL7 1YD, UK; Gould Electronics Ltd, Stanford House, Science Park South, Birchwood, Warrington, WA3 7BH, UK; Gould Inc., 19050 Pruneridge Avenue, Cupertino, CA 95014, USA.

osmium tetroxide, OXKEM Ltd, Mulberry House, Holton, Oxford, OX9 1PY; see also electron microscope equipment suppliers.

Parafilm, TAAB Labs Equip Ltd, 3, Minerva House, Calleva Industrial Park, Aldermaston, Reading, Berkshire, RG7 4QW, UK; American Can Co, Greenwich, CT 06830. USA.

Scottish Antibody Production Unit (SPAU), Law Hospital, Carluke, ML8 5ES, Lanarkshire, Scotland.

shaker, (IKA-VibraxVKR) Satorius Instruments Ltd, 18, Avenue Road, Belmont, Surrey, SM2 67D, UK; Sartorius North America Inc., 140 Wilbur Place, Bohemia, Long Island, New York 11716, USA.

Sigma Chemical Co. Ltd, Fancy Road, Poole, Dorset, BH17 7NH, UK; PO Box 14508, St. Louis, MO 63178, USA.

sterotaxic-frame and manipulators, Clarke Electromedical Instruments, PO Box 8, Pangbourne, Reading, Berkshire, RG8 7HU, UK; D. Kopf Instruments, 7324 Elmo Street, Tujunga, CA 91042, USA.

TAAB Labs Equip Ltd, 3, Minerva House, Calleva Industrial Park, Aldermaston, Reading, Berkshire, RG7 4QW, UK; Normco Inc. Suite 209, 1751 Elton Road, Silver Spring, Maryland 20903, USA.

Transkinetics Systems Inc., Canton, MA, USA.

Vector Labs Ltd, 16, Wilfric Square, Bretton, Peterborough, Cambs., UK; 30, Ingold Road, Burlingame, CA 94010, USA.

vibrating microtomes, (Vibratome) A.R. Howell Ltd, Laboratory and Clinical Supplies, 73, Maygrove Road, West Hampstead, London, NW62 2BP, UK; Technical Products International Inc., St. Louis, MO 63045, USA. (Micro-cut) V.G. Microtech, Bellbrook Business Park, Bell Lane, Uckfield, East Sussex, TN22 1QZ, UK. (Vibroslice) UK Campden Instruments Ltd, King Street, Sileby, Loughborough, LE 12 7LZ. UK; Stoelting, 620 Wheat Lane, Wood Dale, IL 60191. USA.

ultramicrotomes, Leica UK Ltd, Davy Avenue, Knowhill, Milton Keynes, MK5 8LB, UK; Leica Inc., 24 Line Drive, Rockleigh, New Jersey, USA.

Index

Index